S.M.A.R.T. Environments

The book series will cover a broad spectrum of data-driven multivalence in the built environment. The individual volumes will set the stage for understanding multiple ways in which the exponential escalation of digital ubiquity in the contemporary environment is being absorbed, modulated, processed and actively used for enhancing the performance of our built environment.S.M.A.R.T., is used as an acronym for Systems & Materials in Architectural & Urban Research and Technology, with a specific focus on investigating the intricate relationship between information systems and associative material formations at variable scales within the built environment. This is deeply rooted in exploring multi-domain research and design strategies involving nonlinear processes for developing data-driven generative meta-design systems. This book series is relevant to the shaping our Built Environment and will explore novel design and research paradigms.

More information about this series at http://www.springer.com/series/15908

Nimish Biloria
Editor

Data-driven Multivalence in the Built Environment

Springer

Editor
Nimish Biloria
University of Technology Sydney
Sydney, NSW, Australia

ISSN 2523-8469 ISSN 2523-8477 (electronic)
S.M.A.R.T. Environments
ISBN 978-3-030-12179-2 ISBN 978-3-030-12180-8 (eBook)
https://doi.org/10.1007/978-3-030-12180-8

This Springer imprint is published by the registered company Springer Nature Switzerland AG.
The registered company address is: Gewerbestrasse 11, 6330 Cham, Switzerland

Foreword

The city has always been a locus for ideas, engagements and ideals. For most of us, a city is where we encounter other people in our jobs and social lives, but city governments and administrators tend to focus on the material city, its structure and supporting systems. These material systems include an expanding array of digital technologies. These technologies are often focused on making the material city run more smoothly – traffic, water, power, waste management and so on. Such enhancements are usually about the 'business' of the city and a perception of the city as primarily a place of business in its broadest sense – the city as a marketplace. This is an ancient idea being modified for our present digital age. But it is only one important dimension of the city; another sees the city as place for living, not simply surviving but one of flourishing.

A central focus in many critiques of the smart city is the desperate need for a focus on people and not just on the technology. This has become a key part of the contemporary smart cities discussion – how to humanise the smart city and what additional opportunities humanising the smart city might offer? And this raises the idea as to how digitisation might make the city more liveable. Can we effectively go against historical flows and make the city a more people-centric environment using technologies often designed to facilitate the material city and its economic focus? In The Netherlands, for example, some of these ideas are already in play including the option for older people to 'hack' the lights on pedestrian crossings. In this context, technologies can facilitate this process of humanising the city.

One of the central and essential foci of this volume is the place of people in the smart city and the smart city as a place for people of all descriptions. This is important because the twenty-first-century city is a global phenomenon characterised by various forms of migration and associated demographic changes. People come into the city in search of opportunities, as they have always done, while others attempt to leave the city for all manner of reasons ranging from the cost of housing in the globalised city through to a desire to escape the actual and perceived stresses of contemporary urban environments.

Perhaps one of the least smart elements of many contemporary cities is that they are often more disruptive than adaptive for their inhabitants, especially those most vulnerable to rapid changes in urban form and function. In the context of high-income countries, this means looking at the city, smart or not, from the perspective of an ageing population, from those with disability, the very young, the homeless and all those groups whose needs don't fit easily with the high-technology rhetoric of the smart city. The city is dependent on the contributions of people, but in many cases, it does not return that favour in its design or operations. In this sense, we often forget that the city is more than the physical infrastructure and its technology; it is a fundamentally social space – one with an almost unlimited potential and capacity for places of representation and participation. Throughout this volume, this idea is presented to the reader across a variety of national and social contexts.

The issue of 'mobilities' is also addressed because new technologies can be a change in and of themselves (e.g. electric vehicles), but their adoption drives flow-on effects and produces new adaptations (e.g. ride sharing, car sharing and the 'gig' economy) that were previously unanticipated. In addition, conventional wisdoms associated with public and private transport are destabilised, forcing a fresh perspective on the potential of new technologies, digital and analogue, and their implications for established systems and ideas as change unfolds. The speed of new digital technologies and applications, in particular, means that the growth of knowledge in this space is increasingly dynamic.

The smart cities discourse has been given an added momentum by the rapid developments in digital technologies and methods including the incredible hype and potential opportunities associated with 'big data'. The literature in this space is developing rapidly with contributions from the low- to high-income countries increasingly the norm.

What Nimish Biloria and the contributing authors bring to this digital urban environment is a broad-ranging understanding of the history of the smart city, actual and idealised, as well as its intersectional nature with the human domain. The city is clearly not simply a mechanism for business but a dynamic, lived environment. An increasingly important aspect of this lived dynamism is the changing nature of the city's population and the implications of demographic change. If digital technologies and thinking can help humanise the smart city, now is the time as population ageing becomes a global phenomenon. This volume addresses this and a number of related concerns with the idealised, smart techno-city and expands our understanding of the knowledge we need to create a humane, liveable smart city fit for all its inhabitants.

Senior Research Fellow, Faculty of Health
University of Technology Sydney,
Sydney, Australia

Hamish Robertson

Introduction

Data-Driven Multivalence in the Built Environment is the first issue of the 5-year Springer Book Series on S.M.A.R.T. Environments. This issue sets the stage for understanding multiple ways in which the exponential escalation of digital ubiquity in the contemporary environment is being absorbed, modulated, processed and actively used for enhancing the performance of our built environment. S.M.A.R.T., in this context, is thus used as an acronym for Systems & Materials in Architectural & Urban Research and Technology, with a specific focus on interrogating the intricate relationship between information systems and associative material formations at variable scales within the built environment. This interrogation is deeply rooted in exploring multidomain research and design strategies involving nonlinear processes for developing data-driven generative meta-design systems.

Such meta-systems are in turn used to conceive multi-performative architectures, which can respond, reconfigure and adapt to observed contextual data variations in real time. The multi-performative nature of such research-driven social, spatial and technical initiatives is deemed critical in deciphering new realities within which we situate ourselves. Mining and generating informed architectural and urban formations within such a context thus challenge conventional top-down decision-making-driven approaches towards shaping the built environment and instead conceive data-driven design hybrids. Such hybrids evolve from the creative fusion of social and cultural data, ubiquitous computing, computational design systems and place-making policies.

This context implies changes to the manner in which the physical, the human and the digital counterparts formulating the contemporary built environment are inextricably interlinked into complex relational networks. Implications on how different facets of the built environment such as energy, health, mobility, governance, urban design and architecture operate and innovate with this mediated layer of real-time data are thus crucial and are thus captured and exposed via this opening volume's focus on the multivalence of data in the built environment. What is also vital to understand is the relationship between the micro-, mezzo- and macroscales of operation, which collectively build up the so-called 'smart' nature of the built environment. The opening issue of S.M.A.R.T. Environments sets the base for understanding the city as a complex ecosystem wherein the operative term 'smart' is seen as a customised creative response to urban problems residing at the confluence of people, technology, context and economics properties of the city.

The following multifarious domains constituting the built environment are covered under the opening issue: health, mobility, energy, infrastructure and the built environment. The book is accordingly organised in seven parts: Perspectives on the City, Smart Urban Infrastructure, Urban Health and Wellbeing, Urban Living Labs, Disruptive Technologies, Socio-spatial Ecosystems and Conclusions. The book begins with a collection of three chapters under the operative title Perspectives on the City, which creates an overarching narrative around three vital considerations while developing a smart city: firstly, considering economic equity as an important dimension of performance to promote an inclusive environment of wellbeing and democratic growth; secondly, developing guidelines on designing the 'Convenient City' by making use of available technology while harnessing a critical wholistic viewpoint on the current propaganda of smart cities rather than understanding them as technocratic interventions; and thirdly, by acquiring a human-centric perspective, which outlines emerging humanism of urban technologies as a quintessential tool for developing smart and equitable urban environments.

After setting a socio-economic context around the state of the city, the next part focuses on smart urban infrastructure wherein both physical and digital infrastructure are explored for their potential. Smart urban mobility solutions and customer-centric infrastructure planning, big data command and control centres for smart cities and city information models in conjunction with advanced design, analysis and management systems and smart governance frameworks involved in the development of smart infrastructure projects are explored under this book section. The subsequent part focuses on urban health and wellbeing by covering multiple scales of urban health and wellbeing applications, from the object scale, involving customised 3D printing, to socio-technical measures for promoting agile ageing and the use of contemporary ICT-enabled enhancements, both in terms of advanced meta-systems and integrated IoT-based solutions within the built environment. Living labs within urban settings in European as well as Indonesian contexts as evidence-based design-thinking enablers are further discussed via two chapters. These cover two scales: firstly, the design and development of interaction labs, which go beyond conventional scientifically controlled experimental spaces but rather acquire the character of design research labs which predominantly deal with exploring, hacking and tinkering with electronics via messy engineering processes, and secondly, utilising the city as a lab for conducting socio-technical experiments as well as for mapping the biorhythms of the city within dense urban environments in the form of urban living labs.

The Disruptive Technologies part of the book focuses on developing biotechnology-based techniques for developing sustainable energy solutions and creative ways of incorporating image processing-driven visioning and mapping technologies. Both look at intelligent means of collecting, processing and applying urban resources via both software- and hardware-based adaptations to service the urban environment. Evidence driven explorations around the application of algae building technology and the technology transfer-based applications of image processing to map pedestrian and vehicular flows, to develop a new and more abstract understanding of the material nature of the city, are two such promising technologies discussed in the book.

The Disruptive Technologies part is complemented by the Socio-spatial Ecosystems part of the book. Here, the focus moves towards understanding such innovative technologies as entrepreneurial ecosystems and their relationship and impact on smart cities. Apart from this, the part also looks at spatial innovation within today's cultural context and focuses on practical applications within the housing sector by exploring multimodal accommodations in the age of the millennial as well as speculates upon finding suitable ways of measuring urban wellbeing within the contemporary city via interfacing quantitative, qualitative measuring techniques together with citizen science-based participatory methodologies. The book finally concludes with a section on inferences and speculates upon the future of a data-rich wholistic smart environment.

Faculty of Design Architecture and Building
University of Technology Sydney,
Sydney, Australia

Nimish Biloria

Contents

Contributors

Mahmoud AlSaeed Department of Architecture and Urban Planning, College of Engineering, Qatar University, Doha, Qatar

Arry Akhmad Arman Institute of Technology Bandung, Bandung, Indonesia

Nimish Biloria Faculty of Design Architecture and Building, School of Architecture, University of Technology Sydney, Ultimo, Australia

D. Cetindamar School of Information, Systems and Modelling, University of Technology Sydney, Sydney, Australia

Dimitra Dritsa Faculty of Design Architecture Building, University of Technology Sydney, Ultimo, Australia

Fodil Fadli Department of Architecture and Urban Planning, College of Engineering, Qatar University, Doha, Qatar

Yuti Ariani Fatimah Institute of Technology Bandung, Bandung, Indonesia

Hendra Sandhi Firmansyah Institute of Technology Bandung, Bandung, Indonesia

Mathias Funk Department of Industrial Design, Eindhoven University of Technology, Eindhoven, The Netherlands

T. Lammers School of Information, Systems and Modelling, University of Technology Sydney, Sydney, Australia

Jennifer Loy Deakin University, Geelong, Victoria, Australia

Linda Matthews School of Architecture, Faculty of Design Architecture and Building, University of Technology Sydney, Sydney, Australia

Dhrumil Mehta Faculty of Design Architecture Building, University of Technology Sydney, Sydney, Australia

Masi Mohammadi Chair Smart Architectural Technologies, Eindhoven University of Technology, Eindhoven, The Netherlands

Kivi Chair Architecture in Health, HAN University of Applied Sciences, Arnhem, The Netherlands

Nienke Moor Kivi Chair Architecture in Health, HAN University of Applied Sciences, Arnhem, The Netherlands

Ryan Adhitya Nugraha Institute of Technology Bandung, Bandung, Indonesia

Aurobindo Ogra Department of Town and Regional Planning, Faculty of Engineering and the Built Environment, University of Johannesburg, Johannesburg, South Africa

Kas Oosterhuis Qatar University, Doha, Qatar

Technical University Delft, Delft, The Netherlands

Sarbeswar Praharaj Faculty of Built Environment, University of New South Wales, Sydney, Australia

Peter J. Ralph Faculty of Science, C3, University of Technology Sydney, Sydney, Australia

Prasuna Reddy Faculty of Science, Engineering and Technology, Swinburne University of Technology, Hawthorn, VIC, Australia

Rob Roggema Research Centre for the Built Environment NoorderRuimte, Hanze University of Applied Sciences, Groningen, The Netherlands

Somwrita Sarkar Sydney School of Architecture, Design and Planning, The University of Sydney, Sydney, Australia

N. Sick School of Information, Systems and Modelling, University of Technology Sydney, Sydney, Australia

Suhono Harso Supangkat Institute of Technology Bandung, Bandung, Indonesia

Akshay Vij Institute for Choice, University of South Australia, Adelaide, Australia

Sara J. Wilkinson Faculty of Design Architecture and Building, School of Building, University of Technology Sydney, Sydney, Australia

Part I
Perspectives on the City

Chapter 1
Smart Equity: An Australian Lens on the Need to Measure Distributive Justice

Somwrita Sarkar

Abstract This chapter reviews ideas on the multidimensional measurement of wellbeing from economics, and proposes that smart cities must include equity as an important dimension of performance. A city, in order to be smart, should have equitable distributions of opportunities and outcomes driving overall system performance on efficiency, productivity, resilience, or sustainability.

Keywords Smart cities · Social Equity · Infrastructure · Growth · Spatial justice.

1.1 Introduction

Discussions on smart cities frequently focus on questions of making the city more efficient, more productive, more resilient, and more sustainable. The chapter starts with the observation that *planning for equity of opportunities and outcomes*, especially in the urban spatial domain, is not a primary goal in current smart city policies and implementation plans. This is despite the issue garnering a significant amount of academic and scholarly research and community action in several parts of the world. It then proposes the primary postulate that *a smart city* cannot be achieved when inequities are not explicitly measured within a performance framework in the same way as efficient solutions cannot be devised unless the inefficiencies in the system are mapped, measured and monitored. Indeed, a system that appears to be efficient and productive in the aggregate may appear inefficient and unproductive once the distributive aspects related to equity are considered (Sarkar et al. 2018a; Sarkar 2018).

Using lessons from economics, especially the Stiglitz-Sen-Fitoussi framework (2010) on critical reviews of econometric measurements of productivity and wellbeing, and using the current Australian Government framework on the *National Cities Performance Framework* proposed as part of the *Smart Cities Plan* (Australian

S. Sarkar (✉)
Sydney School of Architecture, Design and Planning, The University of Sydney, Sydney, Australia
e-mail: somwrita.sarkar@sydney.edu.au

N. Biloria (ed.), *Data-driven Multivalence in the Built Environment*, S.M.A.R.T. Environments, https://doi.org/10.1007/978-3-030-12180-8_1

Government 2016a, b) and the *Smart London Plan* (Smart London Plan, 2011, Smarter London Together, 2018) as reflection domains, the chapter presents a review of why an equity-based human-centred view on smart cities is critical and urgent. It is shown that existing performance frameworks rest on an underlying assumption that increasing business productivity and efficiency in the aggregate will be beneficial for everyone. However, this focus prevents an explicit consideration of the distributions, especially spatial, of the overall gains in productivity and efficiency. Thus, equity considerations along several measurement dimensions are passive: either dormant, or implicit through the other measures, or not considered at all. I bring out some variables in the existing set which can implicitly shed light on spatial, social and economic inequities, and through an overall qualitative and naïve text analysis, present a set of five recommendations that shape the smart city agenda to include the explicit measurement and monitoring of distributive outcomes. The chapter argues that the assumption that increasing productivity and efficiency at the aggregate level is beneficial to everyone should be reframed to respond to questions of distributive justice and spatial and socio-economic equity explicitly within the smart city agenda.

1.2 The Importance of Correct Measurement: A Lesson from Economics

In the introduction to the book *Mismeasuring our lives: Why GDP doesn't add up* (Stiglitz et al. 2010), Nicholas Sarkozy, the then French President who commissioned the study, says: *We will not change our behaviour unless we change the ways we measure our economic performance*. In this chapter, we rephrase this to say: *We will not change the way we build cities unless we change the ways we measure our systemic spatial socio-economic performance.* The goal to create smart, more efficient, more productive, and more resilient cities rests on the dogma that data and measurement is key – if you can measure it, if you can monitor it, you can plan for the system to be more efficient, productive, resilient and sustainable. However, what if we were measuring the wrong things, or were omitting the measurement of some right things?

The smart cities agenda has something to learn from this focus on the importance of measurement and indicators (Stiglitz et al. 2010; Foster and Sen 1997). The Commission on the Measurement of Economic Performance and Social Progress, commissioned by the then French Prime Minister Nicholas Sarkozy, brought to the fore that statistical indicators driven by data play a key support role for the design and evaluation of public policies as well as assessing and influencing how economic markets work. They note: *What we measure affects what we do; and if our measurements are flawed, decisions may be distorted* (Stiglitz et al. 2010, pg. 7).

In particular, the findings of the Commission say that focussing all measurement on growth and productivity can lead to the neglect of wellbeing, which should be final goal spurred by economic growth. The report makes 12 key recommendations:

- The first 5 recommendations outline why measuring distributions of income and consumption, and the economic value of non-market activities is a better overall measure of wellbeing than aggregate production and wealth generation.
- The next 5 recommendations emphasize how wellbeing at the personal or household level is inherently multi-dimensional, including material living standards (income, consumption, and wealth), health, education, personal activities including work, political voice and governance, social connections and relationships, the present and future conditions of the environment, and the social and economic insecurities that people may face. The recommendations note that all these dimensions shape wellbeing, but are missed by conventional measures almost in entirety.
- The last 2 recommendations focus on sustainability and the environment, pointing to the necessity of a dashboard of indicators that span the multiple dimensions of the costs as well as the benefits of economic growth and its distribution and overall impacts on populations.

What is key here is to note that although the report does not specifically focus on the physical and spatial aspect of the urban built environment (although some indicators proposed in later chapters can only be measured from an explicitly spatial angle), all the dimensions for wellbeing mentioned in the 12 recommendations critically play out in a spatial and physical and now increasingly urban environment. For example, consider the dimensions of where we live, where we work, where we or our children study, how we travel, whether or not we have the agency or power to shape our local environments, whether or not we feel we have a voice in politics and governance, whether we feel connected or disconnected from other parts of the city we live in – we find that all of the multi-dimensional indicators of wellbeing discussed above turn immediately and urgently spatial. Our ease or difficulty of accessing the material, social and economic resources we value for a good life makes a real difference to whether, as citizens, we perceive our city to be "smart". Ultimately, it also makes a difference to whether we are efficient and productive as individuals, and individual efficiencies and productivities, however measured, lead to the collective performance of the system.

1.3 Human-Centred Versus Technology-Centred Views of the Smart City

This human-centred view, the idea of productivity, efficiency, and resilience arising out of equitable interactions of a citizen with their city, is laterally different from the much more common information systems and technology focussed definitions of a smart city.

Batty (2012, 2013) notes that technology, innovation, and information exchanges have always been one of the prominent bases of city building, but what is new is the ever-accelerating scale at which big data, sensor technologies, algorithms, models, and methods are expanding and proliferating through nearly all daily acts of living in a city. In one sense, this paves a whole new way forward to objectively inform the science of cities, that is, our quest to understand how cities are shaped, which processes govern their short- and long-term evolution, and how we might better understand these processes of evolution, onward to predicting possible futures for cities. Measuring, monitoring, understanding, predicting, inferring and forecasting are included in this positive, scientific view.

But, there is also a more direct normative and action-oriented view on the connection between technology and city building. For example, here is Townsend's definition: *Smart cities are places where information technology is wielded to address problems old and new* (Townsend 2013). In this normative view, we not only use the technology of the smart to understand, monitor and map our cities, but we also employ these technological means to intervene and shape the behaviours of citizens and to actively build cities (ranging from the humble smart phone acting as a sensor to entire disruptions of the economic or socio-political space to grand plans for realising entirely new city-machines from scratch). However, in a voice of warning on the equity perspective, Townsend's book is full of examples where the lure of technology and blind belief in its power to bring benefit and wellbeing to people's lives, interventions were designed at grand scales: only to fail dismally (Townsend 2013, Ch. 6).

The term *smart city building* therefore has two parts: (a) the measuring, mapping, and monitoring of what we perceive as important, in order to (b) build a city that fulfils certain normative criteria (e.g., efficiency, productivity, resilience, sustainability). It is here that the human-centred questions on *what we measure* become really critical. In one sense, part (b) informs part (a): what we desire helps us to formulate what we should measure. If we do not perceive equity of opportunities and outcomes as an important normative goal, then our performance frameworks and indicators that measure the success or failure of our smart cities will never include those data points or derived data variables that bring out distributions of wellbeing. With spatial data, this becomes even more crucial, since inequitable outcomes have a spatial inertia of their own: existing spatially embedded outcomes have the power to shape future opportunities of access.

Thus, any proposed indicator set that measures the performance of cities has at least two principal aims. First, it must be able to assess, evaluate and influence collective societal wellbeing. Second, it must be able to assess, evaluate and influence the economic functioning of a city. With this background, we now review the *National Cities Performance Framework* which is part of the *Australian Smart Cities Plan.*

1.4 A naïve Text-Based Analysis of Smart Cities Plans for Australia and London

1.4.1 Method

We perform a naïve word-document analysis of two smart cities plans, one at a national level (Australia) and one at a city level (London). We pair this textual analysis with a qualitative reflection on the contents. We analyze, for both sets of plans, what is at the center or focus, for these plans, and whether equitable growth features either implicitly, or explicitly as a goal in these plans. In doing so, the next section will propose some general recommendations on smart city goals, new classes of data points and indicators, as well as new perspectives on analysis that can inform decision making, and make the whole smart cities agenda more rigorous and more holistic from the conceptual perspective.

The method followed for the analysis was:

- To first list all the words used in a plan
- To remove all noise information (special characters, frequent stop words that do not capture meaning, such as "and", "or", and "the" etc. Lists of these stopwords can commonly be obtained from multiple machine learning type libraries, but instead of automating the process completely, we chose a more qualitative analysis approach. For example, we found that the words "where" or "when" seemed relevant in context, since they were repeated with nearly similar frequencies in plans, and could contain significant action information.
- Sort the words in alphabetical order, and count the frequency of each word being used.
- Generate WordClouds based on this word-frequency list, where the size of the word is scaled to the frequency of its use.

In addition, we also performed an extra search over the three documents for a small representative list of words that could signal equitable growth, either implicitly or explicitly. Further, all the three documents were read carefully, and their overall structures analyzed, including plans and implementations of dashboard design, methods of data processing, data and geography granularity, and the analytical approaches adopted to convert raw data points to actual indicators.

1.4.2 Smart Cities Plan, Australia: Qualitative Reflections

The *Smart Cities Plan* for Australia was released by the Australian Government on 29 April 2016, with the stated aim of "*building an agile, innovative and prosperous nation*". The *National Cities Performance Framework* (NCPF) was released as part of the Smart Cities Plan to help stakeholders and users understand the context of the social and economic performance of cities, to measure this performance, and to support the selection, focus and evaluation of *City Deals* (Australian Government 2016b). These deals are planned to promote collaborations between the local, state, and federal levels of government, in order to bring to fruition "*collective plans for growth and commit to the actions, investments, reforms and governance needed to implement them*" (Smart Cities Plan, 2016).

The introduction to the NCPF notes that *cities reduce poverty, they don't cause it*. If this were true as a blanket statement, we would be in an ideal planet already, and there would indeed be no need for concern, urgency, or action. A couple of thousand years ago, Plato had already responded, providing the famous counter argument: *any city however small, is in fact divided into two, one the city of the poor, the other of the rich*. But, crucially, if this is a starting point for the NCPF, then already the lens of measurement is shifted to not seeing or measuring social and economic disadvantage, poverty, and non-inclusive distributive outcomes. But, a wealth of evidence on inequality and urbanisation research in fact shows that this statement cannot be defended: not only may it prove incorrect in the light of empirical analysis, it also masks many other complex issues. For example, consider the following ethical questions: Even if overall poverty reduces, is it acceptable that inequality increases faster? If there is current inequity embedded in the system, then what spatial decisions will exacerbate this inequity, and which possible actions may prevent and reverse it?

The NPCF is organised into two sets of indicators: (a) a set of contextual indicators, covering overall demographic, social, and economic aspects of the city, and (b) a set of performance indicators, that measure performance of a city along six different policy dimensions. These policy dimensions are described in Table 1.1.

1.4.2.1 Very Few Equity Measures

There are no indicators that explicitly measure equity or inequalities along any of the dimensions (although the contextual indicators do include some variables such as the Index of Relative Socio-economic Disadvantage (IRSD) from SEIFA (ABS, 2018), the share of the bottom income quintile, household income, disability rate, and life expectancy). However, some implicit focus is seen through the access indicators (to jobs, public transport, and green space), and housing indicators (for public and community housing, homelessness, rental/mortgage stress, etc.).

1.4.2.2 Coarse Temporal, Spatial, and Modal Granularities

An overarching observation for all these indicators is the level of spatial, modal or temporal granularity of measurement. Most indicators are measured at the city level, even when they derive from underlying finer scale geographies. Thus, an

Table 1.1 Performance Indicators proposed in the NCPF, Australia

Performance dimension	Final indicators on dashboard and NPCF report
Jobs and skills	Employment growth
	Unemployment rate
	Participation rate
	Educational attainment
Infrastructure and investment	Jobs accessible in 30 min
	Work trips by public and active transport
	Peak travel delay
Liveability and sustainability	Adult obesity rate
	Perceived safety
	Access to green space
	Green space area
	Support in times of crisis
	Suicide rate
	Air quality
	Volunteering
	Greenhouse gas emissions per capita
	Office building energy efficiency
	Access to public transport
Innovation and digital opportunities	Knowledge services industries
	Broadband connections
	New business entrants and exits
	Patents and trademarks
Governance, planning, and regulation	Governance fragmentation
Housing	Public and community housing
	Homelessness rate
	Rent stress
	Mortgage stress
	Housing construction costs
	Dwelling price to income ratio
	Population change per building approval

overall city measure may hide the underlying heterogeneity or variation that exists intra-city on a particular dimension. For example, accessibility to jobs within 30 min, is currently measured only for the automobile mode (not public transit) for the entire city. In contrast, accessibility within a single city has a highly disaggregated and heterogeneous form when measured at the fine spatial scale (and for which data is available). If these indicators are to be truly useful at a level where they can inform policy, they need to be developed at fine spatio-temporal and modal scales, so that meaningful local information on performance may be extracted from them, even while keeping the overall framework of comparison constant. We discuss an example and some possibilities in the recommendations section.

1.4.2.3 Uni-Dimensional Analytics

Another crucial observation that emerges from a qualitative analysis of the indicator framework is that each indicator variable stands on its own, is computed, analysed and visualised as its own independent dimension, both in the NCPF report as well as the dashboard. The dashboard currently presents comparative performance analysis for a set of 22 Australian cities. The cities are all individually presented with an overview and context (overall average measures for a city), and the six major dimensions discussed above.

One of the strengths of this framework is that it presents a stable overarching scheme of organisation against which each city or urban area may be considered. Comparisons are thus made possible between different cities and their performance on the same set of variables. However, care needs to be exercised on this same front, since there would likely be sets of indicators very critical for specific cities arising from their very local contexts, and this would likely be missed if only a standard set of common indicators is measured. Thus, it would be appropriate to extend the standardised set of indicators with local indicators relevant to each city.

Secondly, while each indicator stands on its own and presents a particular "view" of the city, crossing these in a multi-dimensional framework of analysis will bring out more robust insights and empirical evidence bases to inform decision making. We discuss an example and some possibilities in the analysis and recommendation section.

1.4.3 Smart London Plan: Qualitative Reflections

So, if one shifts from a national perspective to a city perspective, and focus on a Smart City Plan focused specifically on a single city, do some of the dilemmas raised above solve themselves? We now briefly discuss the Smart London Plan, which is much more focussed on the Digital and Technological agenda in cities. Two versions will be discussed: (a) the Smart London Plan (Smart London Plan, 2011), and (b) the new Smarter London action map recently released (Smarter London Together, 2018). Table 1.2 shows a summary of the seven dimensions and the success indicators. A particularly interesting format is the layout of the vision statement that is broken down into the seven dimensions.

Table 1.2 Smart London Plan aims and measures of success

Performance dimension	Final indicators on dashboard and NPCF report
Londoners at the core	Increase the number of Londoners who use digital technology to engage in London's policy making.
	Host hackathons to involve Londoners and businesses in solving the city's growth challenges.
	Deliver a pan-London digital inclusion strategy by end 2014.
	Double the number of technology apprenticeships by end 2016.
	1000 people per borough engaged through City Hall's online research community by 2016 [33,000 in total].
With access to open data	Creation and wide dissemination of compelling evidence-based stories to demonstrate the power of open data for Londoners and businesses.
	Increase the number of Londoners who use digital technology to access information about the city.
	Publication of the Mayor's Long-Term Infrastructure Investment Plan, which includes plans for open data release, conforming to open standards by 2015.
	Evolve the London Datastore into a global exemplar platform by 2016.
	Double the number of users on the Datastore and dashboard by 2018.
Leveraging London's research, technology, and creative talent	Invest up to £24 million in the provision of affordable ultrafast broadband to SMEs, and help up to 22,000 SMEs to gain access by 2016.
	Support at least 100 SMEs through a Smart London Export Programme by 2016.
	Support an employment increase to 200,000 technology employees by 2020.
	Support a continued increase in the number of businesses who are 'innovation active' (at least by 10% up to 2020).
Brought together through networks	Establish a Smart London Innovation Network by 2014.
	£200 million levered into London to demonstrate smart city approaches by 2018.

(continued)

Table 1.2 (continued)

Performance dimension	Final indicators on dashboard and NPCF report
To enable London to adapt and grow	Make available the city's performance, consumption, and environmental data as open data (energy, water, waste, pollution).
	By 2016, develop a robust quantitative understanding of the contributions that smart technical solutions and associated services can make to the management of London's transport and environmental infrastructures.
	By 2020, stimulate smart grid services in London to restrict growth in peak electricity demand and associated infrastructure costs, with 10,000 MWh/annum of contracted supply and demand response.
	By 2020 showcase a robust 3-D map of all London's underground assets, accessible and updatable in real-time by all asset owners and works planners.
	By 2020 ensure London has the best air quality of any major world city, which will require significant (c. 50%) reduction in emissions from London's transport sector.
	Work towards a reduction of greenhouse gas emissions to reach 40% below 1990 levels by 2020.
And City Hall to Better Serve Londoners Needs	Increase data sharing between London government (City Hall and boroughs) and stakeholders.
	Conduct research to monetise the efficiencies that can be generated, and how service delivery can be improved.
	Support the continued increase in the number of SMEs winning public sector contracts or supply chain opportunities.
Offering a "Smarter" London Experience for All.	Develop an index to benchmark global progress on digital money (at the city level), and establish a digital money demonstrator by end 2015.
	Ensure London has one of the fastest wireless networks globally by 2016.
	Increase in the number of Londoners who think the use of digital technology has improved London as a city to live in.

1.4.3.1 The Central Focus on Digital Technologies

In the first version of the plan, the overwhelming focus on information technologies, data access and data and technology enabled services is clear, a focus that clearly continues and holds its central position in the new version (Smarter London Together, 2018). Equity or equitable growth do not feature in any central way in the plan, but there is some evidence of a parallel secondary focus on accessibility, environmental quality, health and education. The word "inequality" features once in the document, where it is noted as one of the central challenges faced by the city. Access to digital services and digital inclusion is provided as a solution. There is a big focus on enabling citizens' participation into the process of city building, at least the ways in which the aims and measures of success are written down, which forms a primary difference from the Australian perspective (where the measures sit objectively separated – more on this below).

1.4.3.2 The Central Focus on Open Access to Data

A crucial point to note is the focus on open access to data for businesses, as well as citizens. In comparison to the Australian case, this emerges as a big point of difference, where with the exception of the datasets provided by central and state archive offices, data is in general hard to find, and data access is harder (as compared to the London model). The London Plan makes accessible public data a central aim that is also tied in with its respective measures of success.

1.4.3.3 Action Oriented Plans Versus Performance Tracking Plans

A third interesting point of difference emerges from the structure of the plan – the London Plan is much more focused on the "measuring" being intricately tied with the "doing" and "achieving" of the stated measures of success. The measures of success are themselves worded in action-oriented ways. This sits in contrast to the Australian plan, where the performance indicator set is not directly tied to any specific achievement goals or aims, although overall broad goals are stated.

On the one hand, this is a strength of the London Plan: concretely stated achievements will necessitate the measurement of very specific sets of indicators, and these will then be employed to measure the performance of the stated goals. On the other hand, the Australian Smart Cities Plan shows a much larger set of socio-economic indicators, that at least implicitly, be closer to equitable growth concerns.

Table 1.3 lists out a naïve word count of equity related words in the texts of the three documents discussed above. It becomes quite clear that equity and equitable growth are not central concerns yet in the respective smart city agendas.

Figure 1.1 shows the wordclouds for the texts of the three plans. Infrastructure, investment, transport, economic development, data, and technology emerge as key areas, but any aspects of distributive aspects of such development are clearly missing.

1.5 A Sydney Based Case Study

The discussion in this section engages in a naïve visual exploration of both why distributive concerns need a voice in the smart city agenda, as well as prepare the ground for what possible shapes measurement and data can take if they do.

Table 1.3 A count of a representative key words related to equitable growth in the Australia and London Smart City Plans

	Smart Cities Plan, Australia	National Cities Performance Framework, Australia	Smart London Plan	Adequate measurement of dimension/concept in the Plans?
Equity	2 (with reference to debt and investments only)	0	0	No
Equitable	0	0	0	No
Wellbeing	2	14	1	No
Welfare	1	0	0	No
Inclusion/ Inclusive	0	3,0 (3)	4,1 (5)	No
Access/ Accessibility/ Accessible	25,5,3 (33)	25,6,18 (49)	23,1,8 (32)	Partially
Affordable/ Affordability/ Housing	13,9,35 (57)	2,16,100 (118)	5,0,1 (6)	Partially
Diversity	2 (in relation to biodiversity)	8	1	No
Connectivity	5	2	2	No
Health/Healthy	4,2 (6)	30,3 (33)	20, 0 (includes myhealthonline, telehealth) (20)	Partially
Education/ educated/ educational	3,1,0 (4)	13,3,5 (21)	15,0,2 (17)	Partially
Liveable	6	11	2	Partially
Poverty	0	2	0	No
Homelessness	0	7	0	No

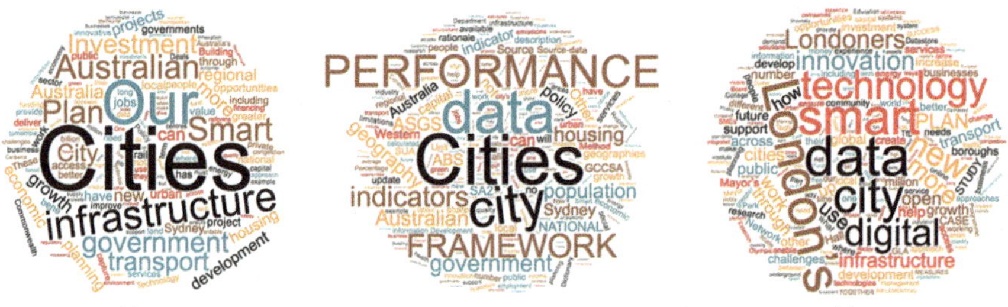

(a) (b) (c)

Fig. 1.1 Frequency based word clouds generated for the Australia and London smart city plans. In each case, all words that have been used at least ten times in each of the documents has been included in the visualization, and the size of the word corresponds to its frequency of use in the document. Appendices A, B, and C, respectively provide the actual count data

1.5.1 Distributions of the Aggregate Are Key to Measuring Performance and Future Planning

The *National Cities Performance Dashboard* presents the computed indicators described Table 1.1, by city. Inter-city comparisons are also presented. However, all the indicators are presented as overall aggregate figures, while the fundamental idea of distribution, especially spatial distributions, but also demographic or other types of sectoral distributions are not measured or presented. As an example, consider that for Sydney, it is reported that 58.2% jobs accessible by car within 30 min. However, this does not tell us anything about which areas of the city perform the best or worst, modal comparisons between public transit and automobile modes, peak hours versus non-peak hour performance, or the distribution of accessibility by demographic, industrial or occupational sectors. Figures 1.2a, b show a derived indicator of how accessible a location is and whether Sydney is really polycentric or continues to be very largely monocentric: using Journey-To-Work (JTW) data at the SA2 level, a derived (normalised) flow based indicator of accessibility is developed (Sarkar et al. 2018b). The maps show, for each SA2, its 30-min accessibility to jobs minus its 30-min accessibility to labour, by SA2, and by automobile and transit modes, by peak hours (7–9 AM). As is seen, especially for the public transport mode, there is a very large accessibility lack for most of the Sydney region, with the singular exception of the cluster formed by the SA2 Sydney- Haymarket – The Rocks, and its surrounding SA2s. Performance evaluation thus must focus on not just the aggregate amount (58.2% workers by car can access work within 30 min), but also on the proportions of workers in the outer fringes who are unable to make the 30 min limit, or the proportions of workers who are unable to make the 30 min limit by public transit, etc. This could be critical when performance analysis is done on how congestion or poor accessibility influence workforce participation and employment, for example, a case that we analyse from a multi-dimensional analysis perspective below.

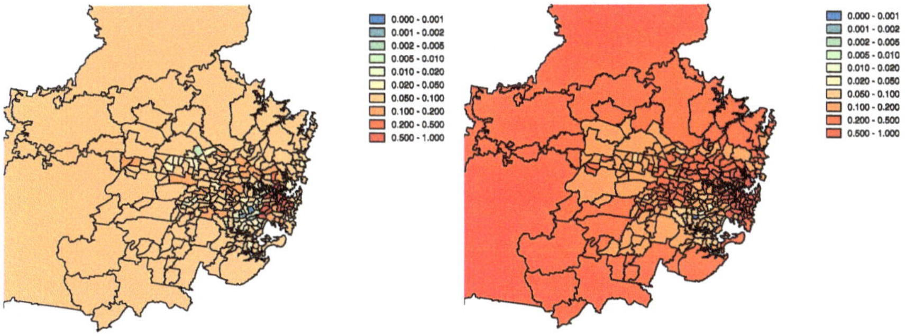

(a) (b)

Fig. 1.2 (**a**, **b**) Accessibility based centricity computed for (**a**) Automobile and (**b**) Public Transit modes computed for the Sydney GMR. The indicator is a normalised measure of 30-min accessibility to jobs minus 30-min accessibility to labour for the same SA2. Higher values correspond to a location being more "central" as a workplace in the city. The maps have been reproduced from (Sarkar et al. 2018b)

1.5.2 *Multidimensional Analyses Are Key to Measuring Performance and Future Planning*

The *National Cities Performance Dashboard* currently organises the presentation of indicators by category and type, along the 6 dimensions shown in Table 1.1, and while inter-city comparisons are enabled through this framework, a multidimensional analysis of a single issue is not. A multidimensional analysis is defined as an analysis on a single focus issue that spans through multiple dimensions. For example, if a relationship between barriers and incentives to workforce participation rates (that ultimately affects and access to public transit was being considered (as increasing workforce participation rate is a smart city goal), then the dimensions of Jobs and Skills and Infrastructure and Investment need to be considered together. Figure 1.3 shows the spatial concentrations of people in a lower middle and very high income category in the Sydney Greater Metropolitan region, alongside proposed new housing supply and transport infrastructure for the region. From a visual

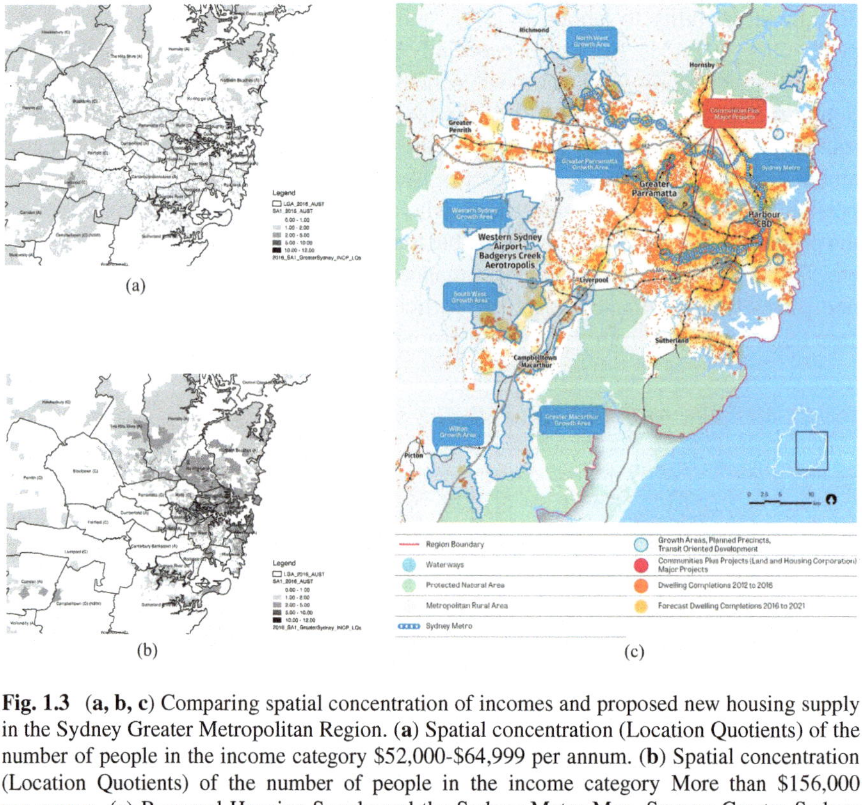

(a) (b) (c)

Fig. 1.3 (**a, b, c**) Comparing spatial concentration of incomes and proposed new housing supply in the Sydney Greater Metropolitan Region. (**a**) Spatial concentration (Location Quotients) of the number of people in the income category \$52,000-\$64,999 per annum. (**b**) Spatial concentration (Location Quotients) of the number of people in the income category More than \$156,000 per annum. (**c**) Proposed Housing Supply and the Sydney Metro Map. Source: Greater Sydney Commission, https://www.greater.sydney/metropolis-of-three-cities/liveability/housing-city/greater-housing-supply comparison of Figs. 1.1a, b we immediately see that while lower and middle income categories are spread more or less over the entire region with a greater concentration towards the west and south, there is a very sharp concentration of the highest income earners in the north and east of Sydney. While this spatial inequality is quite well-established in the literature, when we look at the new housing supply, and very critically the new transport infrastructure lines (the Sydney Metro), it is likely that a high proportion of high income earners are well served by new transport infrastructure, but a high proportion of lower and middle income earners, spatially concentrated in regions that do not come under new transport infrastructure development, lose out on the increases to participation and productivity that they could have contributed to if provided with better access and connectivity opportunities. Further, Fig. 1.4 shows the proportion of unemployed persons as a proportion of the total number of workers, again by SA1: new proposed public transit does not serve areas with the highest unemployment.

While it is likely that density is a major reason for public transit provision (economies of scale and benefits will be realised for public transit investment when the areas are high density), the reverse is also true: once an area is connected by public transit, accessibility, and therefore density will increase. In Sydney's case, the multidimensional analysis of several variables considered together and spatially shows that the north-east and the south-west parts of the city have distinctly uneven geog-

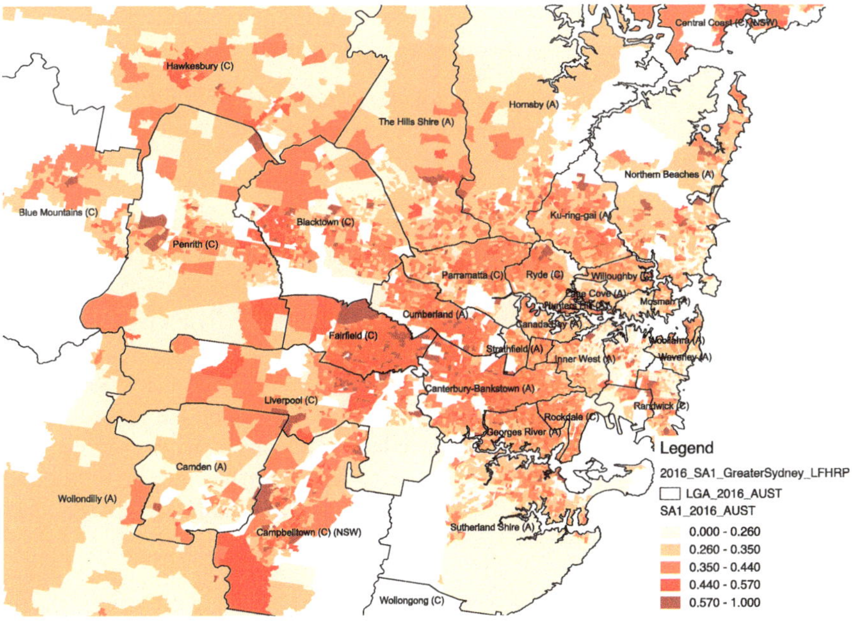

Fig. 1.4 Proportion of unemployed (looking for work full time, looking for work part time) and people over 15 years not in labour force against total number of workers by SA1 in the Sydney Greater Metropolitan region

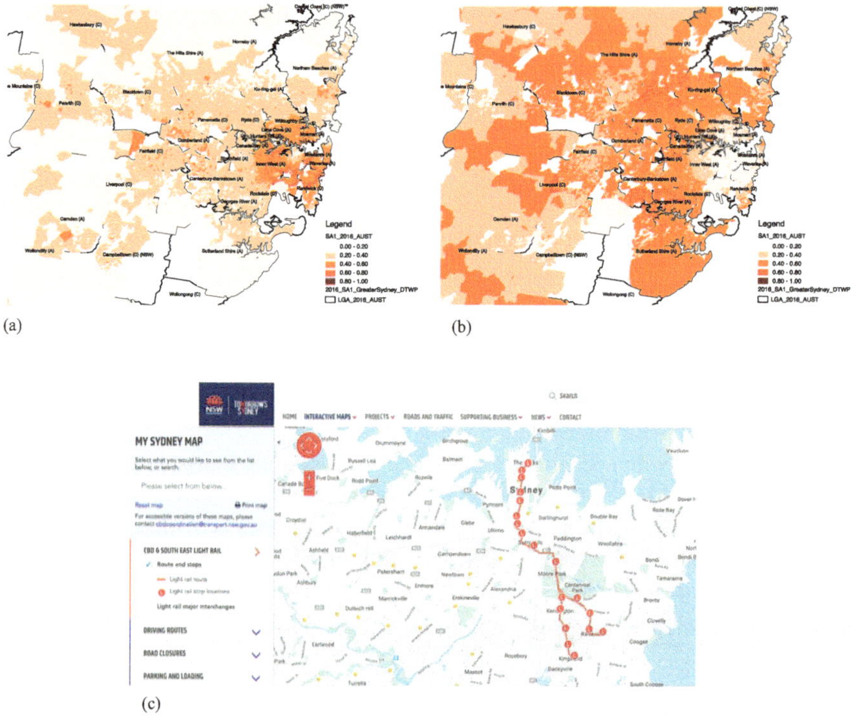

Fig. 1.5 (**a**) Proportion of people travelling from 2.5 km to less than 10 km by SA1. (**b**) Proportion of people travelling from 10 km to less than 30 km by SA1. (**c**) Sydney CBD and South East Light Rail. https://mysydneycbd.nsw.gov.au/interactive-maps?eld_map_ids[0]=54ee46d749c4405 97c611721. (**a**, **b**) Travel to work distance in Sydney, and (**c**) Proposed Sydney CBD and South East Light Rail

raphies of public investment. Figure 1.5 shows, by SA1, the proportion of people travelling from 2.5 km to less than 10 km, and from 10 km to less than 30 km: the accessibility is spatially symmetric, but Figs. 1.3c and 1.5c combined together show significant public transit investment occurring around the Sydney CBD (which already enjoys extremely high access by all public transit modes), the south-east areas close to the CBD, and the north-west. The west and south are clear losers. The economic perspective on inequality measurement and distributive justice (Foster and Sen 1997) will then argue that social welfare is maximised when income transfers occur in the direction of those who need it the most. Instead, income or resource transfers to the already better off groups increase inequality and decrease the social welfare of the entire system.

1.6 Discussion: A Set of Five Recommendations

This paper reviewed ideas on the multidimensional measurement of wellbeing from economics, and proposed the primary thesis that smart cities must include equity as an important dimension of performance. By analysing current examples of Smart City Plans for Australia and London, it brought out that even when an overall productivity, income, wealth or any other aggregate measure rises, if inequalities and uneven geographies of distribution also rise comparably, this might mean more people are worse off, even when the average is rising. Any measurement of smart city performance would consider this critical issue if the smart city is to maximise collective welfare over individual welfare. We provide here a set of five recommendations:

(a) ***Make equity a central, explicitly stated goal for smart cities.***

Aggregate economic development, by itself, cannot be taken to automatically raise wellbeing and collective welfare. By concentrating on distributive issues explicitly, along with the aggregative issues, the smart city agenda can drive its aims for building resilient, sustainable and efficient cities not just for specific groups but for most groups, especially the most disadvantaged whose needs might be greater than others who are better off.

(b) ***Along with positive indicators, develop normative indicators that measure gains and losses of wellbeing and social and spatial welfare***

The issue of measurement is crucial. If we do not measure distribution, we will never record the gains, losses and redistributions of access and equity and local evolution that occur through major global investment decisions. Further, positive indicators must be augmented with normative indicators that can explicitly measure deviations from an acceptable equitable standard of distribution (Foster and Sen 1997; Sen 1992). The two competing models of distribution are discussed in (Foster and Sen 1997): (a) the "needs" based view: the most needy person is considered when distribution is in focus, or (b) the "desert" based view: the most deserving person is considered when distribution is in focus. However, (b) is fraught with difficulties: even though a school teacher's salary is much lower than say a banker's salary, there could be no ethical basis to say that a banker is more deserving of a higher income (or in this case resources and investment directed to where most bankers live). Instead, it could be argued that several low and middle income groups render extremely vital services to the economy, and in the needs based view deserve to be served by a smart city in the same proportion, or in some cases more, than a higher income person. While defining the normative criteria for what is "just" is a difficult question, even beginning to acknowledge wellbeing measurement within smart city frameworks would be a good start.

(c) ***Make analysis of performance multi-dimensional and spatial.***

As the short analysis on Sydney reveals, wellbeing is multidimensional. Smart and the measurement of smart should also be multi-dimensional. This type of analysis and evidence base becomes critical when major public investment decisions are taken – so that wellbeing for the most vulnerable and for those who need access and connectivity the most is maximised. Multidimensional analysis of smart performance should extend to infrastructure (transport, housing), amenities (green space, schools, hospitals), and other dimensions of life that are affected by the physical organisation of cities. Analysis should be spatial, and not aggregate, since the spatial distribution brings out uneven geographies of development that remain hidden when only aggregate measures are considered.

(d) ***Use new types of data for performance evaluation***

Combine and leverage the power of open data sources to traditional data sources to capture new processes of disruption and reorganisation, such as the informal housing market, the informal transport sector, or digital disruptions in the rental market (Gurran and Phibbs 2017, Alizadeh et al. 2018). Capture local voices and local flavours of smart: it is important to have a common framework to understand cities, but it is also important to understand how each city might have its very own local needs and desires based sculpting of smart (Dowling et al. 2018). Develop a new expanded set of indicators that captures new spatial processes unfolding in the smart, technologically framed city.

(e) ***Use real time data for performance evaluation***

Finally, with smart cards and smart apps in smart cities, there is a wealth of data that can be used to measure and understand the performance of the real-time city (Batty 2012, 2013; Townsend 2013). While there are valid privacy concerns, and the ethics on the "surveillance" of citizens to capture personalised data, it can be argued that it is already being captured by private organisations. This data, suitably anonymised, and brought into the public open access data domain ensures that it is accessible to everyone collectively (this should actually be posed as a *fundamental right to data*, especially as it is generated by everyone collectively), and can be used to inform real time city planning. Develop a new expanded set of indicators that captures real time spatial processes unfolding in the smart, technologically driven city.

This chapter has focused on issues of measurement, analysis and data on smart cities. But, the act of measurement itself is a subjective issue – there is no such thing as objective data measurement. Therefore, it becomes even more critical to actively discuss the role of equitable growth and distributive justice: a smart city would give power to those who have the least in the system.

Acknowledgements The author would like to thank her 45 students and 2 tutors, Catherine Gilbert and Carolina Rodriguez, of the *2017 Urban Data and Science of Cities* unit of study at The University of Sydney. The major assessment that the students worked on was to critique, redesign and extend the indicator set proposed on the *National Cities Performance Framework*, with a specific equity focus. The author would like to thank the entire team and acknowledges the stimulating discussions in class.

Appendices

Appendix A: Word Counts (Upto 10 Times) for the Smart Cities Plan, Australia

200	Cities
134	our
92	infrastructure
75	Australian
74	smart
71	plan
64	government
61	investment
59	transport
55	city
44	more
43	Australia
40	can
40	growth
39	new
38	regional
37	economic
36	development
36	projects
35	housing
35	planning
30	have
29	jobs
29	urban
28	Sydney
27	local
26	opportunities
26	project
26	through
25	access
25	governments
25	greater
25	value
25	work
24	has
24	national
24	people
24	rail

23	including
23	public
22	better
22	building
22	deliver
22	these
21	not
21	services
20	improve
20	private
20	sector
20	technology
19	business
19	capture
19	Commonwealth
19	innovative
19	land
19	long
19	need
19	provide
18	energy
18	policy
18	term
18	use
18	where
18	financing
17	Australia's
17	billion
17	capital
17	data
17	deals
17	economy
17	funding
17	they
16	tomorrow
15	approach
15	centres
15	congestion
15	example
15	reforms
14	across
14	between
14	challenges
14	do
14	fund

14	job
14	live
14	major
14	million
14	must
14	population
14	reform
13	environment
13	metropolitan
13	one
13	affordable
13	state
13	such
13	supply
13	support
12	based
12	but
12	Canberra
12	cent
12	ensure
12	green
12	innovation
12	investments
12	levels
12	potential
12	quality
11	areas
11	businesses
11	create
11	drive
11	high
11	make
11	Melbourne
11	needs
11	other
11	regulatory
11	well
11	when
10	area
10	coast
10	cost
10	costs
10	department
10	emissions
10	future

10	governance
10	important
10	increasing
10	involved
10	key
10	Manchester
10	most
10	outcomes
10	report
10	system
10	technologies
10	time
10	up

Appendix B: Word Counts (Upto 10 Times) for the National Cities Performance Framework, Australia

344	cities
293	data
261	city
217	PERFORMANCE
159	FRAMEWORK
140	indicators
116	government
106	Australian
100	housing
100	population
97	geography
90	ASGS
80	can
80	policy
78	ABS
78	Sydney
73	other
72	Australia
72	indicator
70	not
66	capital
65	NATIONAL
62	SA2
62	Western
59	source

56	geographies
55	local
54	will
53	GCCSA
53	no
51	growth
51	people
49	description
49	services
49	SUA
49	Unit
47	rationale
47	update
46	method
46	source-data
46	urban
45	all
45	have
44	economic
44	public
44	regional
43	more
43	share
42	available
40	number
39	limitations
39	social
39	work
38	infrastructure
38	jobs
38	use
36	areas
36	calculated
36	development
36	green
36	information
35	new
35	report
34	dictionary
34	emissions
34	help
33	industry
33	percentage
32	city’s
32	how

32	innovation
32	labour
32	planning
32	quality
32	smart
31	department
31	employment
31	example
31	rate
31	space
31	transport
30	health
30	measure
30	our
29	census
29	community
29	greater
28	align
28	Australia's
28	energy
28	income
28	one
28	research
27	average
27	support
26	across
26	over
26	time
25	access
25	business
25	future
24	change
24	liveability
23	environment
23	estimates
23	five
23	household
23	investment
23	life
23	Melbourne
23	proportions
23	state
22	based
22	better
22	Building

22	economy
22	include
22	level
22	may
22	provide
22	summed
22	understand
22	yearly
21	Council
21	global
21	opportunities
21	they
20	Canberra
20	important
20	key
20	priorities
20	well
19	been
19	force
19	households
19	industries
19	within
18	accessible
18	air
18	area
18	digital
18	governance
18	improve
18	Index
17	different
17	dwelling
17	governments
17	greenhouse
17	measures
17	online
17	water
16	affordability
16	annually
16	contextual
16	institute
16	output
16	size
16	skills
15	aims
15	between

15	businesses
15	cent
15	challenges
15	deals
15	gas
15	including
15	provides
15	range
15	ratio
15	SA4
15	together
15	travel
15	weights
15	years
14	annual
14	city-level
14	comparable
14	congestion
14	dwellings
14	international
14	land
14	levels
14	productivity
14	statistical
14	three
14	updates
14	users
14	wellbeing
14	year
13	centre
13	converted
13	derived
13	disadvantage
13	education
13	frameworks
13	knowledge
13	make
13	minutes
13	person
13	persons
13	proportion
13	reliable
13	sustainable
13	understanding
12	age

12	chart
12	context
12	living
12	objectives
12	only
12	peak
12	progress
12	rates
12	residential
12	science
12	six
12	socio-economic
12	when
12	where
11	coast
11	communities
11	construction
11	consultation
11	costs
11	less
11	liveable
11	made
11	price
11	score
11	should
11	success
11	times
11	University
11	who
10	activity
10	amount
10	association
10	consistent
10	every
10	high
10	higher
10	improved
10	interim
10	many
10	measuring
10	median
10	mesh
10	Perth
10	place
10	statistics

10	sustainability
10	unavailable
10	unemployment
10	updated

Appendix C: Word Counts (Upto 10 Times) for the Smart London Plan

367	LONDON
138	data
132	London's
124	smart
121	city
98	technology
94	digital
85	new
67	innovation
65	Londoners
64	more
52	PLAN
52	use
51	infrastructure
46	open
45	cities
45	work
44	how
41	transport
40	through
40	up
39	public
37	help
36	across
36	growth
34	development
34	global
33	future
33	number
33	support
32	other
31	million
30	challenges
30	STUDY

29	boroughs
29	develop
29	increase
29	investment
28	businesses
28	CASE
28	create
28	Hall
28	Mayor's
28	services
27	better
27	local
27	network
26	opportunities
25	needs
24	different
24	people
24	research
24	their
23	access
23	community
23	one
23	world
22	energy
22	including
22	information
22	what
22	where
21	approaches
21	business
21	ensure
21	GLA
21	our
20	approach
20	enable
20	experience
20	money
20	park
20	planning
20	service
20	TfL
20	time
20	traffic
19	capital
19	change

19	datastore
19	greater
19	online
19	technologies
19	working
18	between
18	make
18	Mayor
18	part
18	scale
18	SUCCESS
18	Tech
17	areas
17	college
17	management
17	need
17	not
17	SMEs
17	solutions
17	system
17	systems
17	term
16	demand
16	free
16	Olympic
16	Programme
16	real
16	TOGETHER
16	waste
16	way
16	ways
15	Board
15	centre
15	companies
15	Education
15	end
15	MEASURES
15	most
15	provide
15	sector
15	set
15	UK
14	assets
14	congestion
14	economy

14	establish
14	identify
14	IMPLEMENTING
14	institute
14	Oyster
14	underground
14	Urban
13	Catapult
13	created
13	Hire
13	integrated
13	meet
13	mobile
13	policy
13	results
12	engage
12	entrepreneurs
12	first
12	fund
12	high
12	ideas
12	NHS
12	out
12	platform
12	population
12	project
12	role
12	sharing
12	SMARTER
12	social
12	standards
12	talent
12	times
11	already
11	authority
11	both
11	build
11	connected
11	costs
11	cycle
11	existing
11	financial
11	firms
11	level
11	live

11	markets
11	NETWORKS
11	schools
11	showcase
11	skills
11	University
11	users
11	your
10	activity
10	bring
10	broadband
10	BUILDING
10	capital's
10	city's
10	deliver
10	efficiencies
10	Elizabeth
10	encourage
10	enterprise
10	European
10	Imperial
10	improve
10	jobs
10	least
10	long
10	market
10	organisations
10	private
10	providers
10	put
10	quality
10	Queen
10	reduce
10	road
10	Scheme
10	talk
10	them
10	two
10	want
10	Wi-Fi

References

Alizadeh, T., Farid, R., & Sarkar, S. (2018). Towards understanding the socioeconomic patterns of sharing economy in Australia: An investigation of Airbnb listings in the Sydney and Melbourne metropolitan regions. *Urban Policy and Research.* https://doi.org/10.1080/08111146.2018.1460269.

Australian Government (2016a) *Smart Cities Plan,* Department of the Prime Minister and the cabinet.

Australian Government. (2016b). *National cities performance framework, smart cities plan.* Department of the Prime Minister and the Cabinet.

Batty, M. (2012). Smart cities, big data. *Environment and Planning B, 39*, 191–193.

Batty, M. (2013). Big data, smart cities, and city planning. *Dialogues in Human Geography, 3*(3), 274–279.

Dowling, R., McGuirk, P., & Maalsen, S. (2018) Realising smart cities: Partnerships and economic development in the emergence and practice of smart in Newcastle, Australia, *Inside smart cities* (pp. 33–47). London: Routledge.

Foster, J., & Sen, A. (1997). *On economic inequality*. Oxford: Oxford University Press.

Gurran, N., & Phibbs, P. (2017). When tourists move in: How should urban planners respond to Airbnb. *Journal of the American Planning Association, 83*(1), 80–92.

Sarkar, S. (2018). Urban scaling and the geographic concentrations of inequality by city size. *Environment and Planning B*, early access online: 2399808318766070.

Sarkar, S., Phibbs, P., Simpson, R., & Wasnik, S. (2018a). The scaling of income distribution in Australia: Possible relationships between urban allometry, city size, and economic inequality. *Environment and Planning B, 45*(4), 603–622.

Sarkar, S., Wu, H., & Levinson, D. (2018b). *Measuring polycentricity via network flows, spatial interaction, and percolation*. Working paper pre-print: http://hdl.handle.net/2123/18792

Sen, A. (1992). *Inequality reexamined*. Oxford: Oxford University Press.

Stiglitz, J. E., Sen, A., & Fitoussi, J.-P. (2010). *Mismeasuring our lives: Why the GDP does not add up*. New York: New Press.

Townsend, A. M. (2013). *Smart cities: Big data, civic hackers, and the quest for a new utopia.* New York: WW Norton & Company.

Chapter 2
The Convenient City: Smart Urbanism for a Resilient City

Rob Roggema

Abstract The surge of smart city technology, thinking, publications and consultancy offerings is significant. This implies there is something seriously developing. But to what extent is this a new development? In this paper the case will be made that urban design has always had to include new technologies and the smart city movement is just another wave of technology that demands inclusion in urban design practice. Nevertheless, city designers and policy makers should make use of the new possibilities on offering. Interactive urban environments could support healthy living, while smart and responsive regulators could minimize our energy use, and anticipative traffic management could help minimising congestion. Further to this, crowd-sensing could smoothen urban mobility and new forms of 3d-printing may re-use and reduce waste. The core of all new technological potential however is still to service people and to make life for urban citizens better. How could people in search for a convenient life be better serviced? Many of them want to have a nice house, a clean, safe and healthy environment, access to resources such as clean water, renewable energy and healthy food, a resilient place that is not vulnerable for all kinds of climate impacts and possibly some room for contemplation. With Maslow's ladder in mind, achieving this not only depends on the availability and use of technology, rather a well-designed and integrated urban plan is asked for. Meeting the needs of contemporary urban citizens must be served by what urban design is supposed to deliver, only now with current available technologies in the back pocket. The paper emphasises how to design the convenient city by making use of the available technology, but it also takes a stand on the relativity of the current hype of smart cities.

Keywords Smart urbanism · Convenience · Resilience · Smart city

R. Roggema (✉)
Research Centre for the Built Environment NoorderRuimte,
Hanze University of Applied Sciences, Groningen, The Netherlands
e-mail: r.e.roggema@pl.hanze.nl

N. Biloria (ed.), *Data-driven Multivalence in the Built Environment*, S.M.A.R.T. Environments, https://doi.org/10.1007/978-3-030-12180-8_2

2.1 Introduction

Your smartphone, yes it gives you all the options to live your live. The invention of the Internet has opened a connected world and exchange of information is now easier than ever. The smart city is under construction, with light bulbs that turn on when you pass, cycle paths that lighten up when you ride over them, energy generating roads and self-charging highways that charge your electric car. We are sensed everywhere and out of our user profiles Google, Facebook, and Microsoft know more about your choices in life than yourself (O'Grady et al. 2016). They use your profiles to predict what is going to happen. Sometimes this creates solutions that make life easier, such as the Rain Sense project (Foresti and Seed 2014; AMS 2014), or more environmental friendly, as the New Raw project illustrates (AMS 2016; Thenewraw undated), but sometimes it is just big data that isn't necessarily essential for the quality of life, such as understanding why Indian cuisine is unique (Jain et al. 2015), or how to grow the ideal Christmas tree (Buckley 2014).

The smart city is all around us, and many prospectuses promise better urban lives supported by loads of technology. High-tech could add to the quality of our urban environments and could help us in daily life. The fridge knows when to order new milk or eggs, the building could respond to our demands, creating more comfortable surroundings. But, is the smart city really novel? Or is it just another phase in human development, a new add-on of technology, just as it always has done, accommodating us to live our (urban) lives. And is the city fundamentally different from the pre-smart city era? There is a broad and solid number of academic outputs available describing the benefits of smart cities, but also questioning its real impact. In this article the role of smartness in conceiving cities is explored. The definitions of smart city and the role new technologies could play in creating a sustainable or resilient city are discussed. Secondly the position of technology in the development of society is illuminated. In the next section a more fundamental question is asked when a city performs well according the SDG's (UN 2015) hence when smart city thinking contributes to establishing a resilient, sustainable city. The article then ends with the conditions for realising a convenient and resilient city, through a design-led, tech-supported collaborative model, before concluding.

2.2 Recent Developments and Thinking About Smart Cities

Urban growth raises a variety of problems that tend to jeopardize the environmental, economic, and social sustainability of cities (e.g. Neirotti et al. 2014). In more detail, rapid urbanization of the world, albeit an emblem of social evolution, gives rise to numerous challenges associated with intensive energy consumption, endemic congestion, saturated transport networks, air and water pollution, toxic waste disposal, resource depletion, social inequality and vulnerability, public health decrease, and so on. In a nutshell, as a dynamic clustering of people, buildings, infrastructures, and resources (Bibri 2013), urbanization puts an enormous strain on urban systems, thereby stressing urban life in terms of the underlying operating and organizing processes, functions, and services (Bibri and Krogstie 2017).

2.2.1 Definitions

In literature a multitude of definitions about smart cities is available without any universally acknowledged definition (Allwinkle and Cruickshank 2011; Chourabi et al. 2012; Hollands 2008; Komninos 2011; Lombardi et al. 2012; Nam and Pardo 2011; Papa et al. 2013; Wolfram 2012). Furthermore, strategic planning for the development of smart cities is still a largely unknown field (ABB 2012; Abdoullaev 2011; Chourabi et al. 2012; Gsma and Cisco 2011; Hollands 2008; Huber and Mayer 2012; Komninos 2011; Nam and Pardo 2011) and the terms 'smart' and 'intelligent' are used interchangeably throughout literature (Hollands 2008; Pardo et al. 2012; Wolfram 2012).

Smart city is defined by two essential attributes. First is the use of technologies to facilitate the coordination of fragmented urban sub-systems (energy, water, mobility, built environment). Becoming 'smart' by improving subsystems is associated with new employment opportunities, wealth creation and economic growth. In a second and more futuristic definition, smart cities are urban places where lived experiences calls forth a new reality (Glasmeier and Christopherson 2015). Several perspectives on smart city are defined:

- A city well performing in a forward-looking way in economy, people, governance, mobility, environment, and living, built on the smart combination of endowments and activities of self-decisive, independent and aware citizens (Giffinger et al. 2007).
- A city that monitors and integrates conditions of all of its critical infrastructures, including roads, bridges, tunnels, rails, subways, airports, seaports, communications, water, power, even major buildings, can better optimize its resources, plan its preventive maintenance activities, and monitor security aspects while maximizing services to its citizens (Hall 2000).
- A city "connecting the physical infrastructure, the IT infrastructure, the social infrastructure, and the business infrastructure to leverage the collective intelligence of the city" (Harrison et al. 2010)
- A city striving to make itself "smarter" (more efficient, sustainable, equitable, and liveable) (Natural Resources Defence Council undated)
- A city "combining ICT and Web 2.0 technology with other organizational, design and planning efforts to dematerialize and speed up bureaucratic processes and help to identify new, innovative solutions to city management complexity, in order to improve sustainability and liveability." (Toppeta 2010)
- "The use of Smart Computing technologies to make the critical infrastructure components and services of a city—which include city administration, education,

healthcare, public safety, real estate, transportation, and utilities—more intelligent, interconnected, and efficient" (Washburn et al. 2010)

The smart city "utilising networked infrastructures to improve economic and political efficiency and enable socio-cultural and urban development" (Hollands 2008, p. 307) has been projected as a panacea to problems related to rapid urbanization and a way to achieve sustainable development (Datta 2015). Information and Communication Technologies (ICTs) are claimed to be at the core of the smart city discourse (Graham and Marvin 2001), which emphasises "enhancing the socioeconomic, ecological, logistic and competitive performance of cities" (Kourtit and Nijkamp 2012, p. 93). It is further articulated that such an aim could be achieved by tapping human capital, infrastructural capital, social capital and the entrepreneurial capital of the city. In a nutshell, the intent of the smart city is to offer its citizens the highest possible quality of urban life (Bakici et al. 2013).

2.2.2 *Smart and Resilient*

In recent years, there has been a shift in cities striving for smart city targets instead of sustainability goals (Marsal-Llacuna et al. 2015). However, smart cities share often similar goals as sustainable cities (Ahvenniemi et al. 2017). And then, there are 'sustainable cities'; 'green cities'; 'liveable cities'; 'digital cities'; 'intelligent cities'; 'smart cities'; 'knowledge cities'; 'information cities'; 'resilient cities'; 'eco cities'; 'low carbon cities' proposed, and even combinations of these, such as 'low carbon eco cities' and 'ubiquitous eco cities'. Each of these terms apparently seeks to capture and conceptualise key aspects of ongoing urban sustainability efforts. Closer examination, however, reveals that policy makers, planners and developers often use the terms interchangeably. If the terms are largely interchangeable this would imply that 'sustainable', 'smart', 'resilient' etc. cities are informed by an overarching common understanding of urban development and regeneration which seeks to interrelate social, economic and environmental dimensions in a balanced and mutually beneficial way (De Jong et al. 2015).

Based on three overarching conceptualisations, sustainable development (Barton 2000; Wheeler and Beatley 2009; Rydin 2010), ecological modernisation (Hajer 1996; Mol 2001; Mol et al. 2009), and regenerative sustainability (du Plessis 2012; Cole 2012; Cole et al. 2012; Mang and Reed 2012; Girardet 2013; Robinson and Cole 2015; Gabel undated) the various city categories mentioned could be understood as implying major overlap: 'intelligent', 'low carbon', 'resilient', 'liveable' cities would essentially all point in the same direction, whereby comprehensive human-supported technological interventions benefit social well-being, economic growth and ecological regeneration in the city (De Jong et al. 2015).

In academic literature, with an interest in knowledge and information development, the meaning of 'smart' covers a range of technological characteristics, such as self-configuring, self-healing, self-protection, and self-optimizing (Nam and

Pardo 2011). In industrial literature with a tendency in business and industrial instruments, "smart" refers to intelligent-acting products and services, artificial intelligence, and thinking machines (Nam and Pardo 2011). Finally, governmental documents, which aim to manage urban development, interpret 'smart' with regard to an urban planning theory, Smart Growth, which emerged in the US in early 90's to avoid urban sprawl (Herrschel 2013), supporting compact, mixed-use and walkable cities and making development decisions predictable, fair and cost effective. It encourages community and stakeholder collaboration (EPA 2014).

The Smart City is a sustainable and efficient city with high 'Quality of Life' that aims to address urban challenges by application of ICT in its infrastructure and services, collaboration between its key stakeholders, integration of its main domains and investment in social capital (Mosannenzadeh and Vettorato 2014). The core, underlying promise is that more information will improve the experience of urban social life and lead to the creation of many useful and efficient services (Rabari and Storper 2015). How does urban form contribute to sustainable development? Relevant questions in this regard involve how these forms should be monitored, understood, analysed, and planned to improve sustainability. The underlying argument is that urban systems have been in themselves complex in terms of their operation, management, assessment, and planning in line with the vision of sustainability. Here comes the role of ICT into play given its foundation on the application of complexity sciences to urban systems and problems (Batty et al. 2012a, b; Bibri and Krogstie 2016). The development of smart city with its various faces has come to the fore in recent years as a promising response to the same challenge (e.g. Al Nuaimi et al. 2015; Batty et al. 2012a, b; Neirotti et al. 2014) by developing smart solutions for sustainability, optimizing efficiency in urban systems, and enhancing the quality of life of citizens. It is in such cities that the key to a better world, which is held by ICT, will be most evidently demonstrated (Batty et al. 2012a, b). The question is, is that promise made to everyone, is the conception of the 'smart city' inclusive or does it, by the very nature of the data it relies upon, exclude important groups in society?

The interlinked development of sustainability awareness, urban growth, and technological development have recently converged under what is labelled 'smart sustainable cities' (Höjer and Wangel 2015). A smart sustainable city', although not always explicitly discussed, is used to denote a city that is supported by a pervasive presence and massive use of advanced ICT, which, in connection with various urban domains and systems and how these intricately interrelate, enables cities to become more sustainable and to provide citizens with a better quality of life. In more detail, it can be described as a social fabric made of a complex set of net-works of relations between various synergistic clusters of urban entities that, in taking a holistic and systemic approach converge on a common approach into using and applying smart technologies that enable to create, disseminate, and to mainstream solutions and methods that help provide a fertile environment conducive to improving the contribution to the goals of sustainable development (Bibri and Krogstie 2017). Smart sustainable cities entail thinking about and conceiving of urban environments as constellations of instruments across spatial and temporal scales that are networked in multiple ways to provide continuous data coming from urban domains, employing pervasive sensing, processing, and networking technologies, in order to monitor, understand, and analyse how cities function and can be managed so as to guide and direct their development towards sustainability (Bibri and Krogstie 2017).

The traditional model of the city, which is founded on the idea of the city as being a stable or constant structure, is rapidly changing, so too are the associated planning approaches in response to the emerging shifts brought by computing and ICT, under-pinned by their foundation on the complexity and data sciences: from focusing on physical and spatial development to including broader principles (e.g. sustainability) and relying on big data analytics, context information processing, intelligence functions, and simulation models, and what these entail in terms of sensing, computing, data processing, and wireless networking technologies (Bibri and Krogstie 2017).

The integrated model of the smart sustainable city works toward the following assets (Angelidou 2015):

- Advancement of human capital: citizen empowerment (informed, educated, and participatory citizens), intellectual capital and knowledge creation (Aurigi 2006; Chourabi et al. 2012; Komninos 2009; Liugailaité-Radzvickiené and Jucevičius 2012; Neves 2009; Ratti and Townsend 2011).
- Advancement of social capital: social sustainability and digital inclusion (Batty et al. 2012a, b; Caragliu et al. 2009; Hodgkinson 2011; Liugailaité-Radzvickiené and Jucevičius 2012).
- Behavioural change—sense of agency and meaning (i.e. the feeling that we are all owners and equally responsible for our city) (Frenchman et al. 2011; Townsend et al. 2010).
- Humane approach: Technology responsive to needs, skills and interests of users, respecting their diversity and individuality (Bria 2012; Lind 2012; Roche et al. 2012; Streitz 2011).

In the smart cities discourse, the conviction that collecting historical data sets will provide the insights for planning and design is often believed in (see e.g. Rathore et al. 2016). However, this is risky as even when big data is collected, for instance through abundant placement of sensors and IoT practice, all relevant data can never be collected. Especially subjective data such as emotions, values and moods of people are difficult to collect and may change considerably over time. Also, the data of the past does not give any certainty about the future. Especially factors such as climate change, migration and economic change will influence the sort of city that is required in the future. The use of data is generally sectoral which might make it useful, but urbanism is integrative for reasons that in the city all different factors are present in conjunction with each other at every given time. A sectoral approach could then solve the traffic problem, while other problems, such as biodiversity or water might increase as result. Finally, design is science with creativity build into its approaches. Creativity implies emergence of unexpected combinations, integration of problems, and the employment of novel propositions.

Paraphrasing Jane Jacobs (Jacobs 1961) social ideas (and laws) shape private investments, which shapes cities, today's planning and procurement practices do not explicitly recognize the value of the Smart City vision, and therefore are not shaping the financial instruments to deliver it (Robinson undated). Urban life comes first, then urban place, before thinking technology.

As is often the case with technological change, the producers can't dream users into existence, but instead uptake requires learning by doing through collaboration and risk sharing. The degree of know-how and collateral resources required to use smart city interventions, assuming that everyone owns a smart phone and knows how to operate it at maximum performance, is often taken for granted, but technology audits are necessary to reveal just how flexible, usable and accessible these technology designs are (Offenhuber 2015). Beyond making cities more liveable because their inner political workings are more accessible, local organisations are building tools to make 'sensibility' real, using devices such as Carlo Ratti's City Lab's algorithm, which integrates crowd sourced data from cell phone users who are seeking to track night life hot spots. But how much of the smart city research is being directed toward questions of groups in society unlikely to be consulted or enabled to use the sophisticated facets of a cell phone? What of the elderly, the disabled, the economically and socially isolated? (Glasmeier and Christopherson 2015). The goal should be to produce morally balanced and socially aware smart city strategies, stakeholder engagement is crucial. Stakeholder engagement can provide valuable insights about the assets and the needs of the city, increase public acceptance of the smart city venture and elevate the 'smartness' of the city to a whole new level, leveraging human capital and collective intelligence (Angelidou 2014).

Therefore, the role of technologies in smart cities should be in enabling sustainable development of cities as suggested by Bifulco et al. (2016), not in the new technology as an end in itself (Marsal-Llacuna and Segal 2016). Ultimately, a city that is not sustainable is not really "smart" (Ahvenniemi et al. 2017). Although smart city technology investments are mainly comprised of upgrades rather than true innovations, on the citizen user side, they potentially offer access to information on local conditions. They can afford communities and interest groups the opportunity to identify negative conditions and the potential to improve the urban experience (Glasmeier and Christopherson 2015). Citizen movements have demonstrated the ability to successfully adopt and adapt the core of smart city technologies to engage in public debate and to advocate for urban improvements (Glasmeier and Christopherson 2015).

The need to develop an inclusive city that is sustainable and supported by technology, is evident. The urban planning process, in several steps from abstract-larger scale, to implementation and smaller scale should therefore be linked with information attributes of smart cities: users (both providers of data and the end-users), services, infrastructure and data (Anthopoulos and Vakali 2012).

2.3 Urban Transitions

Toffler and Toffler (2006), distinguish three global revolutions of wealth. Every period has its own characteristics, and technology attached to it. In the first wave of wealth, agricultural society, farmers used agricultural techniques and tools to cultivate the land, and let things grow. In this period the family was the dominant social unit.

The second period is the industrial society, in which the household became the social entity and mass movements emerged for the production of tangible products in hierarchal organized factories. Land, labour and capital are the main production factors. Within this 'wave of wealth' cities made the transformation from medieval to industrial, with newly developed railways, industrial estates, collective housing for the workers and the instalment of sanitary systems, and from this industrial period through towards the car-based society with its ring roads, high-rise buildings, CBD's and suburbs. This functional city promised a healthy urban life, which was clean and efficient, and supplied with clean nuclear energy, yet it brought an urban metabolism which is completely out of sync (Hajer and Dassen 2014). The third wave of wealth, the prosumer society, is currently emerging and based on knowledge and the individualizing of production, markets and society. Intangible products, based on service, thought, understanding and experience, are produced in connected networks. Socially, a diversity of cohabitation forms exists (Toffler and Toffler 2006). In this time a transformation from the car-based industrialised society to an eco-efficient one need to be made. Smart urban technologies are needed to support this transition in which renewable energy is generated, waste is recycled, traffic is sustainably managed and carbon emissions are rigorously brought down (Hajer and Dassen 2014). Smart urbanism instead of algorithmic urbanism (Swilling 2014), uses these technologies for convenience ánd to become resilient. Were the technologies in former periods mainly applied to produce food, or industrial products, the current technologies are more than a necessity to establish resilience only, as they are also providing convenience.

Angelidou demonstrated that cities use futuristic imagination and possibilities of available and prospective technologies for their planning (Angelidou 2015), such as in the early 1900's with Ebenezer Howards' Garden city movement (Hall 2002), T. Garnier's drawings for 'Une cité industrielle' (Hall 2002), the Futurist movement, such as in Citta Nuova (Da Costa Meyer 1995), The Bauhaus movement (Honour and Fleming 2005), Le Corbusiers' Ville Contemporaine (Fondation Le Corbusier 2014), New Towns (Atkinson 1998; Hall 2002),

In the 1960s Archigram are the 'Plug-in-City', designed by P. Cook and the 'Walking City', designed by R. Herron, both in 1964 (Sadler 2005). Architect T. Zenetos conceived the idea of 'Electronic Urbanism', a city model that embraces networked technology in favor of social equity and creativity, in connection with the natural habitat, economy of energy and time and sustainability. His model calls for tele-working, tele-services and tele-education spaces (Zenetos 1969). Throughout the 1960s 1970s and 1980s there was a significant stream of published work that engaged with the emerging information society on the urban scale in a visionary way (such as Urban planner R. Meier (1962) conceived the 'Communications theory of urban growth', Geographer J. Gottman (1961) 'Megalopolis', and 'Transactional Cities', and Mumford (1961) (re)connecting technology and the natural environment).

By the mid-1990s, many studies featured visions about future cities where ICTs would be the main enabler of democracy and city management (Aurigi 2006). Theorists of the decade 1990–2000 envisaged that the Internet would allow people to access all goods and services from any location in the world. Allegedly all their functions would be transferred to the digital world; thus, physical cities were prone to extinct, as the benefits of spatial agglomeration would disappear (Atkinson 1998; Aurigi and Graham 2000; Crang and Graham 2007; Marvin 2000). Cairncross (1997) even wrote about the 'Death of Distance', suggesting that distance was no longer a limiting factor for communications and transactions 'ubiquitous computing'. M. Weiser, head of the Xerox Palo Alto Research Centre in California was the frontrunner of this idea, having stated that 'the most profound technologies are those that disappear. They weave themselves into the fabric of everyday life until they are indistinguishable from it' (Weiser 1991). Technological ubiquity is rather a condition that we are starting to experience only today, with the broad employment of sensors and actuators throughout the built environment and the Internet of Things. In essence, technology has ever since the industrial era been a major driver of visions about urban futures. These visions involved cities that would use technology to establish modern and healthy living conditions, where perfect democracy would stem from collective digital spaces and where people's needs would be satisfied instantly and intuitively. Some of today's smart city researchers actually acknowledge that the smart cities movement is predominantly a strategic vision for the future, rather than a reality (Komninos et al. 2013; Navigant Research 2011; Schaffers 2012; Wolfram 2012).

A smart city is first and foremost a city, while smartness, gained by cyber-physical intelligence and services, is 'just' another urban asset, which either improves/automates typical functions (transportation, waste management, etc.) or generates jobs and increases citizen satisfaction (from traffic awareness, energy efficiency, etc.) (Anthopoulos 2017). The role of smart technologies is on the one hand side to make our lives more convenient, while on the other hand provide the tools to become more resilient.

2.4 Future City

An estimated 2.6 billion people will move to or be born into urban centres by 2050. Two-thirds of these residents will live in Asia or Africa. Left untouched, many of these cities will emerge out of or swallow-up squatter settlements (New York Times and Shell Oil 2014). Water, sewer, transportation, electricity, telecommunications, housing, health care, education, all of these functions, will have to be built from the ground up. In contrast, the smart city discourse is largely looking into the immediate future and at places already known and functioning. Therefore, the focus on this process of urban transformation should investigate the longer term and unknown places as current characterisation of smart cities will only marginally inform understanding of the real cities of tomorrow. The pace of change is forecast to be so swift that research needs to go beyond current and locally 'sold' technologies. Instead, an intelligent discussion starts with which cities we want in the future and whether and how smart city technologies, and urban design and urbanism, are likely to provide them (Glasmeier and Christopherson 2015).

Intelligence is distributed right across the city, present in sensors, and chips with which the infrastructure, streets and buildings are fitted, as well as in the numerous electronic devices of its inhabitants. The smart city is a city activated at millions of points, thanks to information and communications technology. Since it follows the topography of the networks of streets and buildings as well as the movement of vehicles and its inhabitants, producing a map of urban activity in real time, its intelligence is profoundly spatial (Picot 2015). The critique about the inadequacy of the mechanical tech approach to smart cities is heard from different sides (Greenfield 2013; Sennett 2012; Koolhaas 2014). The tech-driven adagio 'give us your data and we'll give you a techno utopia', the idea that you put sensors out, measure everything, and on that basis make decisions, is biased because all data is crafted (Van Timmeren et al. 2015). Besides such a technology-driven method, a human-driven method (Kummithaa and Crutzen 2017) is equally important. Next to Cyborg City, in which everything is managed the spontaneous collaborative city, in which 'nothing' is managed exists. Both require design, creativity and spontaneity as well as coordinative power (Picot 2015). Sim City (Terzano and Morckel 2016) should not only be seen as a managed calculation, but even so as a creative process of city design.

Smart urbanism goes beyond the mechanical. It is 'A powerful integrative and action-oriented body of thought on cities that emphasises their particular histories, the social composition of cities, analyses the resources it takes to 'run' a city, provides insights into the intricate ways in which design, politics and business interrelate, and helps to think of the institutional formats and practices that can help deliver on the transition needed. The future calls for smart urbanism rather than smart cities' (Hajer and Dassen 2014).

Urbanism aims to deliver a city which provides all its basic functions (shelter, welfare, prosperity, social exchange) and shape it in a way its citizens are serviced and enjoy or consume a convenient life in a sustainable way.

The convenient city provides good houses, a clean, healthy and safe environment, access to resources of clean water, renewable energy and healthy food, social interaction, healthy interactive environments, resiliency/low vulnerability for climate impacts, (intelligent) mobility that guides traffic, mode shifts to new tech and innovative transport (autonomous and air vehicles) and arranges collaboration between the constituencies that shape the city. Smart Urbanism integrates technology, knowledge, governance, citizens, and business hence represent a multidisciplinary field, constantly shaped by advancements in technology and urban development (Angelidou 2015).

The key smart applications enabled by big data analytics and context–aware computing include smart transport, smart energy, smart environment, smart planning, smart design, smart grid, smart traffic, smart education, smart healthcare, and smart safety (Bibri and Krogstie 2016). Big data analytics and context–aware computing and what these entail in terms of digital sensing technologies, cloud computing infrastructures, middleware architectures, and wireless communication networks, will be the dominant mode of monitoring, understanding, analysing, assessing, operating, organizing, and planning smart (and) sustainable cities to improve their contribution to the goals of sustainable development (Bibri and Krogstie 2017).

The big difference for urban planners is they suddenly have access to real time data, which may alternate and differ over time. City makers and urbanists suddenly have to deal with the option of emerging events (Dosse 2010) and spontaneous developments rather than a determined program or future. This requires in strategic design of temporary uses being it events, temporary urbanism (Bishop and Williams 2012) and including voids and redundancy in the urban fabric (Roggema 2018).

The way energy generation and storage can be balanced with real time demand and usage in Smart Grids (Obinna et al. 2017), or how the Living PlanIT in Portugal (Carvalho et al. 2014) and ReGen Villages in the Netherlands (Ehrlich et al. 2015) are monitoring, adapting closing environmental flow cycles are early examples of these urban design applications of combinations of the virtual and physical city.

No matter what digital input cities undergo, in its essence the city remains the same. The design of the city may be inspired by the fluctuating insights data deliver, and new gadgets and shared bike systems may flock the city, meanwhile the urban form has basically not changed, its physical components and purpose remain the same. New cities such as Songdo, Masdar or existing cities such as Rio de Janeiro or Barcelona, all dubbed smart cities, do not look any different than the cities before the digital revolution. One may speak about the rise of a new planning paradigm of the intelligent city, other than virtual spaces (Ishida and Isbister 2000) and digital ecosystems enhancing innovation (Komninos 2015) are not distinguished, leaving current physical urban structures intact. The breadth of street widths, the suite of urban block sizes, these have not changed because of digitisation. The city still consists of a street and a façade, no matter whether these are private, public or when a virtual space over cities is created.

There is one fundamental new opportunity for urban life. The way the city can be 3D-mapped (Picot 2015) is new and allows us to access data and info in real time about mobility services, entertainment, food/restaurants, the environmental quality and leisure of places near us but not physically visible. This provides us with a convenience tool that makes our urban life potentially of a better quality. We can be informed and make better decisions on where what is available in real time, but even this doesn't fundamentally change the physical appearance of the city.

However, smart urbanism could re-emphasise urban planning principles (Hajer and Dassen 2014):

1. To not limit growth of wealth yet at the same time minimise the use of resources in a socially just and safe way.
2. To present a strong persuasive story, 'beyond the smart gadget', for the use of smart technologies, supporting positive social reform and bringing about urban resilience.
3. To use urban metabolism as the central urban planning framework on which to base urban performance decisions on, and focus on the potential transformations, by increasing urban redundancy by including spatial voids in the city to use whenever suitable (Roggema 2018).
4. To develop urban infrastructure that provides shelter, water, energy and contact in a (hyper)localised, small-scale, off-grid way?
5. To establish a symbiosis of smart technologies, social innovation, and business models.
6. To create the technological environment enhancing open politics of continuous learning, using the intelligence of the energetic citizen (Hajer 2011) as part of the search for solutions. Establish a digital democracy and participatory urban planning using urban living labs (Steen and van Bueren 2017).
7. To practice the urbanism of transplantation, searching for the suitable conditionalities to adapt, correct, adopt and create add-ons to the city and transplant solutions in matching contexts.

The urban consumer turns into a smart citizen, 'prosuming' in an intelligent, agonistic and creative way while making use of interoperable and open data sources (Van Timmeren et al. 2015). Smart urbanism in practice could work in a quadruple model in which the innovative company, investing in developing new concepts or products, academia, participating with the brightest minds, the government, allowing the novelty to emerge and be tested in the city, and the urban prosumer, being the primary user and tests the prototypes, come together in an urban ecosystem of exchange, creativity finding new ways of co-design and co-development.

2.5 Conclusion

A smart city is nothing new, as throughout times society has always used the appropriate and available technologies to shape its cities. However, the possibility of integrative collaboration and continuous testing and improving is novel. The density of data allows us to think laterally and use information in real time implying on the daily uses in the city. This can make the city both more convenient to use as well as safer and more resilient.

There are several uncertainties whether this will be effectuated and successful. It is most likely and easy to believe the Homo Ludens (Huizinga 1938) will take up novel smart applications that will make his life easier and more joyful. Most probably, the market for smart gadgets will continue to emerge. More uncertain is whether the smart city movement will be able to enforce the implementation of the urban infrastructure needed for the new urban population for a fraction of the costs of current infrastructure. Secondly, will it be able to deliver on the promise to create the smart technology for the eco-efficiency needed to become really resilient cities?

Apart from these uncertainties directly related to the development and the promise of smart cities, some big questions should also be addressed. Not the least because these questions are an inevitable part of good urbanism, so smart urbanism should as a natural habit contribute to finding solutions for these big questions:

- Will smart cities help to control climate change and keep the earth below a reasonable rise in temperature?
- Can smart city technologies play a role in moderating rapid population growth at global level?
- Is smart urbanism capable of preventing large scale migration, of which a large amount is caused by climate impacts.
- Will the smart city promise also contribute to social justice and equity at world scale?
- Could the smart city provide sufficient healthy food for everyone?
- Could it bring corruption-free democracy everywhere?

Urbanism, not even smart urbanism will instantly pull the switch and solve these and other big issues. But at the same time, it would be a matter of negligence if smart thinking, with the availability of all algorithms, big data and the Internet of Things would not try to make big changes in these fields. This way Smart Cities become a humanitarian effort, bringing a better quality of life for the global population.

References

ABB and European House-Ambrosetti. (2012). *Smart cities in Italy: An opportunity in the spirit of the Renaissance for a new quality of life*. Zurich

Abdoullaev, A. (2011). A smart world: A development model for intelligent cities. In *The 11th IEEE international conference on computer and information technology*, 31 August–2 September 2011, Pafos, Cyprus.

Ahvenniemi, H., Huovila, A., Pinto-Seppä, I., & Airaksinen, M. (2017). What are the differences between sustainable and smart cities? *Cities, 60*, 234–245.

Al Nuaimi, E., Al Neyadi, H., Nader, M., & Al-Jaroodi, J. (2015). Applications of bigdata to smart cities. *Journal of Internet Services and Applications, 6*(25), 1–15.

Allwinkle, S., & Cruickshank, P. (2011). Creating smarter cities: An overview. *Journal of Urban Technology, 18*, 1–16.

AMS. (2014). *Rain sense: Citizens preparing Amsterdam for future weather*. https://www.ams-institute.org/solution/rain-sense/. Accessed 12 July 2018.

AMS. (2016). *3D printing in the circular city*. https://www.ams-institute.org/solution/3d-printing-in-the-circular-city/. Accessed 12 July 2018.

Angelidou, M. (2014). Smart city policies: A spatial approach. *Cities, 41*, S3–S11.

Angelidou, M. (2015). Smart cities: A conjuncture of four forces. *Cities, 47*, 95–106.

Anthopoulos, L. (2017). Smart utopia vs smart reality: Learning by experience from 10 smart city cases. *Cities, 63*, 128–148.

Anthopoulos, L. G., & Vakali, A. (2012). Urban planning and smart cities: Interrelations and reciprocities. In F. Álvarez et al. (Eds.), *FIA 2012* (LNCS 7281) (pp. 178–189). Cham: Springer.

Atkinson, R. (1998). Technological change and cities. *Cityscape: A Journal of Policy Development and Research, 3*(3), 129–170.

Aurigi, A. (2006). New technologies, same dilemmas: Policy and design issues for the augmented city. *Journal of Urban Technology, 13*(3), 5–28. https://doi.org/10.1080/10630730601145989.

Aurigi, A., & Graham, S. (2000). Cyberspace and the city: The "Virtual City" in Europe. In G. Bridge & S. Watson (Eds.), *A companion to the city* (pp. 489–502). Malden: Blackwell.

Bakici, T., Almirall, E., & Wareham, J. (2013). A smart city initiative: The case of Barcelona. *Journal of the Knowledge Economy, 4*(2), 135–148.

Barton, H. (2000). *Sustainable communities: The potential of eco-neighbourhoods*. London: Earthscan.

Batty, M., Axhausen, K., Fosca, G., Pozdnoukhov, A., Bazzani, A., Wachowicz, M., et al. (2012a). *Smart cities of the future* (paper 188). UCL CASA working paper series.

Batty, M., Axhausen, K. W., Giannotti, F., Pozdnoukhov, A., Bazzani, A., Wachowicz, M., et al. (2012b). Smart cities of the future. *The European Physical Journal, 214*, 481–518.

Bibri, S. E. (2013). *ICT for sustainable urban development in the European Information Society: A discursive investigation of energy efficiency technology*. Master Thesis. School of Culture and Society, Malmö University.

Bibri, S. E., & Krogstie, J. (2016, November 15). Big data analytics and context–aware computing for smart sustainable cities of the future. *Norwegian Big Data symposium (NOBIDS)*, Trondheim.

Bibri, S. E., & Krogstie, J. (2017). Smart sustainable cities of the future: An extensive interdisciplinary literature review. *Sustainable Cities and Society, 31*, 183–212.

Bifulco, F., Tregua, M., Amitrano, C., & D'Auria, A. (2016). ICT and sustainability in smart cities management. *International Journal of Public Sector Management, 29*(2), 132–147. https://doi.org/10.1108/IJPSM-07-2015-0132.

Bishop, P., & Williams, L. (2012). *The Temporary city*. Abingdon: Taylor and Francis.

Bria, F. (2012). *New governance models towards an open Internet ecosystem for smart connected European cities and regions*. Open Innovation, Directorate-General for the Information Society and Media, European Commission (pp. 62–71).

Buckley, M. (2014). *Big Data and the science of the Christmas tree*. https://today.uconn.edu/2014/12/big-data-and-the-science-of-the-christmas-tree/. Accessed 12 July 2018.

Cairncross, F. (1997). *A connected world*. http://www.economist.com/node/598895?story_id=598895. Accessed 4 July 2018.

Caragliu, A., Del Bo, C., & Nijkamp, P. (2009). *Smart cities in Europe*. Serie Research Memoranda 0048. VU University Amsterdam, Faculty of Economics, Business Administration and Econometrics.

Carvalho, L., Santos, I. P., & van Winden, W. (2014). Knowledge spaces and places: From the perspective of a "born-global" start-up in the field of urban technology. *Expert Systems with Applications, 41*(12), 5647–5655. https://doi.org/10.1016/j.eswa.2014.02.015.

Chourabi, H., Gil-Garcia, J. R., Pardo, T. A., Nam, T., Mellouli, S., Scholl, H. J., Walker, S., & Nahon, K. (2012). Understanding smart cities: An integrative framework 45th Hawaii international conference on system. *Sciences*, 2289–2297. https://doi.org/10.1109/HICSS.2012.615.

Cole, R. J. (2012). Regenerative design and development: Current theory and practice. *Building Research and Information, 40*(1), 1–6.

Cole, R. J., Busby, P., Guenther, R., Briney, L., Blaviesciunaite, A., & Alencar, T. (2012). A regenerative design framework: Setting new aspirations and initiating new discussions. *Building Research and Information, 40*(1), 95–111.
Crang, M., & Graham, S. (2007). Sentient cities: Ambient intelligence and the politics of urban space. *Information, Communication & Society, 10*(6), 789–817.
Da Costa Meyer, E. (1995). *The work of Antonio Sant'Elia: Retreat into the future*. New Haven: Yale University Press.
Datta, A. (2015). A 100 smart cities, a 100 utopias. *Dialogue in Human Geography, 5*(1), 49–53.
De Jong, M., Joss, S., Schraven, D., Zhan, C., & Weijnen, M. (2015). Sustainable-smart-resilient-low carbon-eco-knowledge cities; making sense of a multitude of concepts promoting sustainable urbanization. *Journal of Cleaner Production, 109*, 25–38.
Dosse, F. (2010). *Renaissance de l'événement: Un défi pour l'historien – entre sphinx et phénix*. Paris: PUF.
Du Plessis, C. (2012). Towards a regenerative paradigm for the built environment. *Building Research and Information, 40*(1), 7–22.
Ehrlich, J., Leifer, L., & Ford, C. (2015). *RegenVillages – Integrated village designs for thriving regenerative communities*. Sustainable Development Knowledge Platform, Department of Economic and Social Affairs, United Nations. https://sustainabledevelopment.un.org/content/documents/622766_Ehrlich_Integrated%20village%20designs%20for%20thriving%20regenerative%20communities.pdf. Accessed 15 July 2018.
EPA (Environmental Protection Agency). (2014). *Smart growth*. http://www.epa.gov/smartgrowth/. Accessed 20 June 2018.
Fondation Le Corbusier. (2014). http://www.fondationlecorbusier.fr
Foresti, L., & Seed, A. (2014). The effect of flow and orography on the spatial distribution of the very short-term predictability of rainfall from composite radar images. *Hydrology and Earth System Sciences, 18*, 4671–4686.
Frenchman, D., Joroff, M., & Albericci, A. (2011). *Smart cities as engines of sustainable growth*. Massachusetts Institute of Technology, prepared for the World Bank Institute.
Gabel, M. (undated). *Regenerative development; going beyond sustainability*. http://www.designsciencelab.com/resources/Regenerative-Development.pdf. Accessed: 21 June 2018.
Giffinger, R., Fertner, C., Kramar, H., Kalasek, R., Pichler-Milanović, N., & Meijers, E. (2007). *Smart cities: Ranking of European medium-sized cities*. Vienna: Centre of Regional Science (SRF), Vienna University of Technology. http://www.smartcities.eu/download/smart_cities_final_report.pdf. Accessed 2 July 2018.
Girardet, H. (2013) Sustainability is unhelpful: We need to think about regeneration. http://www.theguardian.com/sustainable-business/blog/sustainabilityunhelpful-think-regeneration
Glasmeier, A., & Christopherson, S. (2015). Thinking about smart cities. *Cambridge Journal of Regions, Economy and Society, 8*, 3–12. https://doi.org/10.1093/cjres/rsu034.
Gottman, J. (1961). *Megalopolis: The urbanized northeastern seaboard of the United States*. New York: The Twentieth Century Fund.
Graham, S., & Marvin, S. (2001). *Splintering urbanism: Networked infrastructures, technological. Mobilities and the urban conditions*. London: Routledge.
Greenfield, A. (2013). *Against the smart city: A pamphlet*. New York: Verso.
Gsma, Accenture and Cisco. (2011). *Smart mobile cities: Opportunities for mobile operators to deliver intelligent cities*. London
Hajer, M. A. (1996). *The politics of environmental discourse: Ecological modernization and the policy process*. New York: Oxford University Press.
Hajer, M. A. (2011). *The energetic society*. Den Haag: PBL Publishers.
Hajer, M., & Dassen, T. (2014). *Smart about cities. Visualising the challenge for the 21st century urbanism*. Rotterdam/Den Haag: PBL publishers.

Hall, R. E. (2000, September 28). The vision of a smart city. In *Proceedings of the 2nd international life extension technology workshop*, Paris, France. http://www.osti.gov/bridge/servlets/purl/773961-oyxp82/webviewable/773961.pdf. Accessed 2 July 2018.

Hall, P. (2002). *Cities of tomorrow: An intellectual history of urban planning and design in the twentieth century* (3rd ed.). Malden: Wiley-Blackwell.

Harrison, C., Eckman, B., Hamilton, R., Hartswick, P., Kalagnanam, J., Paraszczak, J., & Williams, P. (2010). Foundations for smarter cities. *IBM Journal of Research and Development, 54*(4), 350–365.

Herrschel, T. (2013). Competitiveness AND sustainability: Can "Smart City Regionalism" square the circle? *Urban Studies, 50*, 2332–2348. https://doi.org/10.1177/0042098013478240.

Hodgkinson, S. (2011). *Is your city smart enough? Digitally enabled cities and societies will enhance economic, social, and environmental sustainability in the urban century*. OVUM report.

Höjer, M., & Wangel, S. (2015). Smart sustainable cities: Definition and challenges. In L. Hilty & B. Aebischer (Eds.), *ICT innovations for sustainability* (pp. 333–349). Berlin: Springer.

Hollands, R. G. (2008). Will the real smart city please stand up? *City, 12*(3), 303–320.

Honour, H., & Fleming, J. (2005). *A world history of art*. London: Laurence King Publishing.

Huber, A., & Mayer, I. (2012, August 29–31). Smart cities: An emerging city concept to frame sustainable transitions? In *3rd international conference on sustainability transitions: Sustainable transitions: Navigating theories and challenging realities*, Copenhagen.

Huizinga, J. (1938). *Homo Ludens. Proeve eener bepaling van het spel-element der cultuur*. Groningen: Wolters-Noordhoff.

Ishida, T., & Isbister, K. (Eds.). (2000). *Digital cities: Technologies, experiences and future perspective*. Berlin: Springer.

Jacobs, J. (1961). *The death and life of great American cities*. New York: Random House.

Jain, A., Rakhi, N. K., & Ganesh, B. (2015). *Spices form the basis of food pairing in Indian cuisine*. E-print arXiv:1502.03815.

Komninos, N. (2009). Intelligent cities: Towards interactive and global innovation environments. *International Journal of Innovation and Regional Development, Special Issue: Intelligent Clusters, Communities and Cities: Enhancing Innovation with Virtual Environments and Embedded Systems, 1*(4), 337–355.

Komninos, N. (2011). Intelligent cities: Variable geometries of spatial intelligence. *Intelligent Buildings International, 3*, 172–188.

Komninos, N. (2015). *The age of intelligent cities; smart environments and innovation-for-all strategies*. Abingdon/New York: Routledge.

Komninos, N., Pallot, M., & Schaffers, H. (2013). *Open innovation towards smarter cities*. Open innovation 2013 (pp. 34–41). Luxembourg: European Commission, Directorate-General for Communications Networks Content and Technology.

Koolhaas, R. (2014). *My thoughts on the smart city*. Brussels. https://ec.europa.eu/commission_2010-2014/kroes/en/content/my-thoughts-smart-city-rem-koolhaas. Accessed 16 July 2018.

Kourtit, K., & Nijkamp, P. (2012). Smart cities in the innovation age. *Innovation: The European Journal of Social Sciences, 25*(2), 93–95.

Kummithaa, R. K. R., & Crutzen, N. (2017). How do we understand smart cities? An evolutionary perspective. *Cities, 67*, 43–52.

Lind, D. (2012). Information and communications technologies creating livable, equitable, sustainable cities. In L. Starke (Ed.), *State of the world 2012: Moving toward sustainable prosperity* (pp. 66–76). Washington, DC: Island Press/Center for Resource Economics.

Liugailaitė-Radzvickienė, L., & Jucevičius, R. (2012, May 10–11). An intelligence approach to city development. In *7th international scientific conference "business and management 2012"*, Vilnius, Lithuania.

Lombardi, P., Giordano, S., Farouh, H., & Yousef, W. (2012). Modelling the smart city performance. *The European Journal of Social Science Research, 25*, 137–149.
Mang, P., & Reed, B. (2012). Designing from place: A regenerative framework and methodology. *Building Research and Information, 40*(1), 23–38.
Marsal-Llacuna, M.-L., & Segal, M. E. (2016). The intelligenter method (I) for making "smarter" city projects and plans. *Cities, 55*, 127–138. https://doi.org/10.1016/j.cities.2016.02.006.
Marsal-Llacuna, M.-L., Colomer-Llinàs, J., & Meléndez-Frigola, J. (2015). Lessons in urban monitoring taken from sustainable and livable cities to better address the smart cities initiative. *Technological Forecasting and Social Change, 90*(B), 611–622. https://doi.org/10.1016/j.techfore.2014.01.012.
Marvin, S. (2000). Telecommunications and sustainable cities. In R. Simmonds & G. Hack (Eds.), *Global city regions: Their emerging forms* (pp. 244–248). London: Spon Press.
Meier, R. L. (1962). *A communications theory of urban growth*. Cambridge, MA: MIT Press.
Mol, A. P. J. (2001). *Globalization and environmental reform: The ecological modernization of the global economy*. Cambridge, MA: MIT Press.
Mol, A. P. J., Sonnenfeld, D. A., & Spaargaren, G. (2009). *The ecological modernisation reader: Environmental reform in theory and practice*. London/New York: Routledge.
Mosannenzadeh, F., & Vettorato, D. (2014, June 4–6). Defining smart city: A conceptual framework based on keyword analysis. *TeMA Journal of Land Use Mobility and Environment*. special issue: INPUT 2014 Eighth International Conference INPUT, Naples.
Mumford, L. (1961). *The city in history: Its origins, its transformations, and its prospects*. San Diego: Harcourt, Brace & World.
Nam, T., & Pardo, T. A. (2011). Conceptualizing smart city with dimensions of technology, people, and institutions. In *Proceedings of the 12th annual international digital government research conference*: Digital government innovation in challenging times. ACM, pp. 282–291.
Natural Resources Defense Council. (undated). *What are smarter cities?* http://smartercities.nrdc.org/about. Accessed 2 July 2018.
Navigant Research. (2011). *Smart cities; intelligent information and communications technology infrastructure in the government, buildings, transport, and utility domains* (Research report). http://www.navigantresearch.com/research/smartcities. Accessed 4 July 2018.
Neirotti, P., de Marco, A., Cagliano, A. C., Mangano, G., & Scorrano, F. (2014). Current trends in smart city initiatives – Some stylized facts. *Cities, 38*, 25–36.
Neves, B. B. (2009). Are digital cities intelligent? The Portuguese case. *International Journal of Innovation and Regional Development, 1*(4), 443.
New York Times and Shell Oil. (2014, November 20). Cities energized: the urban transition. *New York Times*. http://paidpost.nytimes.com/shell/cities-energized.html?_r=1. Accessed 4 July 2018.
O'Grady, M. J., Muldoon, C., Carr, D., Wan, J., & Kroon, B. (2016). Intelligent sensing for citizen science. Challenges and future directions. *Mobile Networks and Applications, 21*(2), 375–385.
Obinna, U., Joore, P., Wauben, L., & Reinders, A. (2017). Comparison of two residential smart grid pilots in the Netherlands and in the USA, focusing on energy performance and user experiences. *Applied Energy, 191*, 264–275. https://doi.org/10.1016/j.apenergy.2017.01.086.
Offenhuber, D. (2015). Infrastructure legibility – A comparative analysis of open 311-based citizen feedback systems. *Cambridge Journal of Regions, Economy and Society, 8*, 93–112.
Papa, R., Garguilo, C., & Galderisi, A. (2013). Towards and urban planners' perspective on smart city. *TeMA Journal of Land Use, Mobility and Environment, 6*(1), 5–17.
Pardo, T., Nam, T., & Burke, B. (2012). E-government interoperability: Interaction of policy, management, and technology dimensions. *Social Science Computer Review, 30*, 7–23.
Picot, A. (2015). *Smart cities; a spatialized intelligence*. Chichester: Wiley.

Rabari, C., & Storper, M. (2015). The digital skin of cities: Urban theory and research in the age of the sensored and metered city, ubiquitous computing and big data. *Cambridge Journal of Regions, Economy and Society, 8*, 27–42.

Rathore, M. M., Ahmad, A., Paul, A., & Rho, S. (2016). Urban planning and building smart cities based on the Internet of things using Big Data analytics. *Computer Networks, 101*, 63–80. https://doi.org/10.1016/j.comnet.2015.12.023.

Ratti, C., & Townsend, A. (2011, August 16). Harnessing residents' electronic devices will yield truly smart cities. *Scientific American*. http://www.scientificamerican.com/article.cfm?id=the-social-nexus Accessed 9 June 2018.

Robinson, R. (undated). *Smart city design principles*. https://theurbantechnologist.com/smarter-city-design-principles/. Accessed 18 June 2018.

Robinson, J., & Cole, R. J. (2015). Theoretical underpinnings of regenerative sustainability. *Building Research & Information, 43*(2), 133–142.

Roche, S., Nabian, N., Kloeckl, K., & Ratti, C. (2012, May 14–17). *Are 'smart cities' smart enough?* Global geospatial conference 2012, spatially enabling government, industry and citizens, Québec City, Canada. http://www.gsdi.org/gsdiconf/gsdi13/papers/182.pdf

Roggema, R. (2018, in print). Design *with* voids. How inverted urbanism increases urban resilience. *Architectural Science Review*, (Special issue: Time, Place and Architecture). https://doi.org/10.1080/00038628.2018.1502153.

Rydin, Y. (2010). *Governing for sustainable urban development*. London: Earthscan.

Sadler, S. (2005). *Archigram: Architecture without architecture*. Cambridge, MA: MIT Press.

Schaffers, H. (2012, May 10–11). Empowering citizens to realizing smart cities: Results from FIREBALL Smart city case studies (presentation). *2012 future internet assembly (FIA), "smart cities and internet of things"*, Aalborg. http://www.fi-aalborg.eu/downloads/Session_1.1_Hans_Schaffers.pdf. Accessed 4 July 2018.

Sennett, R. (2012, December 4). No one likes a city that's too smart. *The Guardian*. http://www.theguardian.com/commentisfree/2012/dec/04/smart-city-rio-songdo-masdar. Accessed 16 July 2018.

Steen, K. Y. G., & van Bueren, E. M. (2017). *Urban living labs: A living lab way of working*. Amsterdam: AMS Institute.

Streitz, N. (2011). Smart cities, ambient intelligence and universal access. In C. Stephanidis (Ed.), *Universal access in HCI, Part III, HCII 2011, LNCS 6767* (pp. 425–432). Berlin/Heidelberg: Springer.

Swilling, M. (2014). Towards sustainable urban infrastructures for the urban Anthropocene. In A. Allen, A. Lampis, & M. Swilling (Eds.), *Untamed urbanism*. New York: Routledge.

Terzano, K., & Morckel, V. (2016). SimCity in the community planning classroom. Effects on student knowledge, interests, and perceptions of the discipline of planning. *Journal of Planning Education and Research, 37*(1), 95–105. https://doi.org/10.1177/0739456X16628959.

Thenewraw. (undated). *The new raw*. https://www.thenewraw.org/. Accessed 12 July 2018.

Toffler, A., & Toffler, H. (2006). *Revolutionary wealth. How will it be created and how will it change our lives*. New York: Random House.

Toppeta, D. (2010). The smart city vision: How innovation and ICT can build smart, "Livable", *Sustainable Cities*. The Innovation Knowledge Foundation. http://www.thinkinnovation.org/file/research/23/en/Toppeta_Report_005_2010.pdf. Accessed 2 July 2018.

Townsend, A., Maguire, R., Liebhold, M., & Crawford, M. (2010). *The future of cities, information, and inclusion: A planet of civic laboratories*. Palo Alto: Institute for the Future.

UN. (2015). *Transforming our world: The 2030 agenda for sustainable development*. A/Res/70/1. New York: United Nations.

Van Timmeren, A., Henriquez, L., & Reynolds, A. (2015). *Ubikquity & the illuminated city*. Delft: Delft University of Technology.

Washburn, D., Sindhu, U., Balaouras, S., Dines, R. A., Hayes, N. M., & Nelson, L. E. (2010). *Helping CIOs understand "Smart City" initiatives: Defining the smart city, its drivers, and the role of the CIO*. Cambridge, MA: Forrester Research, Inc. http://public.dhe.ibm.com/partnerworld/pub/smb/smarterplanet/forr_help_cios_und_smart_city_initiatives.pdf. Accessed 2 July 2018.
Weiser, M. (1991). The computer for the 21st century. *Scientific American, 265*(3), 94–104.
Wheeler, S., & Beatley, T. (2009). *The sustainable urban development reader* (2nd ed.). London: Routledge.
Wolfram, M. (2012, May 14–16). Deconstructing smart cities: An intertextual reading of concepts and practices for integrated urban and ICT development. *REAL CORP 2012*, Schwechat. http://www.corp.at/archive/CORP2012_192.pdf. Accessed 4 July 2018.
Zenetos, T. (1969). Electronic urbanism. *Architectural Themes, 3*, 114–125.

Chapter 3
Conceptualization of Smart City: A Methodological Framework for Smart Infrastructure, Smart Solutions and Smart Governance

Aurobindo Ogra

Abstract The concept of 'Smart City' has witnessed widespread applications across several city planning and development domains with specific emphasis on achieving smart sustainable cities. These concepts are seen to have evolved across the horizontal and vertical domains of the city governance, administration, planning and development and among others sectors. The overall approach is aimed at enhancing the efficiency, effectiveness, productivity, financial improvement and among other benefits. Some of these approaches have high technology dependence, while the other ones use a hybrid system which adopts specific measurable frameworks within the city working eco-system. Eventually, these Smart City approaches cuts across several multidimensional domains of city governance, administration and planning systems. This chapter introduces and discusses two concepts around Smart City in terms of conceptualization and measurement of Smart City. First, it discusses a conceptual methodological framework for contextualizing Smart City through a concept/approach of City Life Cycle (CLC). Second, it discusses a conceptual framework for measurement of Smart City which is based on integration of various functional and process-oriented approach across horizontal and vertical layers/dimensions of smart infrastructure, smart solution and smart governance within the broader context of socio-technical regimes. The conceptualized methodological framework for assessing Smart City can be applied at any stage of contextualizing a Smart City or evaluating a Smart City during post implementation of smart programmes and projects.

Keywords Smart city · Smart framework · Smart assessment · Smart infrastructure · Smart solution · Smart governance

---

A. Ogra (✉)
Department of Town and Regional Planning, Faculty of Engineering and the Built Environment, University of Johannesburg, Johannesburg, South Africa
e-mail: aogra@uj.ac.za

N. Biloria (ed.), *Data-driven Multivalence in the Built Environment*, S.M.A.R.T. Environments, https://doi.org/10.1007/978-3-030-12180-8_3

3.1 Introduction

The cities are witnessing a continuous transition period in terms of delivering its functional roles and responsibilities, adapting and adopting to appropriate service delivery mechanisms. Over the period of years, the cities have transitioned from simple manual system to digitalized form of governance and adapting to e-Government, e-Governance, Geospatial, and Location Based System across several domains cutting across at organizational level to people centric approach. The transition has evolved the cities to focus on other thematic concepts such as healthy cities, livable cities, responsible cities and technology oriented with multifunctional cities through the approach of smart cities. The evolution of 'Smart City' can be traced to early 1990s with focused discussed of cities on Information and Communication Technologies (ICTs) in different perspectives. The concepts and emergence of digital city, virtual cities, ICT for democratization, citizen engagements, 2D and 3D cities, WWW, Internet, and networked urban infrastructure had led to the transformation of cities towards Smart Cities.

The term 'Smart City' comes from a lengthy route of urban innovations which tries to re-imagine the city and infuse it with a new tenacity and vision. The Garden City concept, new towns, national capital cities, model neighborhoods, techno-cities, sustainable cities, low-carbon cities, socialist cities, healthy cities and today Smart Cities are all efforts to lay down new forms of utopia (Vinod Kumar 2017). 'Smart Cities' are defined as an urban development vision aimed at assimilating numerous Information and Communication Technology (ICT) solutions in order to control the city's possessions; these possessions include libraries, waste management, water supply networks, local department's information systems, community services and law enforcement (Kwele 2016). Smart cities are further defined as cities that possess the following six elements: smart people, smart living, smart mobility, smart environment, smart economy and smart governance; which are ultimately cities that encourage activities of independence, citizen awareness and self-assurance (Giffinger and Gudrun 2010). Even though smart cities in the developing world are at an honorable advantage, it is important to understand the dimensions and resource limitations of creating smart cities (Odendaal 2003). Smart cities in contrary may lead to problems such as social exclusion, inequality and sustainability issues predominantly in the developing world (Angelakis et al. 2017).

According to the British Standards Institution, a Smart City is an effective integration of physical, digital and human systems in the built environment to deliver a sustainable, prosperous and inclusive future for society. The social element of smart cities is emphasized by Thompson's (2016) argument suggesting that "fundamentally, 'Smartness' should not be determined by how up-to-date or expensive the technology is, but by how we will improve citizens' lives and how we can create better living spaces for all by utilizing all available resources. Cohen (2012) defines smart cities as the cities that employ information and communication technologies to enhance efficiency and effectiveness of services delivered to the inhabitants of the city, subsequently leading to a better quality of life. According to Cruz and Sarmento

(2017), a "Smart City" refers to a city or investment that carries out an action towards decreasing the carbon footprint, or to increasing resilience to disasters, either natural or social. A central element consideration or underlying principle of smart cities is the efficient use of resources, natural, economic and human. Hayat (2016) identifies the following attributes of smart cities: shared ICT, common infrastructure and communication, optical fibre for effective public service delivery, information gathering from sensors like smart meters, monitoring and control from central command center, open government, energy efficient technologies, time optimization, zero emission systems, clean and green environment.

Despite the emphasis of using ICT in smart cities, some scholars argue that while the use of ICT is a central element of smart cities, the use of ICT has to work in tandem with other non-technological elements of smart cities. According to (Batty 2015), for a city to be classified as smart, it has to go beyond the mere extensive use of IT systems and aim for a synthesis of intelligence that transcends mere utilization. Batty argues that this will result in what is called fusion, this forms a city in which information and communications technology (ICT) is merged with traditional infrastructures, coordinated and integrated using new digital technologies, thus making the city more functional and sustainable.

A broader and all-encompassing definition of smart cities is offered by Washburn et al. (2010) who define a smart city as "the use of smart computing technologies to make the critical infrastructure components and services of a city – which include city administration, education, healthcare, public safety, real estate, transportation, and utilities – more intelligent, interconnected, and efficient'. It has also been stated by Meijer and Bolívar (2015), the smartness of a city refers to its ability to attract human capital and to mobilize this human capital in collaborations between the various (organized and individual) actors through the use of information and communication technologies.

3.2 City Life Cycle (CLC) Approach

The conceptualization of Smart City and measuring Smart City are two different contexts. The research on smart cities from the definition context characterizes and highlight the domain of smart cities spanning across: new generation of IT, provision of smart services, effective integration of – physical, digital and human systems, improved quality of life, economic, social and environmental aspects, and aware citizens and among others. The Smart City can be further contextualized in terms of qualitative and quantitative measurements in form of a combination of different domains and indicators spread across horizontal and vertical value chain eco-system within the city functional domains in form of sub-domains and indicators linked to citizen centric good governance (Ogra and Thwala 2014; Sharma et al. 2014).

3.2.1 Existing Frameworks and Approaches

The different frameworks for city functional sectorial measurements such as: Urban Indicators, Global Livable Cities Index (GLCI) (Giap et al. 2012), ISO 37120: 2014 and among others provide a good clarity on the sub-domains and indicators in typical areas of: economy education, energy, environment finance, fire and emergency response, governance, health, recreation, safety, shelter, solid waste, telecommunication, innovation, transportation, urban planning, wastewater, water and sanitation and among other relevant sub-domains.

The standardization approach through indicators such as ISO 37210:2014 has led to some uniformity, however, the approach lacks in terms of relevance of some of the core and supporting indicators across the domains/sub-domains. While it accounts the critical functional areas, but in many instances, it does not portray the weightage and leaves the model/approach to be considered as one size fits for all scenario. The representation of domains and sub-domains by other approaches to standardize or measure smart cities through the indicator system largely helps to contextualize the value system, however, it does not cover sufficiently different socio-technical layers linked within the value chain system and is often representative either on selected domain and sub-domain areas or more biased towards the technology driven approach.

The other approaches such as benchmarking, generic matrix and smartness index based on composite scores of domains/sub-domains requires and is limited to identification of the technologies that possess smart capabilities in their applications. The shortcomings in some of these contextualization and measurement techniques relate to limited focus on selected components, or aggregate scoring without much emphasis on the interlinkages of domains and sub-domains and unit of measurement. The six pillar approach suggested by Joshi et al. (2016) suggests a framework which comprise of developing smart cities in terms of SMELTS framework (Social, Management, Economy, Legal, Technology and Sustainability). The framework places technology, economy, legal and smart city initiative at the core as foundation of smart cities.

Contextualizing Smart City requires a pragmatic multi-pronged and multidimensional approach which can be simplified in terms of an integrated framework recognizing the elements, functions, and processes within the value chain eco-system of internal and external environment. This can be contextualized in terms of people centric technology oriented approach cutting across multiple dimensions and essentially improving the smart eco-system value chain by integration of smart infrastructure, smart solutions and smart governance systems (Lewis and Ogra 2010). The Smart City conceptualizing and its subsequent implementation should be seen in terms of different layered approach depending on the scale of the cities, its status quo in terms of horizontal and vertical domain functional areas, spatial context and among other critical elements like data integration, data management and data analytics (Ogra 2013).

The idea of 'Smart City' advances as a way to accomplish more proficient and sustainable urban areas, even though much more debates are focused on utilizing information and communication innovations to address city problems. Today, cities are getting to be smart regarding automated daily functions, but rather in ways that enable monitoring, understand, scrutinize and plan the city to enhance city performance continuously (Shapiro 2006). The emphasis on social and environmental capital recognizes Smart Cities from an unadulterated innovation driven idea, along these lines improving a multi-dimensional perspective with respect to urban communities.

One of the common approaches adopted by cities in moving ahead for transition towards smart cities is adoption of technologies and measuring it using indicators across representative sectors/functional role areas. This relatively differentiates and help cities in identifying the impacts over the short to long term periods. However, it adopts a uniform and standard measure which is typical in terms of monitoring and evaluation which simply benchmarks the status quo and helps in bridging the gap between the status quo and the vision/objectives across the multi-sectoral city functional dimensions.

3.2.2 City Life Cycle (CLC) Approach

The 'City Life Cycle' context introduces a new methodological approach which is based on approaching the city in terms of demographic dividend within the context of status quo and aiming to structure the city programs and projects smartly. The conventional approach of smart cities is more like a Utopian approach which appears to be far from realistic approach in terms of the requirements – for moving beyond the status quo to the benchmarking system for realizing the city vision (Fig. 3.1).

The cities could be contextualized into four quadrants which reflects the approach for addressing the status quo from conceptual level to advanced level of smart city. The elements of these quadrants can be further analyzed using a suitable simplistic framework to evaluate the level of smartness/further action to be implemented to benchmark the final vision (see Table 3.1).

Each of the quadrants represent a range of target age groups in terms of demographic dividend. Looking at the target group, the typical elements/layers associated with the dimensions associated with smart infrastructure, smart solutions and smart governance would largely get defined based on people centric technology-oriented approach. Each of these typical elements/layers would further require unique as well as common set of smart approaches and solutions to derive maximum integration within the overall value chain network and eco-system. The cities could restructure and direct their strategies based on the representative demographic dividend target groups in areas of smart infrastructure, smart solutions and smart governance (Fig. 3.2).

The dynamic paradigm around Smart Infrastructure, Smart Solutions and Smart Governance can be visualized in terms of critical functional and process-oriented

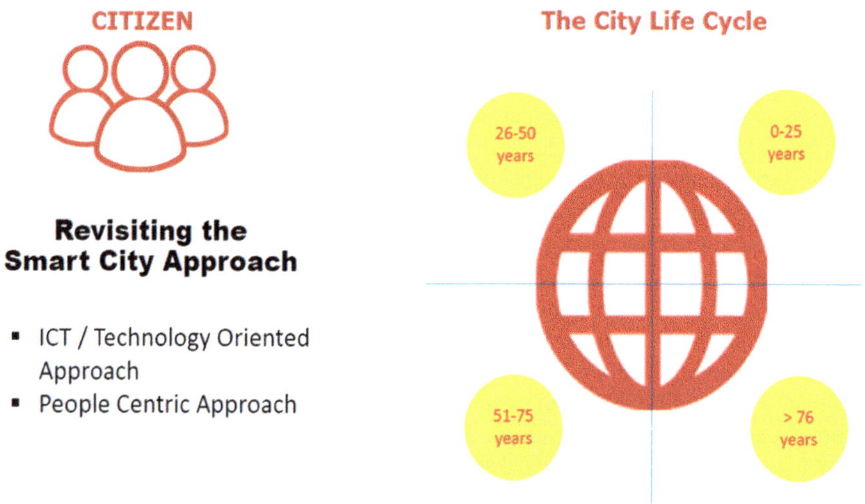

Fig. 3.1 City life cycle (CLC) approach for conceptualization of smart city

Table 3.1 City life cycle (CLC): integrated quadrant approach

Quadrant	Target group	Typical elements/layers	Smart City dimensions
Quadrant-1	0–25 years	Health, education, infrastructure, livelihood, sports, basic social amenities	Smart hospital system, smart social system, smart infrastructure, smart learning, smart spaces, smart mobility, smart environment …
Quadrant-2	26–50 years	Skilled workforce, social infrastructure, economic development, housing, industries, general/social infrastructure	Smart talent, smart housing, smart innovation, smart development, smart entrepreneurs, smart investments, smart mobility, smart environment, smart community …
Quadrant-3	51–75 years	Senior citizens, social amenities, health, general/social infrastructure	Smart health care/medical system, smart mobility, smart open spaces/parks, smart environment, smart safe systems, smart community …
Quadrant-4	> 76 years	Old age/senior citizens, social amenities, health, general/social infrastructure	Smart health care/medical system, smart mobility, smart open spaces/parks, smart environment, smart safe systems, smart community …

applications in areas of planning and development, infrastructure and utilities/service delivery and resource mobilization. These functions and processes are interlinked and have close nexus between the infrastructure and the service delivery domains (see Table 3.2).

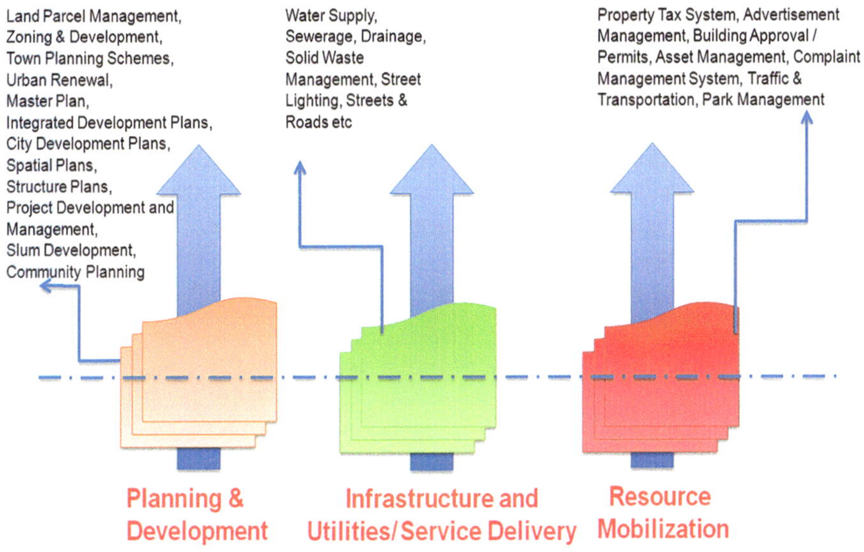

Fig. 3.2 Dynamic paradigm for smart infrastructure, smart solutions and smart governance

Table 3.2 Typical broad contours of smart infrastructure, smart solutions and smart governance (but not limited to)

Smart infrastructure	Smart solutions	Smart governance
Hospitals, health clinics, schools, university, utilities infrastructure (water and sanitation, drainage, waste management, roads & transportation, environmental, energy), city parks, stadiums, libraries, residential accommodation, tourism infrastructure/entertainment & recreation parks, business & industrial parks, age old homes, community centres, agro-processing parks	Integrated health system (hospitals, clinics, doctors, paramedics/emergency response systems, pharmacies); education & learning (literacy, enrolment, learning, skills development); integrated planning & utilities systems (vision, development planning, infrastructure and service delivery, maintenance, safety & surveillance); economic development (business, entrepreneurship, investments, applied science & technology); social development (community development, senior citizens)	Data inventory, data management, data analytics; transparency, accountability, efficiency, effectiveness, good governance and administration, evidence oriented planning; sustainable city: improved quality of life; resource optimization; asset planning, management, and maintenance; food security; climate control; financial sustainability

3.3 Methodological Framework

The smart cities understanding spans across multiple dimensions: it essentially cuts across different sustainability issues in terms of optimization, better quality of life across typical infrastructure and service delivery sectors and services such as but not limited to transportation, energy, water and sanitation, among other horizontal and vertical domain functional and process areas at city level. In order for methodological framework to be conceptualized which could address several dimensions and cuts across horizontal and vertical domains, there are number of questions which had to be taken into account:

- What is the need for measuring/assessing smart cities: preparedness, performance, impact?
- What exactly should we measure to define the smart city context/smartness: infrastructure, service delivery, governance, performance?
- Whose perspectives is highly critical: role players/service providers, receptors/end users, overall eco-system/environment?

The framework could be contextualized in terms of life-cycle of the smart city and can be broadly categorized into planning stage, designing stage and implementation/post implementation stage. The critical elements around each of the stages would largely provide a backdrop for contextualization of the smart cities framework development as provided in Table 3.3.

At a city level, primarily two approaches can be viewed to influence the management of smart cities. These two approaches are largely driven based on the goal and vision of the city and outcomes based on horizontal and vertical functional integration in smart cities conceptualization and implementation. These include:

Table 3.3 Mapping smart dimensions/elements as applicable at planning stage, designing stage, and implementation/post-implementation stage

Planning stage	Designing stage	Implementation/post-implementation stage
Vision, mission and goals	Designing of smart eco-system (value chain elements)	Sectorial approach/incremental approach (infrastructure/services)
Status quo: preparedness analysis/assessment	Framework for smart eco-system/technology architecture	Implementation (PPP/management contract/in-house)
Assessment of value chain: infrastructure, service delivery, technologies, interfaces, drivers/enablers	SWOT (evidence oriented)	Smart technology and service interface
KPAs and KPIs	Measurement matrix, smart tools, dashboard system	Capacity building, re-skilling
Smart strategy		Impact assessment, monitoring and evaluation

- Public sector approach: largely driven in terms of digitalization and service cataloguing, quality of services to citizens, accessibility, transparency and sustainability.
- Private sector approach: largely driven and supported in terms smart applications, technology for infrastructure and services.

The integration, speed, performance, participation, data repository, data management, data reliability and smart analytics remains central to both the public sector and private sector approach.

A typical example in terms of three tiers of governance at national, provincial and local government (see Fig. 3.3) could be linked to: National Priority Plan, Vision, Development Strategy, Development Objectives – Plan, Strategies and Frameworks and the associated key planning tools and instruments such as spatial plans, sectorial plans, economic development plans, spatial development frameworks, master plans, structure plans, vision plans, growth and development strategies and among other development tools and instruments (see Fig. 3.4). The horizontal and vertical sectorial integration should be seen as backdrop to the three tiers of governance.

The principles of good urban governance can be considered as one of the critical layers of conceptualization of smart cities methodological framework. The other larger overarching principles which are grounded in the existing development frameworks, tools and instruments would be equally critical in conceptualization framework. In terms of good urban governance these include: public participation, accountability, transparency, responsiveness, effectiveness and efficiency, equity and inclusivity, rule of law, strategic vision, sustainability, security, citizenship, and integrated governance. In the context of South Africa, as per Spatial Planning and Land Use Management Act (2013), the principles relate to Spatial Sustainability, Spatial Efficiency, Spatial Resilience, Spatial Justice and Good Administration (see Fig. 3.5).

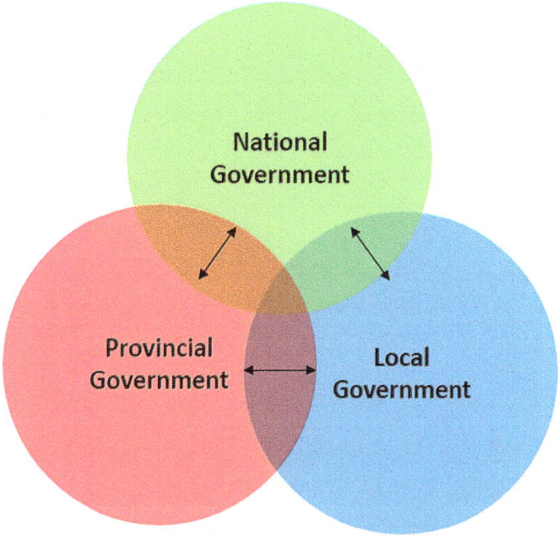

Fig. 3.3 Connected spheres of three tiers of governance

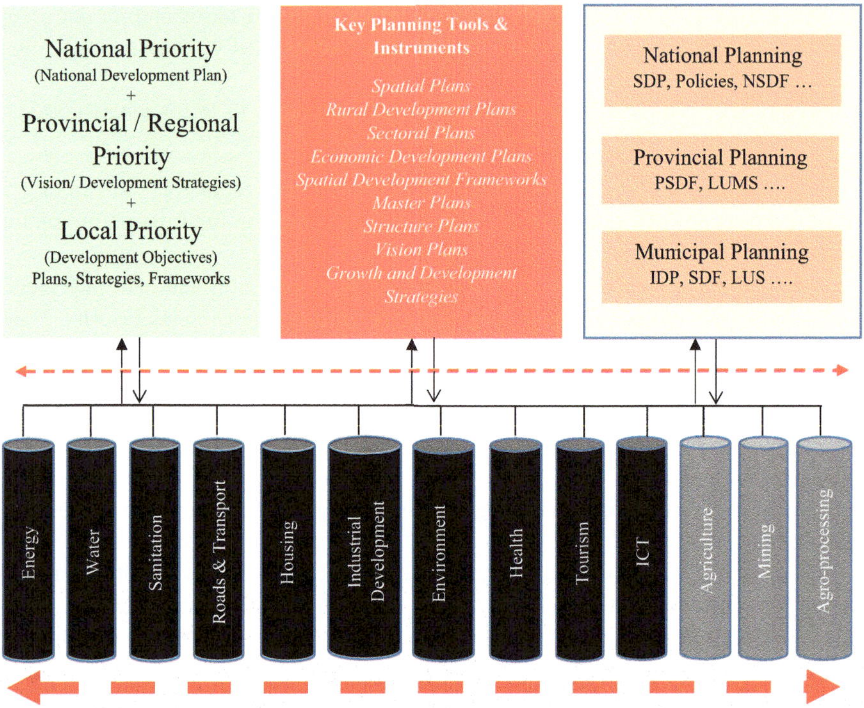

Fig. 3.4 Dimension layers/elements of horizontal and vertical integration

Fig. 3.5 Principles of Spatial Planning and Land Use Management Act

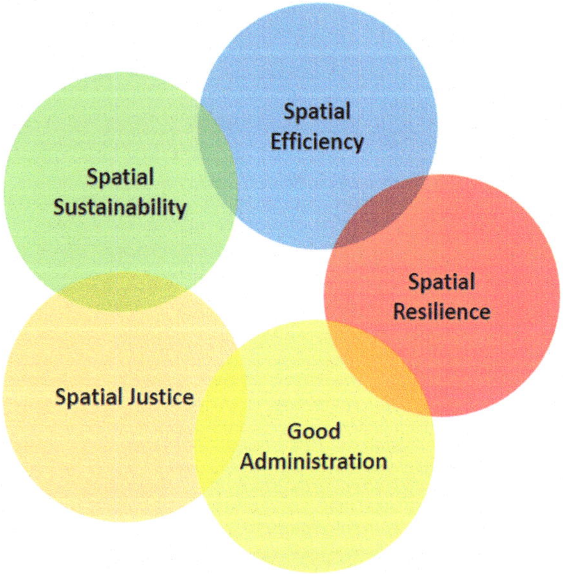

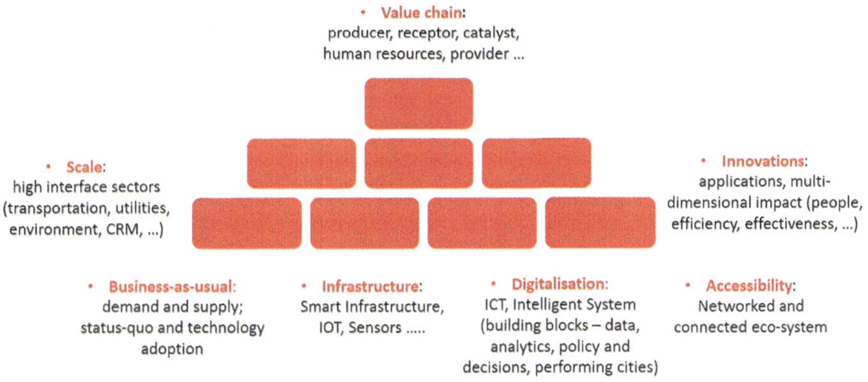

Fig. 3.6 Building blocks for conceptualizing, designing and implementation of smart cities

The building blocks for effective Smart City should essentially account the eco-system in terms of value chain, scale, business-as-usual, infrastructure, digitalisation, accessibility, innovations and among others (see Fig. 3.6).

There are number of key challenges that cities are facing globally, which comes in several dimensions forms but are not limited to specific sectors such as environmental degradation, inadequate service delivery provisions, and lack of land use integration with public transport, infrastructure and social imbalances and among others (Hollands 2008). Cities are experiencing various challenges leading to complex system, the system comprises of distinct network and various elements of urban infrastructure, built environment communication flow, social, cultural, political and economic structure.

3.3.1 Development Approach

The integrated framework for Smart City development could essentially encompass not be to smart service cataloguing, smart technology integration, value chain stakeholders environment in terms of smart systems for G2C, G2G, G2B, smart data integration, smart data interface, smart visual analytics for decision making to capitalize larger diffusion of spin-offs linked to domain, sub-domain functions and processes (see Fig. 3.7).

The methodological framework for conceptualization of smart cities requires an integration approach which cuts across the dimensions of organizational level to city wide level dimensions. Using the City Life Cycle (CLC) approach, these dimensions could be unpacked in terms of strategic measurable KPAs and the corresponding KPIs across several cross-cutting and overarching horizontal and vertical functional and process dimensions encompassing the internal as well as external aspects of the value chain/eco-system. Using these KPAs and KPIs, the framework should be further detailed in terms of evidence-oriented SWOT analysis which

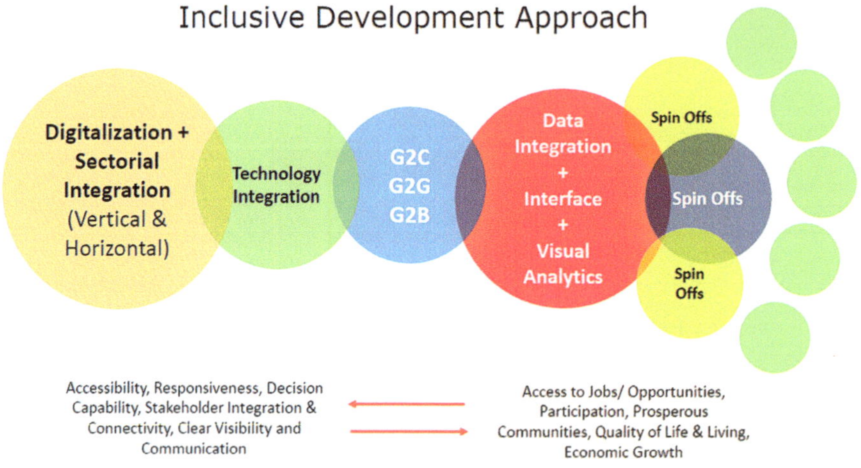

Fig. 3.7 Inclusive development approach for vertical and horizontal sectorial integration

Vision	+	**KPAs/ KPIs**	+	**SWOT analysis**	+	**Score / Weightage**	=	**Smart Rank**

Fig. 3.8 Integrated methodological smart framework: evidence oriented integrated KPAs/KPIs, SWOT approach

should quantify and benchmark the status quo in the identified dimensions. Based on the evidence oriented quantified dimensions, the KPAs and KPIs could be clustered in terms of value-oriented scoring system which could be rationalized based on the priority and relevance of the theme or could be rationalized based on weightage. The overall exercise should lead to ranking based on the specific score achieved (see Fig. 3.8, Tables 3.4a and 3.4b).

The approaches to conceptualize the framework could be based on hybrid system of KPAs, KPIs, and analysis using a simplistic method of SWOT analysis.

The above matrix provides a high-level summarized information about the framework/tool which can be used at various stages of conceptualization of the smart cities or evaluating the smartness of the cities broadly classified/categorized in three specific clusters: smart infrastructure, smart solutions and smart governance. Each of these clusters would be composed of sub-clusters which comprises of relevant measurable KPAs and KPIs. Based on the status quo, each of these KPAs and KPIs can be scored for its strengths, weaknesses, opportunities and threats based on the level of adequacy using a simplistic five-point Likert Scale, along with a customizable weightage. The composite smart score can be evaluated using the

Table 3.4a Conceptual methodological framework for smart cities development and assessment

City Life Cycle	KPA/ KPIs	Strengths	Weaknesses	Opportunities	Threats
Quadrant-1 (0-25 years)	Example: smart health infrastructure				
	– Access to state-of-art general hospitals and clinics within proximate distance – Access to multi-speciality hospitals – Number of hospital beds	90% of the current city population covered.	– Average distance to reach hospitals/clinics is high (15 kms) – The city has limited multi-specialty hospitals (number). – Limited bed capacity of multi-specialty hospitals (per capita)/number of beds.	Provision of accessible hospitals and clinics within 5 kms distance	Lack of funding commitment from stakeholders.
	Smart Health Solutions				
	– Integrated health care system/health information system. – Smart investment management system – Crowd sourced participatory analytics	30 different healthcare portfolio's/services available to the communities.	– High management/ technology costs. – Per capita affordability is high (average cost/person)	Affordable healthcare system.	– Rapid change of technological system. – Data security and privacy.
	Smart Health Governance				
	– Health education. – Doctors and specialists – Beneficiaries' coverage. – Urban poor/ vulnerable communities.	Reputed academic institutions offering medical programmes (number of institutions).	Limited number of specialized programme offerings (number of programmes at undergraduate, postgraduate, short course level)	International and national collaborations.	– Lack of participation from citizens/ doctors. – Lack of political will and private sector participation.

Table 3.4b Conceptual methodological framework for smart cities development and assessment (composite dashboard score and ranking)

Layers/dimensions	S	W	O	T	Score	Weightage (%)	Composite smart score	Smart rank
Example of broad categorization of clusters								
Smart infrastructure	3	2	1	1	1	40	30	2
Smart solutions						30		
Smart governance						30		

overall score and weightages to provide an idea of the status quo and benchmarking levels for a city to be attained in terms of considering/designating a city to be smart city. The smart ranking would be based on comparative score within the cluster and sub-cluster to provide an idea about the priority of the layers/dimensions for an intelligent decision-making process. The matrix fairly provides a customizable dashboard system which can be linked to various customizable horizontal and vertical sectorial functions and process analytical reports at an early stage of conceptualization or during the state of program/project implementation or post implementation stage for monitoring and evaluation of any smart city.

3.4 Discussion

The dynamic context of cities and the challenges encountered by them are generally similar. However, they vary in terms of degrees of differences such as fiscal, spatial, functional, governance, technological and among others. The cities face unique conditions and challenges to meet the expectations of citizens in services and development. In-spite of several efforts, the cities are often found in the vicious cycle of coping with challenges and provision of services to the citizens. The challenges often relate to the issues that arise from internal as well as external environments. This vicious cycle results in poor delivery of services to citizens, which in turn results in lowering of service level benchmarks, financial resources and sustainability. The smart technology, smart infrastructure, smart solutions and smart governance brings functional and process integration within the challenging eco-system at city level.

The infrastructure and service nexus within the dynamic context of Government to Citizen, Government to Government, and Government to Business is critical for smart performance across the three tiers of governance to integrate planning and development, infrastructure, utilities and service delivery and resource mobilization. The smart city understanding spans across multidimensional facets of human settlements: physical systems, environmental, human interactions, system elements, temporal and among other dimensions. This multidimensional dynamic paradigm in not limited to smart infrastructure, smart technology and solutions, smart services, smart planning, smart design, smart management, smart citizens, and smart citizens as enablers of smart city.

The integrated approach of methodological framework for conceptualizing and measuring the Smart City can become complex as its dependent on several socio-technical layers, associated dimensions within the broader contours of planning, designing, implementation and post implementation stages. The clustering approach in terms of CLC quadrant approach helps in quantifying the Smart City status quo and benchmarking for enabling smart transition based on the evidence-oriented status quo. The cities can customize and adopt suitable solution specific to overall broader structure within smart infrastructure, smart solution and smart governance cluster or benchmark specific socio-technical layer as per the requirements and impact depending on the smart scoring system. From conceptual level to advanced level, the approach remains flexible irrespective of the size of the city and any limiting constraints. Further critical evaluation of cities can be done by comparing the performance/benchmarking of cities based on other frameworks and using the CLC approach to see if there are any major differences appearing in terms of city priorities at various stages of city dynamic paradigm. The scoring system of smart city would require further in-depth understanding of structuring city into basic, intermediate and advanced level of smart city depending on the qualifying score which should be representative of the domains, sub-domains, KPAs, and KPIs.

3.5 Conclusions

Sustainable Smart City requires a pragmatic approach for taking into account the business-as-usual, digitalization, accessibility, infrastructure, innovations, scale, and overall value chain dynamics. The context of demand and supply, status-quo and technology adoption will play a critical part in leveraging several building blocks for contextualizing the Smart City. The next critical area would be digitalization approach which requires closer integration and implementation of ICT, intelligent systems, data analytics and performance driven smart governance among other approaches like innovative dashboard interfaces linked to predictive analytics using Artificial Intelligence (AI), Machine Learning (ML), and among other systems. The intrinsic nature of multidimensional issues would demand greater accessibility and infrastructure across the different socio-technical regimes/overall environmental value chain. The scalability would require the seamless integration and innovation driven horizontal and vertical integration linked to multidimensional internal and external impact. The most critical of the conceptualizing and measurement of Smart City is visualizing the integration of several dimensions in forms of various socio-technical layers, KPA, KPIs within the overall value chain and leveraging on it based on data integration and analytics.

References

Angelakis, V., Tragos, E., Pohls, H. C., Kapovits, A., & Bassi, A. (2017). *Designing, developing, and facilitating smart cities: Urban design to IoT solutions* (pp. 17–32). Cham: Springer.

Batty, M. (2015). *Urban informatics and big data: A report to the ESRC Cities Expert Group.* http://www.spatialcomplexity.info/files/2018/05/Urban-Informatics-and-Big-Data.pdf

Cohen, B. (2012). What exactly is a smart city? *Fast Company.* https://www.fastcodesign.com/1680538/what-exactly-is-a-smart-city

Cruz, C., & Sarmento, J. (2017). Reforming traditional PPP models to cope with the challenges of smart cities. *Competition and Regulation in Network Industries, 18*(1–2), 94–114.

Giap, T. K., Thye, W. W., Yam, T. K., Low, L., & Aw, E. L. G. (2012). *Ranking the liveability of the worlds, major cities – The Global Liveable Cities Index (GLCI).* Singapore: World Scientific.

Giffinger, R., & Gudrun, H. (2010). Smart cities ranking: An effective instrument for the positioning of cities? *ACE: Architecture, City & Environ, 4*(12), 7–25.

Hayat, P. (2016). Smart cities: A global perspective. *India Quarterly: A Journal of International Affairs, 72*(2), 177–191.

Hollands, R. G. (2008). Will the real smart city please stand up? *City, 12*, 303–320. https://doi.org/10.1080/13604810802479126.

International Standard ISO 37120: 2014. (2014). *Sustainable development of communities – Indicators for city services and quality of life.* Geneva: ISO.

Joshi, S., Saxena, S., Godbole, T., & Shreya. (2016). Developing smart cities: An integrated framework. 6th international conference on advances on computing & communications, ICACC 2016, 6–8 September, 2016. *Procedia Computer Science, 93*(2016), 902–909.

Kwele, L. (2016). *Enterprise mobility forum 2016 "smart city: Future Tshwane".* [Online] Available at: http://enterprisemobilityforum.co.za. Accessed 15 Oct 2018.

Lewis, M. P., & Ogra, A. (2010). An approach of geographic information system (GIS) for good urban governance. *Conference proceedings of 18th international conference on Geoinformatics 2010*, Beijing, China, ISBN: 978-1-4244-7302-1, IEEE Catalog Number: CFP1032H-ART.

Meijer, A., & Bolívar, M. (2015). Governing the smart city: A review of the literature on smart urban governance. *International Review of Administrative Sciences, 82*(2), 392–408.

Odendaal, N. (2003). Information and communication technology and local governance: Understanding the difference between cities in developed and emerging economies. *Computers, Environment and Urban Systems, 27*(6), 585–607.

Ogra, A. (2013). Mobile solutions and application for smart government. *Proceedings of the 8th international forum on knowledge asset dynamics (IFKAD 2013): Smart growth organizations, cities, and communities*, (pp. 1708–1722) ISBN: 978-88-96687-01-07/ISSN 2280-787X.

Ogra, A., & Thwala, W. D. (2014). E-government perspectives: Evolution, strategies and practices, published in the *Proceedings of international conference on eBusiness, eCommerce, eManagement, eLearning and eGovernance (IC5E 2014).* https://edlib.net/2014/ic5e/ic5e2014011.html.

Shapiro, J. (2006). Smart cities: Quality of life, productivity, and the growth effects of human capital. *Review of Economics and Statistics, 88*(2), 324–335.

Sharma, V., Gutto, D., & Ogra, A. (2014). Next generation citizen centric e-services, IST Africa 2014. Published in *Conference Proceedings by IEEE Explore.* https://doi.org/10.1109/ISTAFRICA.2014.6880672 (Print ISBN: 978-1-905824-43-4).

Thompson, E. (2016). What makes a city 'smart'? *International Journal of Architectural Computing, 14*(4), 358–371.

Vinod Kumar, T. M. (2017). *Smart economy in smart cities.* Singapore: Springer.

Washburn, D., Sindhu, U., Balaouras, S., Dines, R. A., Hayes, N. M., & Nelson, L. E. (2010). *Helping CIOs understand 'smart city' initiatives: Defining the smart city, its drivers, and the role of the CIO.* Cambridge, MA: Forrester Research.

Part II
Smart Urban Infrastructure

Chapter 4
Development Challenges for Big Data Command and Control Centres for Smart Cities in India

Sarbeswar Praharaj

Abstract The 100 Smart Cities Mission in India have received significant attention from the researchers and policymakers globally. This chapter examines the imposing challenge of development of command and control centres that are at the focal point of the smart cities discourse in India with as many as 83 cities investing substantially to capture and use big data through such technologically advanced facilities. A thorough account of the genesis of the Smart Cities Mission in India is presented here to establish the context behind the development of centralised big data command and control centres. This chapter presents the very first analysis of the technical architecture and systems being adopted by the Indian smart cities for creating the command and control centres and highlights their innovations in collecting and integrating big data through a range of audio, video, sound, sensing and crowdsourcing devices. While identifying the domain and application areas incorporated within the command and control centre projects, this research reveals that the focus by the Indian smart cities is more on controlling and surveilling rather than improving the delivery of public services. This chapter also critically assesses the potential of building synergy between different local and state agencies through the command and control centres and how much they can influence the urban planning processes in rapidly growing Indian cities. The outcomes from the research suggest that the command and control centres in Indian smart cities are predominantly privatised and there is an inclination towards big data corporatisation. The chapter argues for public ownership over these big data and command and control centres so that publicly funded high-value datasets can be made openly available for use by the app developers, businesses, innovators, startups and citizens that could open up opportunities for creative collaborations and the development of a data-driven innovation ecosystem.

Keywords Big data · Smart cities · Command and control centre · Smart Cities Mission in India

---

S. Praharaj (✉)
Faculty of Built Environment, University of New South Wales, Sydney, Australia
e-mail: s.praharaj@unsw.edu.au

N. Biloria (ed.), *Data-driven Multivalence in the Built Environment*, S.M.A.R.T. Environments, https://doi.org/10.1007/978-3-030-12180-8_4

4.1 Introduction

A new wave of technocratic imaginations is reshaping the processes of urban planning and governance in India with the current development of 100 smart cities. The Government of India defines smart cities as the ones that create 'smart solutions' by the intelligent use of technology, information and data to improve infrastructure and services (GoI 2015). The select cities under the Smart Cities Mission (SCM) have begun to embed an extensive network of sensors, surveillance cameras, smart water and energy meters into the fabric of urban environments and infrastructure to monitor, manage and regulate city flows and processes in real-time. This paradigm aims to advance a 'smart mentality' (Vanolo 2014) which envisages the city as what Kitchin (2014) calls the 'constellations of instruments' across multiple levels and scales of the built environment that produce data to support the design, operation and governance of urban systems.

A high majority of the 100 smart cities in India have set out ambitious plans to develop 'Integrated Command and Control Centres' (ICCC) for connecting, integrating and analysing the information streamed by the digitally instrumented devices plotted across the city. As many as 83 cities are creating such structures anticipating that the data deluge will transform the knowledge and urban governance with a much more sophisticated, fine-grained and real-time understanding and control of urbanity. The ICCC projects are somewhat embracing the model of data-driven networked urbanism (Townsend 2013) which is based on the premise that rich seams of data can be used to better capture, model and predict the urban processes (Batty 2012) and guide the design of future urban policies and interventions. The first impressions from the recently unveiled command centres of Ahmedabad, Bhopal and Bhubaneswar in India refreshes our memories of the classic smart city set up of Rio de Janeiro in Brazil (see Gaffney and Robertson 2016). Much like the Centro De Operacoes Prefeitura Do Rio (Rio Operations Center), the ICCC in these cities shows off a flashy large wall of video screens with rows of desks and computer terminals facing them (Fig. 4.1). These centralised urban monitoring systems in India have several nomenclatures, such as the smart city operations centre, integrated command and control centre and intelligent city operations and management centre. However, the motivations behind such developments and their functions are identical.

With the upcoming of such massive, technologically driven urban management systems a new era of 'governance through code' (Söderström et al. 2014) has verged on the Indian public discourse. However, little information and research exist outlining the motivations, appropriateness and feasibility of the development of big data superstructures in the Indian cities that have struggled to cope up with digital reforms and change in the past (Chatterji 2017). This chapter aims to uncover the agendas, assumptions and possibilities surrounding the ICCC projects in select Indian cities. The study evaluates the smart city plans to capture the technologies and frameworks of the control centres and critically summarises their scope and potential impacts on transforming urban governance in India. The research also

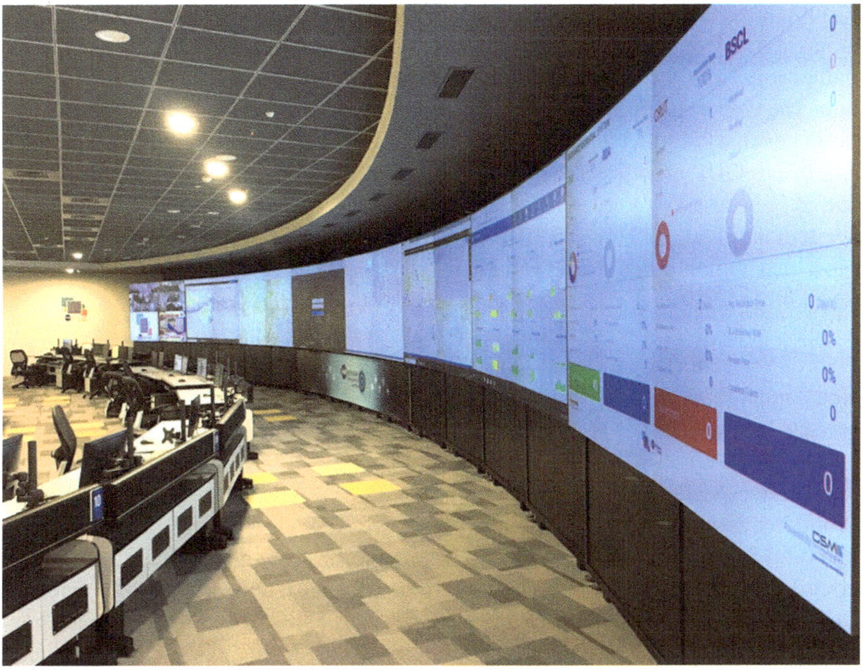

Fig. 4.1 Intelligent City Operations and Management Centre (ICOMC) in Bhubaneswar, India. (Source: Author)

identifies the most significant challenges and barriers to data-driven city operations and policymaking and echoes a word of caution for the cities under investigation. The analysis in this chapter builds a much-needed scholarly ground for vital conversations on urban future and smart cities that are increasingly influenced by big data infrastructure.

4.2 Familiarising with the Smart Cities Mission in India

Dynamic and resilient economic growth as an impact of accelerated economic reforms since the 1990s has unleashed rapid urbanisation in India. The country has added over 200 million population over the last two decades, taking the urban populace to 460 million in 2018 (United Nations 2018). Mckinsey Global Institute estimates suggest that by 2030, India's urban population could soar up to 590 million, adding nearly 270 million net increase in the working-age group (Sankhe et al. 2010). India had 61 cities with a population over one million in 2018, whereas entire Europe hosts 35 such urban agglomerations today. The three megacities of India: Mumbai, Delhi and Kolkata together account for nearly a population of 56 million which is twice the population of Australia.

India's urbanisation has been instrumental in keeping the country's growth momentum alive. In the year 2010, 64% of the Gross Domestic Product (GDP) in India came from the urban areas which house only 31.2% of the country's population. The Government of India appointed High Powered Expert Committee (HPEC) estimates that if India handles its urban expansion efficiently, it could add as much as 1.5% to GDP growth, taking it near the double-digit rate. Such robust economic output is necessary to create adequate jobs for the 270 million additional working age Indians expected between 2010 and 2030. The HPEC (2011) recommendations show that Indian cities possess the capacity to generate 70% of the country's net new jobs by 2030, produce more than 70% of GDP, and stimulate a near-fourfold increase in the per capita incomes across the nation. In this background, the Strategic Plan of the Ministry of Urban Development (2011) argued that the local governments must think innovatively and transform the urban planning, management and service delivery models to ensure the competitiveness of cities in future.

The Smart Cities Mission in India was pitched in 2015 as a response to the need for greater speed in policy decision-making and driving innovation in the cities. While highlighting the purpose and suitability of the initiative, the program guideline (GoI 2015) stated that the concept of smart cities relying on the foundations of urban innovation, creative policies and Information and Communication Technology (ICT) had attracted the significant attention of the political class. The central government document also added that the city leadership in India would use smart technologies as a response to solving persistent tangled and wicked problems congenital in the rapid urbanisation. The primary aim of the mission is to drive economic growth and improve the quality of life for people in 100 selected cities by enabling local development and harnessing technology as a means to create smart solutions for citizens (NITI Ayog and CSTEP 2015). However, a more critical review of the guideline suggests that the objective behind the initiative was to enhance the competitiveness of cities and improve their credit ratings to enable them leveraging investments from the private sector and borrowings from the global financial institutions (Praharaj et al. 2018a, b). The publication of Ease of Living Index by the Indian government in 2018, ranking the 100 cities on a range of parameters re-enforced such intent.

The initial idea of building smart cities in India was expressed in the pre-election manifesto of the Bhartiya Janta Party led by India's current Prime Minister Narendra Modi. The declaration stated, "We will initiate building 100 new cities; enabled with the latest in technology and infrastructure – adhering to concepts like sustainability, walk to work etc. and focused on specialised domains" (Bharatiya Janata Party 2014, p. 18). The initial idea of building smart cities evolved and changed drastically after the newly elected government on August 2014 asked the state governments to identify existing towns for development under the SCM. This marked a shift in focus from green-field development to brown-field development and from the construction of '100 new smart cities' to 'making existing cities smart' (Bhattacharya et al. 2015). The central message that emerges from the discussion is that the Smart Cities Mission in India although appears as a strategic response to the country's urbanisation challenges, the initiative was primarily pushed as a political-economic agenda.

The distribution of the selected smart cities across the Indian States and Union Territories (UT) was proportionate to the total number of statutory towns within the regions. The Government of India in partnership with Bloomberg Philanthropies conducted a 'Smart Cities Challenge' that developed a mechanism for evaluating the capacity of cities and the robustness of the smart city proposals before funds were disbursed. A 30% weight was given for city-level evaluation and 70% weight for smart city proposal-level evaluation. The city-level assessment looked into two aspects. First, the credibility and performance of the urban local body (ULB) over the last 3 years (including operational efficiency improvement in transport scenario, administrative efficiency and user charges collection ratio). Second, the city vision and strategy, including clarity in overall urban vision, articulation of how the information and communication technologies will be used and the potential impact of the vision on the economy, sustainability and inclusiveness. The smart city proposal-level evaluation assessed the feasibility of the proposal, its cost-effectiveness, innovation and scalability issues and the depth of citizen engagement in developing the plan. In the first round of the challenge, a total of 33 smart city proposals were approved which include 20 lighthouse cities and 13 fat-track cities. The lighthouse cities were adjudged as the top performing centres that also had developed an outstanding plan that can inspire other cities. The 67 cities that did not receive approvals were invited to revise their smart city proposals and participate in the second round of the challenge. A total of 27 cities excelled in this round. The subsequent third and fourth rounds of the challenge approved a total of 40 smart city proposals. The location of the 100 smart cities and their selection rounds are mapped in Fig. 4.2.

The Smart Cities Mission Statement and Guideline (2015) proposes a development model that recommends each city to implement at least two projects: one that will focus on area-based development, and the other that can have a city-wide impact. The proposed area-based development is seen as an agent of transformation of the existing areas through retrofitting or redevelopment strategies, to improve the liveability of the precinct. These select areas will then act as lighthouses for other parts of the city, as a best practice model. The guideline also proposes greenfield development as an alternative model of area-based development that can take place in the peripheral areas of cities to accommodate the expanding population in urban areas. The second project which is conceived to impact the entire city population are aimed at the application of 'Smart Solutions' through the use of technology, information and data to improve infrastructure and services. The typical smart solutions proposed in the approved proposals include projects such as the city-wide video surveillance network, real-time monitoring of environmental quality, wide-scale installation of smart energy and water meters and the development of intelligent transport and traffic solutions. The most popular city-scale project was the creation of Integrated Control and Command Centre with as many as 83 Indian municipalities outlining such developments in their smart city proposals.

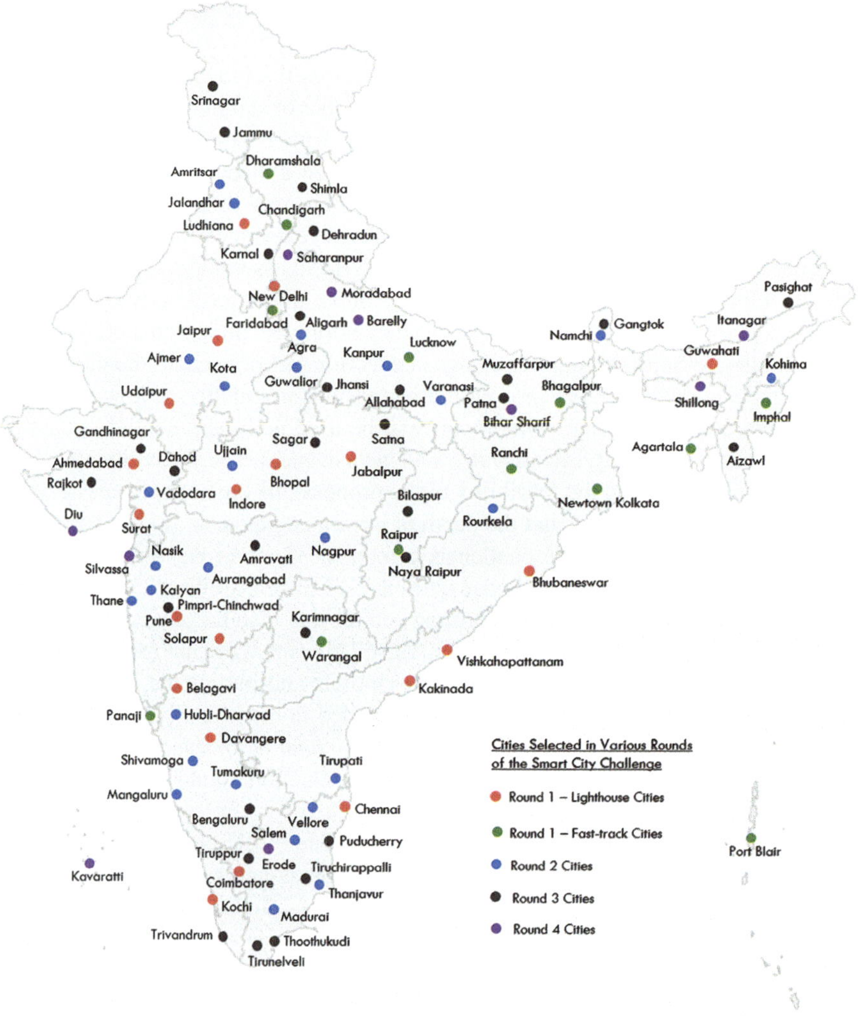

Fig. 4.2 Location of 100 cities selected under the Smart Cities Mission. (Source: Author)

4.3 Uncovering the Emerging Command and Control Centres in the Indian Cities

The discourse on the development of smart city control centres in India first surfaced at the Ministry of Housing and Urban Affairs sponsored "Cross Learning and Experience Sharing Workshop on Integrated Command Control Centre" held at the Yashwantrao Chavan Auditorium in Mumbai on the 22nd September 2017. Key authorities from four cities, including Pune, Bhubaneswar, Kakinada and Bhopal expressed their intentions to set up such structure and presented a preliminary architecture of ICCC. A review of those presentations (Available at http://smartcities.gov.in/content/presentation.php) undertaken as part of this research reveals that the primary motivation behind the ICCC projects was to leverage big data and real-time information for improved monitoring and delivery of services. The assumption here was that the flow of data from the sensors and actuators would allow the urban authorities to gain insights from the natural environment and the built infrastructure. Those streams of information will supposedly then enable the agencies to react to events and also predict phenomenon at the earliest. The workshop discussions laid significant emphasis on the need for the control centres as a supporting instrument for governance in the Indian cities that are currently grappling with shortages in human resource and capacities to deal with tremendous urban growth. The ICCC projects were also pitched as a medium to generate dynamic datasets on physical infrastructure and city operation that could pare the over-reliance on the archaic decennial census that has limited legitimacy for urban planning.

The debate around the ICCC in India intensified with the physical launch of the Integrated Command and Control Centre in Ahmedabad on 23rd February 2018. The project rapidly gained momentum and popularity and was awarded by the Government of India as the most innovative smart city project on the third anniversary of the SCM in July 2018. The direct encouragement inspired other cities to undertake similar ventures of big data centres. The "First Apex Conference of Smart City CEOs" in May 2018 which took place in Bhopal was dominated with the discussion on ICCC projects with as many as 24 lighthouse and fast-track cities showing strong commitment to such development (GoI 2018). The sparking control centres with gigantic screens soon became the unique selling proposition of the smart cities in India. A massive 59 out of the 67 cities that participated in the Smart Cities Challenge in Round 2, 3 and 4 emulated the leading cities by proposing the development of ICCC.

This study examined the technical architecture of the smart city control centres in seven selected cities, including Ahmedabad, Bhopal, Bhubaneswar, Vishkahapattanam, Kakinada and Vadodara. As discussed earlier, these cities are the early establishers of ICCC among the 100 cities selected under the SCM. An in-depth review of the scope of the work outlined in the bidding contracts which otherwise known as Request for Proposal (RFP) was undertaken to illustrate the proposed systems and their domain and application focus. The RFP was accessed from the Government of India operated Smartnet website available at https://smartnet.niua.org/. A summary of the architecture of the ICCC and the different layers and sub-components within the system is diagrammatically presented in Fig. 4.3. The diagram synthesises the key frameworks proposed in the seven cities for a general understanding.

This research finds that a four-layer architecture is typically designed in Indian cities to run the ICCC operations. The 'Applications and Devices Layer' sits at the top of the ladder performing two crucial functions. First, deployment of sensors and edge level devises (such as camera, emergency call boxes) within this layer helps the city administration gather information about the ambient city conditions. Second, the bi-directional output field devices, including variable message display

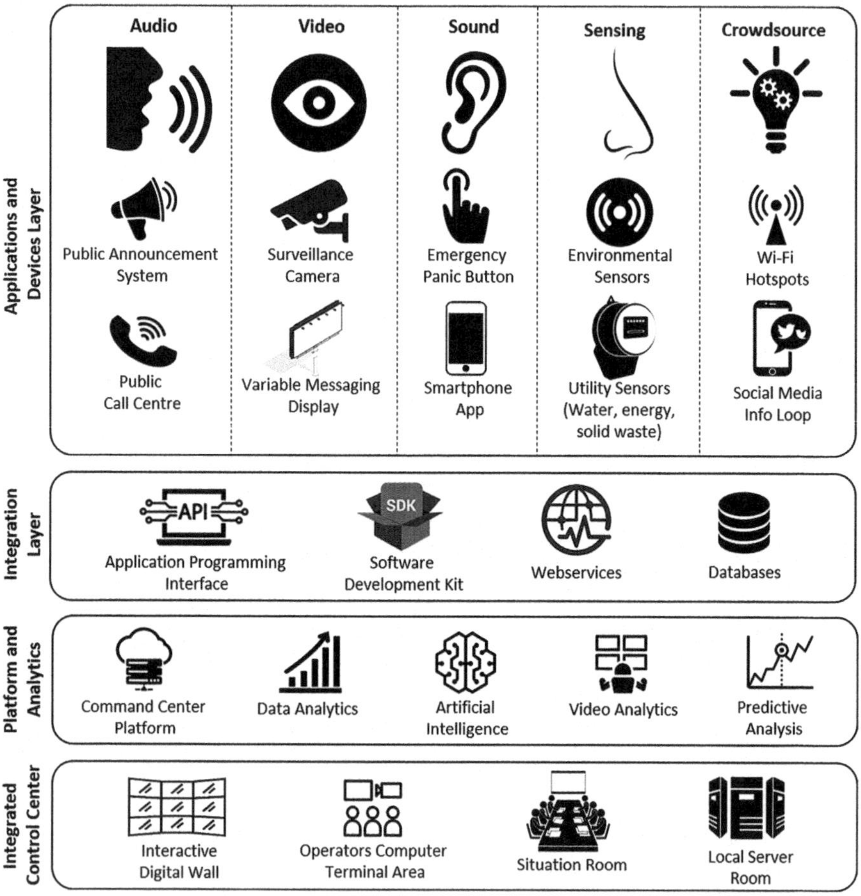

Fig. 4.3 Typical architecture of the integrated command and control centre in Indian cities. (Source: Author)

boards, public announcement system, digital messaging boards support the authorities to provide actionable information that is consumed by citizens. This layer collects and produces five types of information – audio, video, sound, sensing and crowdsourcing through a range of devices as illustrated in Fig. 4.3. Secured network connectivity within this layer serves as the backbone for the project and provide connectivity to gather data from sensors and communicate messages to Wi-Fi services, display devices and actuators. The second layer of the ICCC is the 'Integration Layer' that is used to aggregate the different streams of data and synergise the APIs for different urban services for processing large quantities of information. This layer also deploys a software development kit to enrich applications with advanced functionalities bringing together data from payment gateways, Email and SMS gateways, emergency services and a whole range of platforms. The existing databases and the non-digital information from government departments (such as police department, meteorological department, street lights and transport organisations) and non-government agencies will be linked through this integration layer.

The third layer within the frameworks of ICCC is the 'Platform and Analytics Layer' that include the command centre platform and a variety of analytic approaches. While a majority of the cities are developing smart city platforms for use within their defined territories, in Madhya Pradesh a common cloud-based platform is being deployed for all the eight urban centres of the state that received funding under the SCM. The platform being designed by the Indian smart cities are aiming at cutting-edge data analytics of both statistical, locational data and video feeds to support real-time and predictive analysis. These analytic processes are expected to produce dashboards and reports on urban conditions and operational efficiency. The fourth layer is the physical structures of the control centre that have a large video wall and a series of computer terminals for operators. The smart city Bhubaneswar command centre has massive video walls with a 16 × 2 configuration with 70-inch panels. The centre also hosts the data server room and provide conference and situation management rooms for collaborative responses to emergencies. The data hosting services within the physical ICCC building include servers, storage, ancillary network equipment elements, security devices and corresponding management tools. Cities such as Ahmedabad and Gwalior are simultaneously developing an App that can act as a virtual control centre providing with widgets and viewing tools for understanding the ambient city conditions.

The domain focus of the control centres significantly varies across the seven cities analysed in this study. Table 4.1 presents the targeted application areas of the ICCC projects in the cities and highlights the different interests and motivations behind the developments. The urban transport and surveillance are the two domains that appear to be the typical target of the control centres with each of the studied cities outlining proposals to integrate the data and information from the public transport, traffic signals and CCTV cameras under the ICCC project. Several cities are also focusing on combining the data from various utilities, including smart solid waste bins, garbage truck, SCADA water sensors and smart street light poles with the city control rooms. Such approaches are likely to improve urban infrastructure management and operational efficiency. However, the applications such as flood monitoring and disaster management were linked only by a few cities with the

Table 4.1 The domains and application areas of the ICCC projects in select Indian cities

Domain	Applications	Ahmedabad	Bhopal	Bhubaneswar	Vizag	Pune	Kakinada	Vadodara
Mobility	Public transport	■	■	■	■	■		■
	Traffic management & Signalling	■	■	■	■	■	■	■
	Parking management	■	■	■			■	
Utilities	Solid waste management	■	■	■	■	■	■	
	Water supply management	■	■			■		■
	Street lighting	■	■		■		■	
Environment	Environmental monitoring	■	■	■	■	■	■	■
	Flood monitoring					■		
	Disaster management & response		■		■			■
Safety and Security	Video Surveillance	■	■	■	■	■	■	■
	Wi-Fi Operation	■	■	■	■	■	■	■
Citizen services	Public Announcement System				■	■	■	■
	Grievance redressal/call centre	■	■		■			
	Emergency panic button & call box			■	■	■	■	■
Commercial	App services	■	■		■			■
	Digital Signage	■	■			■		

ICCC frameworks. The findings are surprising as the very project (Rio Operations Center) that acted as a catalyst and inspiration for the Indian command centres was primarily focused around disaster response. The review also indicates that a moderate level of emphasis is laid on integrating citizen services such as public announcement system, grievance redressal with the newly developed command and control offices. Four out of seven cities analysed in Table 4.1 remained non-committed to linking matters related to citizen grievance and call centres with the digital control centres.

This research analysed the investments allocated for the development of ICCC by the 100 smart cities to establish the scope and varying level of significance attached by the municipalities to such projects. The information on budget allocations was retrieved from the smart city proposals available at https://smartnet.niua.org/. Arc GIS software is used to produce Fig. 4.4 that classifies the 100 cities based on the funding outlined for the ICCC project. The analysis shows that the degree of

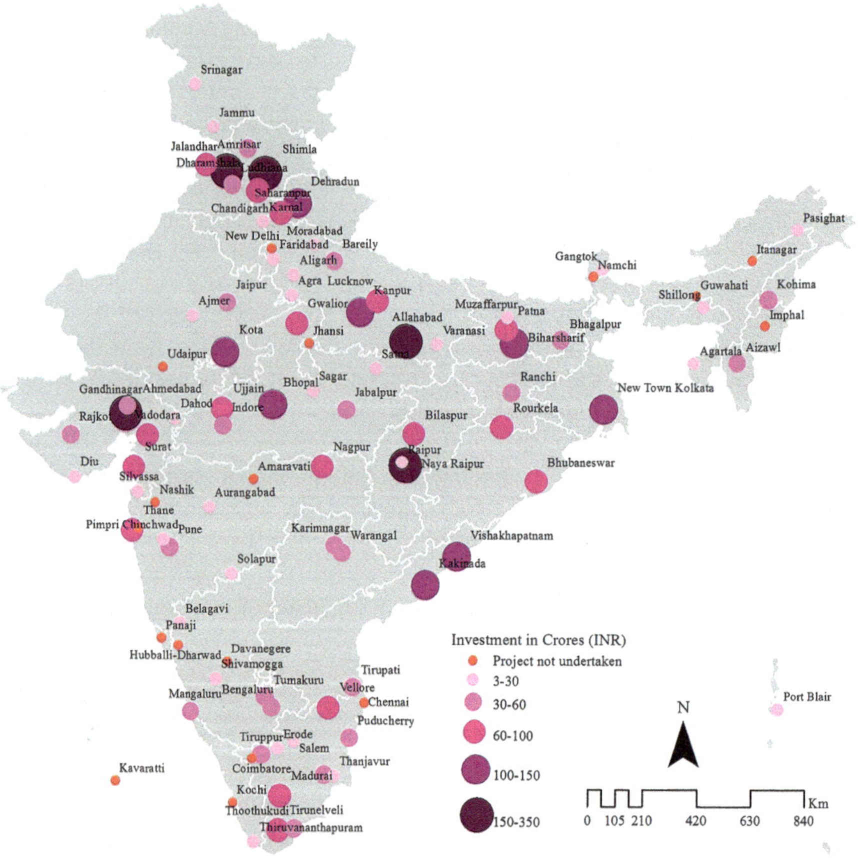

Fig. 4.4 Investments outlined by cities for the development of smart city control centres. (Source: Author)

investments significantly varies across cities. Allahabad allocated the highest outlay for ICCC project worth of INR350.15 crores which is 16% of the total funds estimated in the smart city proposal. The second highest allocation of INR203 crores was made by Ahmedabad that is approximately 9% of the total funds committed by the city under the SCM. Naya Raipur, Shimla, Jalandhar and Bhopal have also allocated substantial funding in the range of INR150–170 crores for the development of smart city control centres. On the other hand, cities such as Erode, Solapur, Port Blair, Shillong and Varanasi assigned a meagre amount ranging between INR3–10 crores. These cities allocated less than 0.5% of the overall smart city development cost for the ICCC project. The significant difference in the investment pattern reflects the degree of emphasis laid and the nature of applications that are conceived under the project. The cities that have adopted a piecemeal approach by covering a handful of applications and services under the ICCC shown minor investments. The ones that have made substantial financial commitments for ICCC project have engaged more comprehensively with the system by linking a range of services and domains. Also, the scale of the proposed physical control centre and the equipment's, such as video walls and data warehouses have influenced the cost differentials.

4.4 A Critical Note on the Potential Challenges and Considerations for Action

The Indian big data urbanism aspirations realised through the smart city control centres does appear to be inherently a good thing, seeking to make city safer, congestion free, efficient and so on by employing innovative technologies that capture, process and analyse massive quantities of data from a range of urban sub-systems. The success of these interventions and their impact on the ground, however, rests on how the cities address the more structural issues and transform their current governance models.

A primary motivation behind the development of command and control centre is to build synergy between different local and state agencies that deliver urban services and infrastructure. The control rooms are being designed to integrate the data from urban systems such as transport, water supply, solid waste management and emergency services that are currently delivered by different agencies in Indian cities. These agencies often operate in silos under the authorities of either local, regional or state government resulting in a complex hierarchy of institutional mandates (Praharaj et al. 2018a, b). The development, operation and management of the smart city control centres are, on the other hand, left with the special purpose vehicles (SPV) being developed as a joint venture company. How the newly imagined smart city SPVs will coordinate with the various agencies to bring them under one roof is a matter of serious contention. Much of the success of the ICCC projects, therefore, will be determined by whether the Indian cities can reform their local governance by empowering the municipal corporation with critical functions that are currently performed by the state agencies. Bringing the SPVs under the direct ambit of the local corporation is also a crucial step towards integrating governance processes and ensuring institutional convergence under the smart city control centres.

Alongside the integration of internal government structure, Indian cities would require collaboration and partnership with external organisations and citizens to extract benefits from the development of big data centres potentially. As Kitchin (2014) says, control and command systems can centralise power and decision making into a select set of offices armed with giant screens and cutting-edge algorithms. But, at the same time, they can also make a vast amount of information publicly available for use by a variety of interested parties, such as the app developers, businesses, innovators, startups and citizens. The Indian cities currently lack mechanisms for opening up of data, and there is a lack of emphasis by the smart city proposals on the establishment of open data platforms. A lot will depend on the degree of openness by the cities in terms of sharing the big data if they have to make a significant impact on the innovation ecosystem. The open sharing of data can potentially support harnessing the collective intelligence and creativity of the local citizens and stakeholders that can shape collaborative smart governance (Meijer and Bolívar 2016). The challenge, therefore, is of maintaining a delicate balance between deploying new forms of digital technologies to monitor and measure cities and opening up critical datasets from the government to ensure transparency and boost creativity.

The smart city control centres will indeed produce vast streams of data on a range of subjects, like the movements of people and vehicles, environmental quality, energy usage, solid waste generation, parking and flooding. But the critical factor in all of this is what is being done with these big datasets and how much they can influence the urban planning processes in rapidly growing Indian cities. As Wiig (2015) states, 'smart' is often equalled with 'efficient' and 'beneficial' in the literature and the promotional smart city materials. Instead of taking such slogans at face value, it is essential to map out and openly report the degree of efficiency, who benefited and where in a city those benefits are located. Several global best practices exist in this regard that can guide the measurement of change across city systems. The Boston 'CityScore' platform (https://www.boston.gov/cityscore) is a leading example that uses data to grade how well the city is performing on a daily, weekly, monthly and annual basis. It provides a "nearly real-time" indication of what's happening in the city across areas such as transport, urban safety, health and human services, and utilities. The city metrics allows the local authorities to take immediate action to improve city services, track improvements and better plan future investments. Similarly, the Indian cities through the big data superstructures have the opportunity to set up measurement processes that can assess how much impact the smart city and urban infrastructure projects have on improving base level scenarios on congestion, the reliability of public transport, energy efficiency, reduction in crime rate and so on. Beyond the mere surveillance of urban assets and spaces, the control centres can potentially play a more constructive role in establishing a municipal performance monitoring system with a feedback loop linked to strategic planning, accurate forecasting and preparedness to emergencies.

Development of strategic policies and investment decisions based on the evidence produced by big data should, however, require a cautious approach. The giant video screens within the command rooms, as Kitchin (2014) says are complex socio-technical systems that do not simply reflect the world but actively produce it. While it is true that big data that are stored in the ICCC is big in quantity, and sometimes exhaustive, but as with all data they are a selective sample and are framed within a thought system. The CCTV cameras for example that are installed in selected locations might provide a good understanding of the people's movements and security situations of those places, but they are by no means all-encompassing to inform city-wide policies on urban safety. Not only where the data capturing devices are deployed in cities that have bearings on the quality and biases in datasets, but factors such as who uses the space or media while the data is recorded, the technology, platform and ontology employed to process, calibrate and visualise information also have serious implications. While using the big data as evidence for designing policies, it must be acknowledged that they may not have been tailored to answer specific questions. Furthermore, the linking of big data directly with the responses to urban issues is problematic as it portrays a technocratic view that assumes that complex social situations can be captured through sensing, data and computation. Such 'instrumental rationality' (Mattern 2013) betrays the very idea of cities, the composite entities they are that we can feel and experience.

The upcoming of high-tech control rooms and a drive towards governance by code (Barns 2016) is throwing up demands for new-type capacities and managerial techniques within the local governments in India. The question is, do the Indian municipal agencies have the desired knowledge and human resource to deal with these challenges? To answer this question objectively, this research considered their performance in implementing the e-governance reforms during the Jawaharlal Nehru National Urban Renewal Mission (JnNURM) that was operational before the SCM came into effect. An analysis by Kundu (2014) has shown that 38 out of the 67 JnNURM cities have failed to develop an e-governance portfolio. The small towns particularly struggled to deal with such ICT-driven service delivery models exposing severe lack of technical capacity and resources within urban local bodies in India. These small towns have allocated significant budget for building command centres under the SCM leading to apprehensions regarding how they will develop technological capacities and knowledge needed for operating the advanced digital structures. Academic collegium, such as the Housing and Land Rights Network (Housing and Land Rights Network 2017) argued that a lack of expertise and know-how could drive the municipal staff away from these big data superstructures that could turn them into ghostly places.

Acknowledging the capacity deficit, a majority of the 100 smart cities have proposed public-private partnerships (PPPs) for the development, operation and management of the city command and control centre. Ahmedabad, which is an early-establishers of the ICCC, for example, has not only hired a private agency for supplying and installation of sensors, cameras and other edge devises, the smart city

SPV has also delegated the responsibility of project commissioning, maintenance of the city-wide ICT infrastructure and the control centre operations. Such privatisation, neo-liberalisation of city management and marketisation of public services are a matter of significant concern wherein Hollands (2008) argues city functions are directed for private profit. The technological lock-in by the corporate vendors through the deployment of specific platforms and secret algorithms threatens to create a monopoly position rather than fostering collaboration among agencies that the smart city control centres are meant for. The evolving nature of quantified, smart urbanism in India, in this regard, appears to be big for business, leading cities to a dangerous corporate path dependency that Bates (2012) contends cannot easily be undone or diverted. While the competitive engagement of the vendors can realistically allow cities to deploy and benefit from the best-available technology solutions in the market, Indian municipal agencies need critical measures for capacity building of its staff to own, manage and operate the digital infrastructure efficiently.

4.5 Conclusion

The opportunities around the use of ICT and data-driven processes for urban operations and planning is unprecedented. These technologies, as Yigitcanlar (2015) observes will increasingly play a vital role in determining how we gain insights into urban problems and address them. The manoeuvre by the Indian cities to build a technological architecture to collect, integrate and use big data to address urbanisation challenges is, therefore, a timely and essential move. However, it is not the novelty of such exercise that this chapter raises aspersion on, but who designs them, own the proprietorship and operates the big data projects has been highlighted as a matter of contention here. The arguments presented here do not question the core philosophy of integrating different urban systems and institutional actors that the smart city control centres are said to be designed for, but critically analyses the potential of Indian cities to achieve them. The chapter, in essence, provides a reality check for the development of big data command and control centres under the Smart Cities Mission in India.

While outlining the genesis of the SCM, this research delved into the various stages of the city selection under the mission and recognised the integrated command and control centre projects as the epicentre of the smart city proposals. The study found that on an average 7% of the total smart city investment was allocated for building the big data centres by the 83 out of 100 municipalities that undertook such developments. Some of the more ambitious cities, such as Allahabad and Ahmedabad have even budgeted for more than one-tenth of the overall smart city funding for ICCC developments. A summary of the technical architecture of the smart city control centre presented in this chapter developed new insights into innovative approaches being adopted by the Indian cities for capturing and integrating data through a range of audio, video, sound, sensing and crowdsourcing devices. The discussions also highlighted key trends in the motivations and focus areas of the

ICCC operations. There was a significant emphasis on surveillance of spaces and monitoring of transport and traffic through the big data centres. However, most cities stayed away from linking a range of citizen services and disaster management and response systems with the ICCC frameworks. The results suggest that while there was a great level of enthusiasm shown by the Indian cities to attract the best-in-class technology through massive investments, the selection of application domains shows exclusivity. Such approaches lead us to believe that the focus of the Indian smart cities was more on controlling and surveillance rather than delivering of citizen services. Findings from this chapter advance arguments developed by Gaffney and Robertson (2016) who in the context of Rio de Janeiro's smart operations centre pointed out that layers of hardware and software, not the people dominate the technological discourse of such classic smart city.

The big data revolution is fast intruding into the global south with the urban policymakers in the region actively looking for innovative approaches to public management. Indeed, big data and centralised operations facilities support governments with near-real-time report of what is unfolding in the city, leading to the development of extraordinary capacities within local authorities to respond to and address the needs of their constituencies. However, the privatisation and corporatisation of such data assemblage and monitoring facilities and superseding of their operations over the democratic municipal institutions poses a severe challenge. It brings us to a stage where cities and their population are vulnerable to manipulation for commercial gains. Such emerging smart city models rather than enabling collaboration through technology create fractures within the governance system. Instead of engaging the local authorities more, they can sideline their interests and that of their electorates. Further research and development, to this end, is critical to inform a working business model of the smart city control centres that place the city government at its operational core, enabling them to stitch creative collaborations with public authorities, businesses and local citizens through big and open data.

References

Barns, S. (2016). Mine your data: Open data, digital strategies and entrepreneurial governance by code. *Urban Geography, 37*(4), 554–571. https://doi.org/10.1080/02723638.2016.1139876.

Bates, J. (2012). "This is what modern deregulation looks like": Co-optation and contestation in the shaping of the UK's Open Government Data Initiative. *The Journal of Community Informatics*, 8(2).

Batty, M. (2012). Smart cities, big data. *Environment and Planning. B, Planning & Design, 39*(2), 191–193. https://doi.org/10.1068/b3902ed.

Bharatiya Janata Party. (2014). *Election Manifesto- BJP*. Retrieved February 12, 2016, from http://www.bjp.org/images/pdf_2014/full_manifesto_english_07.04.2014.pdf

Bhattacharya, S., Rathi, S., Patro, S. A., & Tepa, N. (2015). *Reconceptualising smart cities: A reference framework for India. CSTEP-report-2015-03.* Retrieved from http://niti.gov.in/writereaddata/files/document_publication/CSTEP Report Smart Cities Framework.pdf

Chatterji, T. (2017). Digital urbanism in a transitional economy–a review of India's municipal e-governance policy. *Journal of Asian Public Policy, 11*, 1–16.

Gaffney, C., & Robertson, C. (2016). Smarter than smart: Rio de Janeiro's flawed emergence as a smart city. *Journal of Urban Technology, 25*, 1–18.
GoI. (2011). *Strategic plan of ministry of urban development for 2011–16*. New Delhi: Ministry of Urban Development/Government of India. Retrieved from http://www.indiaenvironmentportal.org.in/files/file/Strategic_Plan_draft_new[1].pdf.pdf
GoI. (2015). *Smart Cities Mission statememt and guidelines. Ministry of urban development, Government of India*. Retrieved from http://smartcities.gov.in/content/innerpage/guidelines.php
GoI. (2018). *First Apex Conference of Smart City CEOs*. Retrieved October 21, 2018, from https://smartnet.niua.org/content/ab71da5a-3ee6-4695-bec2-3d04946af3f6
Hollands, R. G. (2008). Will the real smart city please stand up? *City, 12*(3), 303–320. https://doi.org/10.1080/13604810802479126.
Housing and Land Rights Network. (2017). *India's smart cities mission: Smart for whom? Cities for whom?* New Delhi. Retrieved from http://hlrn.org.in/documents/Smart_Cities_Report_2017.pdf
HPEC. (2011). *Report on Indian Urban Infrastructure and Services. High Powered Expert Committee, Government of India*.
Kitchin, R. (2014). The real-time city? Big data and smart urbanism. *GeoJournal, 79*(1), 1–14. https://doi.org/10.1007/s10708-013-9516-8.
Kundu, D. (2014). Urban development programmes in India: A critique of JNNURM. *Social Change, 44*(4), 615–632.
Mattern, S. (2013). Methodolatry and the art of measure: The new wave of urban data science. *Places Journal*, (November).
Meijer, A., & Bolívar, M. P. R. (2016). Governing the smart city: A review of the literature on smart urban governance. *International Review of Administrative Sciences, 82*(2), 392–408. https://doi.org/10.1177/0020852314564308.
NITI Ayog, & CSTEP. (2015). *Transforming urban India: Creating smart and sustainable cities*. Bangalore: Center for Study of Science Technology and Policy (CSTEP).
Praharaj, S., Han, J. H., & Hawken, S. (2018a). Towards the right model of smart city governance in India. *International Journal of Sustainable Development and Planning, 13*(2), 171–186. https://doi.org/10.2495/SDP-V13-N2-171-186
Praharaj, S., Han, J. H., & Hawken, S. (2018b). Urban innovation through policy integration: Critical perspectives from 100 smart cities mission in India. *City, Culture and Society, 12*, 35–43. https://doi.org/10.1016/j.ccs.2017.06.004.
Sankhe, S., Vittal, I., Dobbs, R., Mohan, A., & Gulati, A. (2010). *India's urban awakening: Building inclusive cities sustaining economic growth*. New Delhi: McKinsey Global Institute. Retrieved from https://www.mckinsey.com/~/media/McKinsey/GlobalThemes/Urbanization/Urban awakening in India/MGI_Indias_urban_awakening_full_report.ashx
Söderström, O., Paasche, T., & Klauser, F. (2014). Smart cities as corporate storytelling. *City, 18*(3), 307–320.
Townsend, A. M. (2013). *Smart cities: Big data, civic hackers, and the quest for a new utopia*. New York: WW Norton & Company.
United Nations. (2018). *World urbanization prospects 2018*. Retrieved October 31, 2018, from https://population.un.org/wup/
Vanolo, A. (2014). Smartmentality: The smart city as disciplinary strategy. *Urban Studies, 51*(5), 883–898.
Wiig, A. (2015). IBM's smart city as techno-utopian policy mobility. *City, 19*(2–3), 258–273.
Yigitcanlar, T. (2015). Smart cities: An effective urban development and management model? *Australian Planner, 52*(1), 27–34.

Chapter 5
Understanding Consumer Demand for New Transport Technologies and Services, and Implications for the Future of Mobility

Akshay Vij

Abstract The transport sector is witnessing unprecedented levels of disruption. Privately owned cars that operate on internal combustion engines have been the dominant modes of passenger transport for much of the last century. However, recent advances in transport technologies and services, such as the development of autonomous vehicles, the emergence of shared mobility services, and the commercialization of alternative fuel vehicle technologies, promise to revolutionise how humans travel. The implications are profound: some have predicted the end of private car dependent Western societies, others have portended greater suburbanization than has ever been observed before. If transport systems are to fulfil current and future needs of different subpopulations, and satisfy short and long-term societal objectives, it is imperative that we comprehend the many factors that shape individual behaviour. This chapter introduces the technologies and services most likely to disrupt prevailing practices in the transport sector. We review past studies that have examined current and future demand for these new technologies and services, and their likely short and long-term impacts on extant mobility patterns. We conclude with a summary of what these new technologies and services might mean for the future of mobility.

Keywords Future mobility · Autonomous vehicles · Electric vehicles · Shared mobility · Travel behaviour

---

A. Vij (✉)
Institute for Choice, University of South Australia, Adelaide, Australia

N. Biloria (ed.), *Data-driven Multivalence in the Built Environment*, S.M.A.R.T. Environments, https://doi.org/10.1007/978-3-030-12180-8_5

5.1 Introduction

The transport sector has not seen this much disruption since Henry Ford invented the Model T in 1908. Privately owned cars that operate on internal combustion engines have been the dominant modes of passenger transport for much of the last century. Recent advances in transport technologies and services, such as the emergence of shared mobility services, the invention of connected and autonomous vehicles, and the commercialization of electric vehicle technologies, hold profound implications for future patterns of transport and land use behavior.

As Cortright (2016) writes, "The optimists see a world where parking spaces are beaten into plowshares, the carnage from car crashes is eliminated, where greenhouse gas emissions fall sharply and where the young, the old and the infirm, those who can't drive have easy access to door-to-door transit. The pessimists visualize a kind of exurban dystopia with mass unemployment for those who now make their living driving vehicles, and where cheap and comfortable autonomous vehicles facilitate a new wave of population decentralization and sprawl."

In the face of such uncertainty between these widely divergent scenarios, it becomes particularly salient that we understand how consumers will engage with these new systems and services, and what will be the consequent economic, social and environmental impacts of their decisions. Over subsequent sections, this chapter introduces the technologies and services most likely to disrupt prevailing practices in the transport sector, namely shared mobility services, connected and autonomous vehicles, and electric vehicles. We review past studies that have examined current and future demand for these new technologies and services, and their likely short and long-term impacts on extant mobility patterns. We follow this discussion with a review of other potential disruptors to the transport sector that might emerge in the future, such as unmanned aerial vehicles, 3D printing and hyperloop transport. Finally, we conclude this chapter with a summary of what these new technologies and services might mean for the future of mobility.

5.2 Shared Mobility Services

A number of recent 'megatrends' are disrupting the provision of transport services worldwide and reshaping the broader mobility landscape (JPI Urban Europe 2017; Corwin et al. 2014). Major advances in information and communication technologies (ICTs) have created a digital economy, where new web-based services, such as e-commerce platforms, video messaging services, digital health services, online distance learning portals, etc., are changing the need and desire for travel (Cohen-Blankshtain and Rotem-Mindali 2016). Many of these same advances have conspired to result in the emergence of new forms of shared mobility services, as represented by short-term carshare services such as ZipCar and GoGet, rideshare services such as Uber and Lyft, and public bikesharing services such as Capital

Bikeshare and oBike, that are changing how consumers use the transportation system (Shaheen et al. 2017).

The rise of collaborative consumption and the growth in business and consumer interest in shared mobility services reflects a broader transition from an ownership-based economy to an access-based economy, particularly with regards to personal mobility (Belk 2014). For example, in Australia alone, a country with a total population of roughly 24 million, carshare services have 66,000 members and offer access to 2200 vehicles, rideshare services employ 72,000 active driver-partners and serve 3.3 million active ride seekers, and bikeshare services offer access to 7000 bicycles nationwide. However, consumer interest has in some cases lagged behind: in a 2018 survey of 3985 Australians nationwide, 12.4% reported using rideshare services a few times a month or more, but the corresponding numbers for carshare and bikeshare services were significantly lower at 5.6% and 4.7%, respectively (ITS Australia 2018).

The transition away from private car ownership has been aided by concurrent economic and demographic shifts. The turn of the twenty-first century has seen suggestions of "peak car" (Goodwin and Van Dender 2013), with stagnant or declining levels of private car use across much of the developed world, including Australia. For example, between 2001 and 2016, per capita vehicle kilometres travelled decreased by 6% nationally, and licensing rates for people under 25 dropped by more than 10% in Victoria and New South Wales. Studies have ascribed the apparent decline in private car dependence to a combination of economic factors, such as a recessionary global economy and rising oil prices, and demographic factors, such as an ageing population, rising higher education enrolment rates, an increase in the average age of entry into the labour market, and the decision to start a family at a later age (see, for example, Vij et al. 2017 and McDonald 2015).

Over subsequent sections, we review rideshare, carshare and public bikeshare services. We introduce formal definitions for each of these services; we review their current and expected future status across different global markets; and we review consumer preferences for these different services.

5.2.1 Rideshare Services

Ridesharing services refer to transportation network companies (TNCs) that use smartphone applications to match individuals wishing to make a trip from a specified origin to a specified destination with individuals willing to drive them there in their personal cars (Rayle et al. 2016). Like taxis, ridesharing services too offer point-to-point transportation. However, there are some key differences between the two: (1) individuals wishing to request or provide rides must register with the ridesharing service before they can use it; (2) rides are crowdsourced from a pool of available drivers that consists largely of part-timers, usually not licensed to drive commercial vehicles, looking to supplement their incomes from other jobs; (3) the ridesharing service employs location-based smartphone technology and data mining algorithms to reduce waiting times, increase reliability and adjust fares in real-time; (4) payments for each trip are processed online using billing information provided at the time of registration by the individuals requesting and providing the ride; and (5) after the trip, the individual who requested the ride can leave feedback about the individual who provided the ride, and this information is visible to other users of the service.

These differences independently may appear marginal at best, but together they have helped create a new paradigm for transportation. Uber, DiDi and Ola Cabs have emerged perhaps as the preeminent ridesharing services currently operating in the world: Uber offers ridesharing services in 633 cities worldwide; DiDi in 400 cities across China; and Ola Cabs in 110 cities in India. Both DiDi and Ola Cabs have plans for expansion into overseas markets, with the latter having recently launched in Australia. Traditional taxi and bus services are adopting some of the same service-based principles championed by ridesharing services. For example, ongoing on-demand public transport trials in Newcastle, New South Wales offer potential passengers the option of booking services through a smartphone app. Similarly, apps like GoCatch and InGoGo allow users to make taxi bookings through smartphone interfaces that are similar to those used by ridesharing services. Increasingly, the boundaries between ridesharing, taxis and public transport services are becoming less clear.

The competition between traditional taxi services and newer ridesharing services has prompted several academic enquiries. Most studies agree that ridesharing services have had the greatest impact on existing taxi services. For example, Pymynts (2016) finds that the annual number of taxi trips in Los Angeles declined from 8.4 million in 2013 to 6.0 million in 2015. Similarly, Hu (2017) reports that, "for the first time, more people are using Uber in New York than the city's fabled yellow cabs. In July [2017], Uber recorded an average of 289,000 rides each day compared with 277,000 taxi trips." Some studies have found that ridesharing services have also been used to substitute trips that would otherwise have been made using public transport services or privately-owned cars. For example, Rayle et al. (2016) find in their survey of 380 intercepted rideshare users in San Francisco that at least half of the ridesharing trips were replacing modes other than taxi, including public transport and driving.

By and large, studies have found that users of rideshare services tend to be young, well-educated, high-income, employed individuals, with low levels of car ownership, living in dense urban environments (e.g. Dias et al. 2017; Rayle et al. 2016). Studies that have examined consumer preferences for different rideshare service attributes are rarer in the literature. In their analysis of 3985 Australians nationwide, Vij et al. (2018) find that while consumers are willing to pay, on average, 0.28$/km more to avoid sharing a vehicle with other passengers and 0.17$/km more for door-to-door service, cost is the most important determinant of rideshare use. For a rideshare service that costs roughly the same as UberX's ridesharing service ($1.15 per km), and offers comparable level-of-service, the study predicts that 17% of the national population could be expected to use the service a few times a week or more.

However, if the same service could be provided at a much lower cost of $0.30 per km, through potential advances in electric, connected and autonomous vehicle technologies, a significantly larger 31% of the national population could be expected to use the service a few times a week or more.

5.2.2 Carshare Services

Carshare services are short-term car rental services that offer consumers access to a private car when and where they need one, without the costs associated with ownership or maintenance. While carsharing has existed in different forms since the earliest days of the automobile, it has only become widely available as a mode of transport since 2000, enabled in large part by the internet (for a comprehensive discussion on the origins of carsharing, the reader is referred to Shaheen and Cohen 2013).

Carshare services may offer access to cars through both peer to peer (P2P) and business to consumer (B2C) models. The P2P model matches individuals wishing to rent their privately-owned cars with individuals needing short-term access to one, with the sharing system operated by a third-party. The B2C model is similar to traditional car rental companies, where a single organization offers customers access to a fleet of vehicles owned by the organization itself at one or more stations, but differs in the following critical ways: (1) customers wishing to access cars must register with the carshare service, and in most cases they must also pay a monthly or yearly subscription cost to have access to the service; (2) vehicles may be rented by the minute, the hour or the day, depending on the service, and fuel costs are inclusive; (3) vehicles are typically distributed across the service area at popular points of departure, either at fixed stations or free floating within designated areas; and (4) customers can usually access and return cars any time of day, and they can track vehicles and make reservations in real time. Carshare service operators might offer roundtrip services, where customers must pick-up and drop-off cars at the same location, or one-way services, where customers may pick-up and drop-off cars at different locations.

The size of the global carsharing market was estimated to be USD 1.5 billion in 2017, and is expected to grow to USD 11 billion by 2024 (Global Market Insights, Inc. 2018). In North America alone, as of 2017, B2C carsharing services had roughly 1.9 million members and a combined fleet of 24,629 vehicles across 39 operators (Shaheen et al. 2018c), and P2P carsharing services had roughly 2.9 million participating individuals and a combined fleet of 131,336 vehicles across six operators (Shaheen et al. 2018a). Future growth is expected to be led by newly industrializing countries like China and India. The Chinese B2C carsharing market already has a combined fleet of 26,000 vehicles, and is projected to grow at 45% per annum until 2025 (Roland Berger 2018).

Notwithstanding this growth, profitability continues to be a concern globally, particularly for B2C carshare service operators with high capital and operating costs, and recent years have seen a number of carshare service operators withdraw from specific markets (e.g. Deschamps 2018; Jackson 2017). Many national and regional governments have offered support to carshare service operators to help them sustain operations locally. For example, most Chinese operators still "rely on government subsidies and are still not running profitable and sustainable business models" (Roland Berger 2018). In Australia, support from regional and local governments has been lacking in many cases, and some have blamed this limited support for low use (Phillip Boyle & Associates 2016).

Carshare members tend to be young and highly educated, frequently university students or white-collar professionals, and often part of moderate-income non-traditional households (see, for example, Becker et al. 2017a, b; Efthymiou and Antoniou 2016; Schmöller et al. 2015; Cervero et al. 2007). Additionally, carshare members are likely to have low levels of car ownership and high levels of public transport patronage, leading studies to conclude that carsharing services act as substitutes to private car ownership and complements to public transport. For example, in a survey of 6281 carshare members in North America, Martin et al. (2010) find that 25% of their sample reduced their level of car ownership after membership, and an additional 25% postponed their decision to purchase a car. Based on further analysis, the study concludes that a single shared car has the capacity to replace between 9 and 13 privately owned cars, and a more recent Australian study corroborates this finding (AECOM 2016). In their analysis of carshare users in Toronto, Canada, Costain et al. (2012) find that carsharing is most often used for off-peak period travel or on weekends, when public transport service is poor. Their findings are echoed by similar studies conducted in Switzerland (Becker et al. 2017a), Italy (De Luca and Di Pace 2015) and the United States (Zoepf and Keith 2016) that find carsharing services are often used by customers to plug gaps in existing public transport services.

In terms of service attributes, one-way services are found to be more popular than round-trip services, often by a factor of three to four (see, for example, Schmöller et al. 2015 and Le Vine et al. 2014). Carsharing costs, and how they compare with alternative modes of travel, are found to be strong determinants of use, as evidenced by findings from North America (Burkhardt and Millard-Ball 2006), Europe (De Luca and Di Pace 2015) and Asia (Yoon et al. 2017). Guaranteed access to a vehicle is found to have a strong positive effect on membership (Kim et al. 2017), and the number of vehicles in the carshare service network is found to increase frequency of use (Habib et al. 2012). Surprisingly, most studies do not find access distance to carshare vehicles to be a significant determinant of carshare use (Yoon et al. 2017), and "that customers are willing to accept a substantially longer access walk to the car-sharing vehicle than for public transportation" (Becker et al. 2017b). Similarly, in their analysis of members of a North American carshare service, Zoepf and Keith (2016) find that customers are willing to pay only USD 2 per hour more in terms of rental costs to reduce access distance by one mile. However, most of these studies surveyed existing carshare users, and it is very likely that individuals who currently do not use carshare services have very different preferences.

5.2.3 Bikeshare Services

Bikeshare services are bike rental companies that offer customers short-term access to bicycles. While bikeshare services have been around since the 1960s, like other shared mobility services, their popularity too has really surged in the last decade due to advances in ICTs. For a recent comprehensive review of the academic literature on bikeshare programs across the world, the reader is referred to Fishman (2016).

In terms of service design, bikeshare services share many features with carsharing services: (1) customers wishing to access bicycles must register with the service, and in some cases monthly or yearly subscription costs and initial registration fees might apply; (2) bicycles may be rented by the minute, the hour or the day, depending on the service; (3) bicycles are typically distributed across the service area at popular points of departure, either at fixed stations, often referred to as 'docks', or fully free floating, resulting in the more recent model of dockless bikeshare services; and (4) customers can usually access and return bicycles any time of day, and they can track available bicycles and make reservations in real time.

The number of cities with bikeshare services has grown to over 2000, and most major metropolitan regions in the world currently have one or more bikeshare services in operation (Meddin and DeMaio 2018). The number of bicycles available through these services worldwide has increased commensurately, from 700,000 in 2013 to 2.3 million in 2016 (Bernard 2018). However, again like carsharing services, profitability continues to be a concern, and many bikeshare service operators have been compelled in recent months to close operations (Tchebotarev 2017). In many cities, the public sector has actively supported bikeshare services, either by taking on the role of service provider through government-run operations, or more frequently, through public-private partnerships.

Greater public sector involvement has typically been motivated through the benefits that increased bicycling can offer, in terms of its impacts on car use and traffic congestion on one hand, and population health outcomes on the other (Fishman 2016). For example, in their analysis of bikeshare programs across five cities in Australia, Europe and the US, Fishman et al. (2014b) find that the programs reduced car use in four of the five cities. However, their analysis also finds that bikeshare services are more frequently used to substitute public transport and walking, than they are to substitute driving, and their finding is supported by other studies as well (e.g. Zhu et al. 2013). In terms of impacts on health and physical activity, in their analysis of bikeshare users in London, Woodcock et al. (2014) find that mean physical activity increased by an average of 0.06 MET hours (or 0.06 kcal per kg in bodyweight) per week per person as a result of joining the bikeshare service. As the authors argue, "although this is small on average at the individual level, it led to notable modelled gains in health at population level."

Bikeshare users tend to have higher incomes (Fishman et al. 2015; Woodcock et al. 2014), are more educated (Fishman et al. 2014a; LDA Consulting 2013; Shaheen et al. 2013), and more likely to be employed (Woodcock et al. 2014). Some studies have also reported gender and racial differences between bikeshare users and general populations, with bikeshare users being more likely to be male and white (Fishman et al. 2014a, b; Goodman and Cheshire 2014; Buck et al. 2013).

Barriers to greater use of bikeshare services centre primarily around concerns for safety, and relatedly, mandatory helmet laws, though some studies have also highlighted lengthy registration processes as additional impediments (Fishman 2016). Despite these concerns, there is no clear agreement on the impacts of bikeshare services on road safety and traffic accidents. For example, in their analysis of hospital injury data from five US cities with bikeshare services and five without, over a 3 year period that extended 2 years before the service first started and 1 year after, Graves et al. (2014) find that the proportion of head injuries among bicycle-related injuries increased in cities with bikeshare services, from 42% before the service to 50% after, leading the authors to conclude that "steps should be taken to make helmets available with PBSPs [public bicycle share programs]." However, Cowling (2014) and Salomon et al. (2014) have contested the validity of these conclusions. Based on their own analysis of the same data, the two studies find that annual *total* bicycle injury rates decreased by 28% in the cities with bikeshare services (despite the increase in the *proportion* of head injuries), leading them to conclude "that overall bike safety improves with PBSPs, possibly because of increased driver awareness or improved biking infrastructure" (Cowling 2014).

5.3 Connected and Autonomous Vehicles

Connected vehicles are vehicles that use ICTs to communicate with the driver, other road users, roadside infrastructure and other wireless services. Autonomous vehicles are vehicles where one or more primary driving controls, such as steering, acceleration and braking, do not require human input for sustained periods of time. Together, connected and autonomous vehicles (CAVs) have the capacity to offer a number of social benefits that include increased road safety, higher traffic flows, greater travel time productivity, improved energy efficiency, greater accessibility, etc. The technology is currently being trialled all across the world, including Australia, both on public roads and more controlled, 'closed-loop' conditions, such as university campuses and retirement villages. The first commercially available fully autonomous car is expected to be available by 2020.

Many of these CAV technologies will likely be offered to potential consumers as both products and services. For example, car companies such as Tesla and Ford are planning to integrate automated features within existing car models. Concurrently, carsharing and ridesharing companies such as Uber are investing in these technologies with the intention of integrating them within existing services. It is anticipated that CAV technologies will enable on-demand door-to-door transport services as a new form of micro public transport, which combines the benefits of existing mass public transport services and private modes of motorized transport, but does not suffer from the same drawbacks (Wong et al. 2017). Compared to mass public transport services that require large catchment areas in order to be feasible, and consequently suffer from first and last mile connectivity problems, micro public transport can offer door-to-door services. Compared to private modes of motorized transport, where high parking costs and frequent congestion can limit access and use, micro public transport is expected to be cheaper, faster and more convenient. Therefore, any analysis of the potential impacts of CAVs must necessarily account for ongoing and future competition between ownership-based and sharing-based models of mobility.

Numerous studies have sought to understand public perceptions of CAVs (Menon et al. 2016; Duncan et al. 2015; Kyriakidis et al. 2015; Payre et al. 2014; Rodel et al. 2014; Schoettle and Sivak 2014; Casley et al. 2013; Howard and Dai 2014). Commonly identified perceived benefits include greater safety, better fuel economy, and more productive use of travel time. And commonly identified concerns include equipment and system failure, cyber security, data privacy, legal liability in case of crash, and loss of control.

From an ownership standpoint, on average, studies find that consumers are willing to pay roughly $3000 for partial automation, and roughly $5000–$7500 for complete automation (e.g. Daziano et al. 2017; Bansal et al. 2016). However, as mentioned previously, shared CAVs could erode current consumer willingness to pay for private CAV ownership. While private ownership will still likely appeal to niche segments, such as families with young children, tradespeople with heavy equipment, etc., shared CAVs could help a significant proportion of the general population transition from owning two cars to one car, and potentially even to no cars. On average, privately owned cars are not in use 95% of the time (Shoup 2017). With automation, it can be expected that many of these cars will likely be available for short-term rental through P2P carshare services, further diminishing the need for private ownership.

Consequently, traditional car manufacturers are looking to replace potential revenue lost because of reduced car sales by taking on the role of transport service providers themselves. For example, BMW already operates carsharing services in North America and Europe, and General Motors plans to commence its own rideshare services in 2019 using self-driving cars developed in house. Simultaneously, existing shared mobility service providers such as Uber, in addition to investing heavily in the development of CAV technology, are continuing to subsidize their current services, with a long-term view towards holding on to their present advantage within the point-to-point transport market.

In light of these developments, several studies in recent years have examined the latent demand for shared CAV services. Krueger et al. (2016), in their survey of 435 Australians nationwide, find that service attributes such as travel time, waiting time and fares will be significant determinants of consumer adoption of shared CAV services, and young travellers will likely be the early adopters. Bansal et al. (2016), in their survey of 347 residents of Austin, Texas in the United States, find that only 13% of survey participants would be willing to give up personal vehicles and rely exclusively on shared CAVs that cost roughly $1/mile, and at least 35% of survey participants would be unwilling to use shared CAV services at all, regardless of their costs. Haboucha et al. (2017), in their survey of 721 individuals living across Israel and North America, find that consumers are still hesitant to embrace CAV technology, and that even if shared CAV services were completely free, 25% of their sample would still be unwilling to use the service. Hao and Yamamoto (2017), in their case study on Meito Ward, Nagoya in Japan, predict that up to 30% of total trips conducted in the region could be served by shared CAVs in the future.

Given both the uncertainty that still surrounds CAVs (in terms of the technology itself, the supporting infrastructure, and the regulatory framework) and consumer unfamiliarity (consumer surveys have repeatedly found that significant proportions of the general population are unfamiliar with CAV technology and how it will likely function; see, for example, Schoettle and Sivak 2014), any research on the potential demand for private CAV ownership and shared CAV use has had to be, by necessity, somewhat speculative. Predicted adoption rates from these studies will likely change as the technology matures and as consumers become more familiar with corresponding services.

5.4 Electric Vehicles

Electric vehicles (EVs) have existed for more than a hundred years, and were among the earliest cars available to the general public. In 1900, prior to the emergence and subsequent dominance of internal combustion engines, EVs comprised roughly one-third of the American car fleet (DoE 2014). Rising oil prices and climate change concerns have fuelled a twenty-first century resurgence. It began with the introduction of Toyota Prius in 1997, a hybrid electric vehicle (HEV) that has an electric drive system and battery, but cannot be plugged in to the electric grid. This was followed by the creation of Tesla Motors in 2003 with the explicit objective of accelerating consumer adoption of EVs. Tesla's creation spurred other car manufacturers to develop their own EVs. In 2010, General Motors launched the Chevrolet Volt, a plug-in hybrid electric vehicle (PHEV) which, like HEVs, has a gasoline engine that supplements its electric drive once the battery is depleted, but unlike HEVs, can be plugged in to the electric grid to recharge the battery. That same year, Nissan launched its Leaf model, a battery electric vehicle (BEV) that is all-electric, does not depend on petrol and produces no tailpipe emissions. Two years later, in 2012, Tesla launched its Model S, also a BEV. Today, there are 35 PHEV and 36 BEV models available on the global market.

Notwithstanding this interest from industry in the production of EVs, consumer demand has been slower to catch up. High costs, low driving ranges, long charging times and limited public charging infrastructure continue to be major impediments to adoption, though most experts agree that the electrification of our transport infrastructure is not a question of if, but when (for a comprehensive recent review of consumer preferences for EVs, the reader is referred to Liao et al. 2017). In 2017, BEVs and PHEVs comprised only 1.7% of total passenger car sales worldwide. However, while total sales remain low, year-on-year growth has averaged 30–40% in the last 5 years, and this rate of growth is expected to continue over coming years (Scutt 2018).

The growth in EV sales has been led by burgeoning demand in China and parts of Europe. In both cases, government support has been essential to stimulating and sustaining consumer demand. In the case of China, government support has been motivated in terms of industrial development. The Chinese government has taken an active interest in positioning China at the forefront of EV research and development activities, and a large local market could help Chinese car manufacturers progress along the global value chain. The Chinese government wants EVs to account for 12% of total car sales by 2020, compared to 3.7% in 2017 (Lee 2018). In its attempt to achieve this ambitious target, the government has been offering subsidies to EV buyers of up to 110,000 yuan (or USD 16,000) per unit. To promote local development of EVs with higher driving ranges, subsidies have been set to be higher for EVs with greater driving ranges (Dixon 2018). Additionally, the government plans to have 500,000 public charging stations nationwide by 2020, up from roughly 200,000 at the end of 2017 (Fusheng 2018), to further support consumer adoption.

In the case of more developed European nations, government support has been motivated by concerns around climate change and oil dependence. Norway in particular has led the way in consumer adoption. The country has the highest market penetration per capita in the world, with roughly 5% of all vehicles on Norwegian roads being PHEVs or BEVs (Manthey 2018), EVs comprised a remarkably high 39% of total car sales in 2017 (Knudsen and Doyle 2018). Local adoption has been helped by high fuel prices, cheap electricity, and most significantly, generous government incentives. Until 2017, EVs were exempt from "value added tax and purchase tax, which on average in Norway add 50% to the cost of a vehicle. They are also exempt from road tolls, tunnel-use charges, and ferry charges. And they get free parking, free charging, and the freedom to use bus lanes" (Mirani 2015). However, national and local governments have indicated that some of this support will be withdrawn over coming years, as the market has matured and subsidies and incentives are no longer deemed necessary to sustain further growth (Nelson 2017).

5.5 Other Potential Disruptions to the Transport Sector

The coming years could see additional disruptions in the form of unmanned aerial vehicles (UAVs), 3D printing, and hyperloop transport. Most of these technologies are still in their research and development phase, with few, if any, commercial applications to date.

UAVs, or drones, are perhaps the most developed of these new technologies. Large drones could potentially displace existing long-distance air, rail and freight shipping industries. Companies like Natilus plan to start testing drones with capacities of up to 100 tons by 2020. Commercialization is still likely at least 5–10 years away, but if and when the technology is market ready, it could reduce long-haul shipping costs by as much as half (Terdiman 2017). Smaller drones could similarly displace urban delivery services. Several companies working in the space of logistics, retail and food, such as United Parcel Service (UPS), Amazon and Domino's, are currently testing drone delivery systems. Regulators and policy-makers in North America and Europe are reacting to these developments accordingly. For example, the Federal Aviation Authority (FAA) in the United States recently launched its Unmanned Aircraft System (UAS) Integration Pilot Program (IPP) as "an opportunity for state, local, and tribal governments to partner with private sector entities, such as UAS operators or manufacturers, to accelerate safe UAS integration". Studies that have examined public perceptions of drones report that privacy and security concerns will likely be major barriers to consumer adoption (see, for example, Chang et al. 2017).

3D printers have become increasingly commercially available in the last decade, but mainstream adoption is yet to happen. Unlike current manufacturing processes that rely on high production volumes to achieve optimal economies of scale, 3D printers could potentially usher in a more distributed and small-scale approach to manufacturing. As Lim and Nair (2017) write, "The advent of 3D printing opens the way for manufacturers to significantly reduce the production cost of their goods by eliminating many steps in the manufacturing process, such as casting and welding metal. It also reduces the complete production process to no more than three to four key players. With 3D printing, what would have initially been a series of stages of production could be cut down to a designer at one end, and the printer or "manufacturer" at the other. The middle players would most likely be suppliers of raw materials or 'ink'… Such reductions in the manufacturing process could affect both regional and international production networks, possibly resulting in reduced capital requirements, warehousing and other logistics and transportation needs." In essence, 3D printing could shorten supply chains by allowing goods to be manufactured closer to the end consumer, and therefore, reduce delivery distances of products (Shaheen et al. 2018b).

A hyperloop is a sealed tube or system of tubes through which a pod may travel free of air resistance or friction conveying people or objects at high speed (Musk 2013). Hyperloop transport could do for long-distance inter-city travel what CAVs promise to do for short-distance urban and regional travel. For example, Musk's original paper conceives "a hyperloop system that would propel passengers along the 350-mile (560 km) route at a speed of 760 mph (1,200 km/h), allowing for a travel time of 35 min, which is considerably faster than current rail or air travel times". However, most experts express scepticism about the technology and its purported potential (see, for example, Taylor et al. 2016), and in the absence of real-world implementations, it is hard to anticipate what impacts, if any, the technology might portend for the future of mobility.

5.6 Preparing for the Future of Mobility

The future of passenger transport is predicted to be electric, autonomous, and increasingly shared (Firnkorn and Müller 2015). Each of these changes by themselves would be potentially disruptive; together they are expected to be transformative, with far-reaching economic, social and environmental ramifications. For example, a 2015 report by the Committee for Economic Development of Australia (CEDA) on Australia's future workforce estimated that 3.28 million Australians employed nationally had jobs that involved driving. "If we assume that over the next 20 years all vehicles become autonomous, these job categories will need to change into something completely different as the human skill of driving a vehicle is no longer the essential part of the job" (CEDA 2015). Electric vehicles could lead to significant reductions in oil consumption and GHG emissions, contributing to the creation of a more sustainable transport system. However, they will require significantly more energy than the electricity grid can currently provide, and provision of appropriate public charging infrastructure to support consumer adoption. Shared mobility services have already been credited with reduced private car ownership and use in some parts of the developed world (Martin et al. 2010). In conjunction with CAVs, they could help accelerate an ongoing transition from two-car households to one-car households, and potentially even to zero-car households, for at least a subset of the population. However, they could also potentially increase net vehicle kilometres travelled, due to greater suburbanization as enabled by reduced travel costs.

If as engineers, planners and policy-makers, we are to influence the process to produce societally optimal outcomes, we must better comprehend the determinants of individual behaviour. In the past, both industry and government have failed to anticipate the rate and scale of change with regards to similarly new technologies and services. For example, the rapid diffusion of rideshare services such as Uber in Australia has caught both taxi providers and transport planners by surprise. State governments have been forced to introduce expensive bailouts to keep local taxi industries afloat and compensate taxi plate owners for their losses. Legislation has had to be amended to allow rideshare companies like Uber to operate legally, following pressure from consumer advocacy groups. New regulations are under review to address concerns around unfair employment practices, inadequate insurance coverage, and lax security measures with regards to the provision of these services. Some of this disruption could have been avoided had the public and private sectors been appropriately prepared.

The impacts of connected, autonomous and electric vehicles, and the accompanying disruption, will only be greater, but we seem to be making the same mistakes. Consider, for example, the ongoing Sydney light rail (SLR) project. Initial plans were announced in 2011 – as a way to connect Sydney's eastern suburbs with the urban centre. The service will commence operation in 2019, and is projected to transport 5,300 inbound and 4,100 outbound passengers per hour during the morning peak period by 2021 (TfNSW 2013; pp. 9–36). However, these projections do not account for shared CAVs which could emerge in the near future as a feasible new form of public transport. From an engineering standpoint, the SLR might be the most efficient means of transport in terms of throughput (i.e. number of passengers moved through a corridor). However, from a consumer standpoint, mass public transport services like the SLR require large catchment areas in order to be feasible, and consequently suffer from first and last mile connectivity problems. In contrast, shared CAVs could enable on-demand door-to-door public transport services that are likely to be much more attractive to customers. The SLR business case does not account for potential loss in demand due to these new technologies and services (TfNSW 2013), which could seriously undermine the project's long-term economic viability and profitability, and render the project obsolete well in advance of planned end-life dates.

The case of ridesharing serves as an excellent example for why we need better tools for understanding consumer response to new transport technologies and services; modelling and forecasting their consequent impacts; and identifying ways in which industry and government can best prepare themselves for these imminent transformations, in an attempt to produce outcomes that are economically efficient, socially equitable and environmentally sustainable.

References

AECOM. (2016). Transport on demand: Accelerating Australian cities. *An AECOM Brilliant Cities Report.*

Bansal, P., Kockelman, K. M., & Singh, A. (2016). Assessing public opinions of and interest in new vehicle technologies: An Austin perspective. *Transportation Research Part C: Emerging Technologies, 67*, 1–14.

Becker, H., Ciari, F., & Axhausen, K. W. (2017a). Comparing car-sharing schemes in Switzerland: User groups and usage patterns. *Transportation Research Part A: Policy and Practice, 97*, 17–29.

Becker, H., Ciari, F., & Axhausen, K. W. (2017b). Modeling free-floating car-sharing use in Switzerland: A spatial regression and conditional logit approach. *Transportation Research Part C: Emerging Technologies, 81*, 286–299.

Belk, R. (2014). You are what you can access: Sharing and collaborative consumption online. *Journal of Business Research, 67*(8), 1595–1600.

Bernard, Z. (2018). The bike-sharing economy is shaking up the transportation market worldwide. *Business Insider Australia*, published April 13, 2018.

Buck, D., Buehler, R., Happ, P., Rawls, B., Chung, P., & Borecki, N. (2013). Are bikeshare users different from regular cyclists? A first look at short-term users, annual members, and area cyclists in the Washington, DC, region. *Transportation Research Record: Journal of the Transportation Research Board, 2387*, 112–119.

Burkhardt, J., & Millard-Ball, A. (2006). Who is attracted to carsharing? *Transportation Research Record: Journal of the Transportation Research Board, 1986*, 98–105.

Casley, S., Jardim, A., & Quartulli, A. (2013). A study of public acceptance of autonomous cars. *Worcester Polytechnic Institute.*

CEDA (Committee for Economic Development of Australia). (2015). *Australia's future workforce?* July 2015.

Cervero, R., Golub, A., & Nee, B. (2007). City CarShare: Longer-term travel demand and car ownership impacts. *Transportation Research Record: Journal of the Transportation Research Board, 1992*, 70–80.

Chang, V., Chundury, P., & Chetty, M. (2017, May). Spiders in the sky: User perceptions of drones, privacy, and security. In *Proceedings of the 2017 CHI conference on human factors in computing systems* (pp. 6765–6776). ACM.

Cohen-Blankshtain, G., & Rotem-Mindali, O. (2016). Key research themes on ICT and sustainable urban mobility. *International Journal of Sustainable Transportation, 10*(1), 9–17.

Cortright, J. (2016). *The price of autonomous cars: Why it matters.* Retrieved from http://cityobservatory.org/price-of-autonomous-cars/

Costain, C., Ardron, C., & Habib, K. N. (2012). Synopsis of users' behaviour of a carsharing program: A case study in Toronto. *Transportation Research Part A: Policy and Practice, 46*(3), 421–434.

Corwin, S., Vitale, J., Kelly, E., & Cathles, E. (2014). The future of mobility: How transportation technology and social trends are creating a new business ecosystem. *Deloitte*.

Cowling, K. (2014). Net effects of bicycle share programs on bike safety. *American Journal of Public Health, 104*(11), E6.

Daziano, R. A., Sarrias, M., & Leard, B. (2017). Are consumers willing to pay to let cars drive for them? Analyzing response to autonomous vehicles. *Transportation Research Part C: Emerging Technologies, 78*, 150–164.

De Luca, S., & Di Pace, R. (2015). Modelling users' behaviour in inter-urban carsharing program: A stated preference approach. *Transportation Research Part A: Policy and Practice, 71*, 59–76.

Deschamps, T. (2018). Car2Go to shutter Toronto operations; service presents different parking issues in Vancouver. *The Canadian Press*, published May 24, 2018.

Dias, F. F., Lavieri, P. S., Garikapati, V. M., Astroza, S., Pendyala, R. M., & Bhat, C. R. (2017). A behavioral choice model of the use of car-sharing and ride-sourcing services. *Transportation, 44*(6), 1307–1323.

Dixon, T. (2018). *Chinese electric vehicle subsidy changes in 2018 — The details. EV Obsession*, published January 6, 2018.

DoE (Department of Energy). (2014). *The history of the electric car*. Retrieved from https://www.energy.gov/articles/history-electric-car

Duncan, M., Charness, N., Chapin, T., Horner, M., Stevens, L., Richard, A., Souders, D., Crute, J., Riemondy, A., & Morgan, D., 2015. *Enhanced mobility for aging populations using automated vehicles* (No. 035048).

Efthymiou, D., & Antoniou, C. (2016). Modeling the propensity to join carsharing using hybrid choice models and mixed survey data. *Transport Policy, 51*, 143–149.

Firnkorn, J., & Müller, M. (2015). Free-floating electric carsharing-fleets in smart cities: The dawning of a post-private car era in urban environments? *Environmental Science & Policy, 45*, 30–40.

Fishman, E. (2016). Bikeshare: A review of recent literature. *Transport Reviews, 36*(1), 92–113.

Fishman, E., Washington, S., Haworth, N., & Mazzei, A. (2014a). Barriers to bikesharing: An analysis from Melbourne and Brisbane. *Journal of Transport Geography, 41*, 325–337.

Fishman, E., Washington, S., & Haworth, N. (2014b). Bike share's impact on car use: Evidence from the United States, Great Britain, and Australia. *Transportation Research Part D: Transport and Environment, 31*, 13–20.

Fishman, E., Washington, S., Haworth, N., & Watson, A. (2015). Factors influencing bike share membership: An analysis of Melbourne and Brisbane. *Transportation Research Part A: Policy and Practice, 71*, 17–30.

Fusheng, L. (2018). China has the most public EV charging stations worldwide. *China Daily*, published January 11, 2018.

Global Market Insights, Inc. (2018). *Car sharing market trends – Global 2018-24 industry size report*.

Goodman, A., & Cheshire, J. (2014). Inequalities in the London bicycle sharing system revisited: Impacts of extending the scheme to poorer areas but then doubling prices. *Journal of Transport Geography, 41*, 272–279.

Goodwin, P., & Van Dender, K. (2013). 'Peak car'—Themes and issues. *Transport Reviews, 33*(3), 243–254.

Graves, J. M., Pless, B., Moore, L., Nathens, A. B., Hunte, G., & Rivara, F. P. (2014). Public bicycle share programs and head injuries. *American Journal of Public Health, 104*(8), e106–e111.

Habib, K. M. N., Morency, C., Islam, M. T., & Grasset, V. (2012). Modelling users' behaviour of a carsharing program: Application of a joint hazard and zero inflated dynamic ordered probability model. *Transportation Research Part A: Policy and Practice, 46*(2), 241–254.

Haboucha, C. J., Ishaq, R., & Shiftan, Y. (2017). User preferences regarding autonomous vehicles. *Transportation Research Part C: Emerging Technologies, 78*, 37–49.

Hao, M., & Yamamoto, T. (2017, October). Analysis on supply and demand of shared autonomous vehicles considering household vehicle ownership and shared use. In *Intelligent transportation systems (ITSC), 2017 IEEE 20th international conference on* (pp. 185–190). IEEE.

Howard, D., & Dai, D. (2014). Public perceptions of self-driving cars: The case of Berkeley, California. In *Transportation research board 93rd annual meeting* (No. 14–4502).

Hu, W. (2017). Uber, surging outside Manhattan, tops Taxis in New York City. *The New York Times*, published October 12, 2017.

ITS Australia. (2018). *Mobility as a Service in Australia: Customer insights and opportunities.*

Jackson, C. V. (2017). Enterprise CarShare is officially pulling out of most Chicago locations. *Chicago Tribune*, published June 28, 2017.

JPI Urban Europe. (2017). Stimulating a transition to sustainable urban mobility.

Kim, J., Rasouli, S., & Timmermans, H. (2017). Satisfaction and uncertainty in car-sharing decisions: An integration of hybrid choice and random regret-based models. *Transportation Research Part A: Policy and Practice, 95*, 13–33.

Knudsen, C., & Doyle, A. (2018). Norway powers ahead (electrically): Over half new car sales now electric or hybrid. *Reuters*, published January 3, 2018.

Krueger, R., Rashidi, T. H., & Rose, J. M. (2016). Preferences for shared autonomous vehicles. *Transportation Research Part C: Emerging Technologies, 69*, 343–355.

Kyriakidis, M., Happee, R., & De Winter, J. C. F. (2015). Public opinion on automated driving: Results of an international questionnaire among 5000 respondents. *Transportation Research Part F: Traffic Psychology and Behaviour, 32*, 127–140.

LDA Consulting. (2013). *2013 capital bikeshare member survey report*. Washington, DC: Commissioned by Capital Bikeshare.

Le Vine, S., Lee-Gosselin, M., Sivakumar, A., & Polak, J. (2014). A new approach to predict the market and impacts of round-trip and point-to-point carsharing systems: Case study of London. *Transportation Research Part D: Transport and Environment, 32*, 218–229.

Lee, A. (2018). China's electric car market is growing twice as fast as the US: Here's why. *South China Morning Post*, published April 27, 2018.

Liao, F., Molin, E., & van Wee, B. (2017). Consumer preferences for electric vehicles: A literature review. *Transport Reviews, 37*(3), 252–275.

Lim, C. H., & Nair, T. (2017). How 3D printing could disrupt Asia's manufacturing economies. *The Conversation*, published January 10, 2017.

Manthey, N. (2018). Norway's EV share at over 5 percent and rising. *Electrive*, published March 26, 2018.

Martin, E., Shaheen, S., & Lidicker, J. (2010). Impact of carsharing on household vehicle holdings: Results from north American shared-use vehicle survey. *Transportation Research Record: Journal of the Transportation Research Board, 2143*, 150–158.

McDonald, N. C. (2015). Are millennials really the "go-nowhere" generation? *Journal of the American Planning Association, 81*(2), 90–103.

Meddin, R., & DeMaio, P. (2018). *The bike-sharing world map*. Retrieved January 26, 2014, from http://www.bikesharingworld.com

Menon, N., Pinjari, A. R., Zhang, Y., & Zou, L. (2016). Consumer perception and intended adoption of autonomous-vehicle technology: Findings from a university population survey. In *Transportation research board 95th annual meeting* (No. 16–5998).

Mirani, L. (2015). Norway's electric-car incentives were so good they had to be stopped. *Quartz*, published May 7, 2015.

Musk, E. (2013). Hyperloop alpha. *SpaceX*.

Nelson, E. (2017). Norway is planning to pull the plug on its wildly successful electric-car incentives. *Quartz*, published October 13, 2017.

Payre, W., Cestac, J., & Delhomme, P. (2014). Intention to use a fully automated car: Attitudes and a priori acceptability. *Transportation Research Part F: Traffic Psychology and Behaviour, 27*, 252–263.

Phillip Boyle & Associates. (2016). The impact of car share services in Australia. *International Car sharing association.*

Pymynts. (2016). *Ride-sharing Kills LA's Taxi Industry*. 18 April 2018.

Rayle, L., Dai, D., Chan, N., Cervero, R., & Shaheen, S. (2016). Just a better taxi? A survey-based comparison of taxis, transit, and ridesourcing services in San Francisco. *Transport Policy, 45*, 168–178.

Rödel, C., Stadler, S., Meschtscherjakov, A., & Tscheligi, M. (2014, September). Towards autonomous cars: The effect of autonomy levels on acceptance and user experience. In *Proceedings of the 6th international conference on automotive user interfaces and interactive vehicular applications* (pp. 1–8). ACM.

Roland Berger. (2018). *Car-sharing in China: How to operate a successful business.*

Salomon, A., Kimbrough, G., & Bershteyn, A. (2014). The safety of public bicycle share programs in North America. *American Journal of Public Health, 104*(11), E4.

Schmöller, S., Weikl, S., Müller, J., & Bogenberger, K. (2015). Empirical analysis of free-floating carsharing usage: The Munich and Berlin case. *Transportation Research Part C: Emerging Technologies, 56*, 34–51.

Schoettle, B., & Sivak, M. (2014). *A survey of public opinion about autonomous and self-driving vehicles in the US, the UK, and Australia* (No. UMTRI-2014-21).

Scutt, D. (2018). Global electric vehicle sales are booming. *Business Insider Australia*, published January 22, 2018.

Shaheen, S. A., & Cohen, A. P. (2013). Carsharing and personal vehicle services: Worldwide market developments and emerging trends. *International Journal of Sustainable Transportation, 7*(1), 5–34.

Shaheen, S., Cohen, A., & Martin, E. (2013). Public bikesharing in North America: Early operator understanding and emerging trends. *Transportation Research Record: Journal of the Transportation Research Board, 2387*, 83–92.

Shaheen, S., Cohen, A., & Zohdy, I. (2017). Shared mobility resources: Helping to understand emerging shifts in transportation. *Policy Briefs, 2017*(18).

Shaheen, S., Martin, E., & Bansal, A. (2018a). *Peer-To-Peer (P2P) carsharing: Understanding early markets, social dynamics, and behavioral impacts.*

Shaheen, S., Totte, H., & Stocker, A. (2018b). *Future of mobility white paper.*

Shaheen, S., Cohen, A., & Jaffee, M. (2018c). *Innovative mobility: Carsharing outlook.* eScholarship, University of California.

Shoup, D. (2017). *The high cost of free parking: Updated edition.* Routledge.

Taylor, C. L., Hyde, D. J., & Barr, L. C. (2016). *Hyperloop commercial feasibility analysis: High level overview* (No. DOT-VNTSC-NASA-16-01). John A. Volpe National Transportation Systems Center (US).

Tchebotarev, E. (2017). With hundreds of millions of dollars burned, the dockless bike sharing market is imploding. *Forbes*, published December 16, 2017.

Terdiman, D. (2017). A Startup's plan to cut air freight costs in half with 777-size drones. *Fast Company*, published March 27, 2017.

TfNSW (Transport for New South Wales). (2013). CBD and south east light rail project: Environmental impact statement.

Vij, A., Gorripaty, S., & Walker, J. L. (2017). From trend spotting to trend'splaining: Understanding modal preference shifts in the San Francisco Bay Area. *Transportation Research Part A: Policy and Practice, 95*, 238–258.

Vij, A., Ryan, S., Sampson, S., & Harris, S. (2018). *The Australian market for on-demand transport.*

Wong, Y. Z., Hensher, D. A., & Mulley, C. (2017). *Emerging transport technologies and the modal efficiency framework: A case for mobility as a service (MaaS).*

Woodcock, J., Tainio, M., Cheshire, J., O'Brien, O., & Goodman, A. (2014). Health effects of the London bicycle sharing system: Health impact modelling study. *BMJ, 348*, g425.

Yoon, T., Cherry, C. R., & Jones, L. R. (2017). One-way and round-trip carsharing: A stated preference experiment in Beijing. *Transportation Research Part D: Transport and Environment, 53*, 102–114.

Zhu, W., Pang, Y., Wang, D., & Timmermans, H. (2013). *Travel behavior change after the introduction of public bicycle systems: Case study in Minhang District, Shanghai* (No. 13-0764).

Zoepf, S. M., & Keith, D. R. (2016). User decision-making and technology choices in the US carsharing market. *Transport Policy, 51*, 150–157.

Chapter 6
Smart Interactive Cities [SICs]: The Use of Computational Tools and Technologies [CTTs] as a Systemic Approach to Reduce Water and Energy Consumption in Urban Areas

Fodil Fadli and Mahmoud AlSaeed

Abstract The traditional thinking of cities as the compilation of their land, buildings and, infrastructure is no longer accurate to study their foundation components. Conventional urban planning is not sufficient anymore to solve city related issues. Moreover, there is an important need to integrate technology through its smart computational systems, to the City Information Modeling [CIM] concepts in order to solve those everlasting re-occurring issues. The design and development of a systemic approach in urban design processes is a necessity to face the various threats to our current and future world. Some of these major threats strongly tied up to reducing water and energy consumption rates, as well as designing and developing a smart interactive city that can maintain and sustain itself. Most importantly, this Smart Interactive C City [SIC] would also strengthen the connections between humans, machines and spaces.

The aim of this explorative innovative work is to enable us as designers, architects and planners, to design and develop our cities in a smart way. Cities will become a digital platform with infinite data floating in and out of their physical and metaphysical structures. This information comes from every element we use and we live with. These data need to be collected in one place that is accessible and usable by all users and stakeholders to enable the resolution of predicting future scenarios and managing existing issues. This can be enabled via the use and integration of the principles of City Information Modelling [CIM] and Computational Tools and Technologies [CTTs].

Keywords Smart city · City Information Modelling [CIM] · Computational systems · Urban design · Technology · Energy & water consumption reduction

F. Fadli (✉) · M. AlSaeed
Department of Architecture and Urban Planning, College of Engineering, Qatar University, Doha, Qatar
e-mail: f.fadli@qu.edu.qa; ma1604309@student.qu.edu.qa

N. Biloria (ed.), *Data-driven Multivalence in the Built Environment*, S.M.A.R.T. Environments, https://doi.org/10.1007/978-3-030-12180-8_6

6.1 Introduction

The powerful attractions of cities had driven 54.5% of the world's population to live in urbanized area by 2016, a figure that is expected to reach 60% in 2030 (UN. 2016). This population shift toward urbanized areas comes with many side effects; at a basic level, it causes a serious depletion in natural resources—mainly water and energy—because of the rapidly growing demand on the same, which causes a series of damages to the natural environment.

In 2003, global energy consumption reached 9200 Mtoe, which is equal to 106,996 TWh/y (terawatt-hours per year); this had increased to 125,000 TWh/y by 2015 (IEA 2016). Our world consumes approximately 4 trillion cubic meters of fresh water every year, (Hoekstra and Chapagain 2006). Meanwhile, the buildings sector alone consumes 34% of total energy consumed and 25% of total water used (Council 2016; Jadhav 2016).

Today, technology has reached a new level of creativity and has become more sophisticated, objective, and universally available. The adjectives "smart" and "intelligent" can be applied to a single building and expanded to encompass the entire city (Cocchia 2014); however, why do we need to create smart cities and integrate the technology in urban design and planning? First, studies have shown that using commercially available technology and computer programs can significantly reduce energy consumption by 30–80% and water usage by 10–40% at the scale of the buildings (EIA 2011; Jadhav 2016). Second, cities must move from a passive to an interactive state (De Paula 2013); the growing interest in smart technology suggests that urban planning for smart cities, using technology to resolve various issues, will be an important field in the near future. With that in mind, conventional urban design is no longer sufficient to create future cities and resolve the existing urban issues of increasing demands on energy and water. The use of computational design technologies integrated to City Information Modeling (CIM) provides an adequate applied tool to provide relevant design solutions. It will for sure deliver efficient smart solutions via the use of the related CIM apps to an inevitable future of urban design and planning. This is aimed to attain the ultimate goals of smart sustainable cities that enhance the quality of life for its inhabitant and maintain the valuable resources (energy and water) without compromising the development capacity.

6.2 Research Design and Strategy

The global consumption rates of energy and water are rising with no clear predictions where they will stop. The increasing consumption rate driven by the consumption culture and behaviors has reached a new critical level of damaging the natural resources, suggesting that the new global conflicts will be on natural resources. At the same time, scholars are working hard to identify the issues that cause such increase to create new methodological ways to reduce the consumptions of such resources.

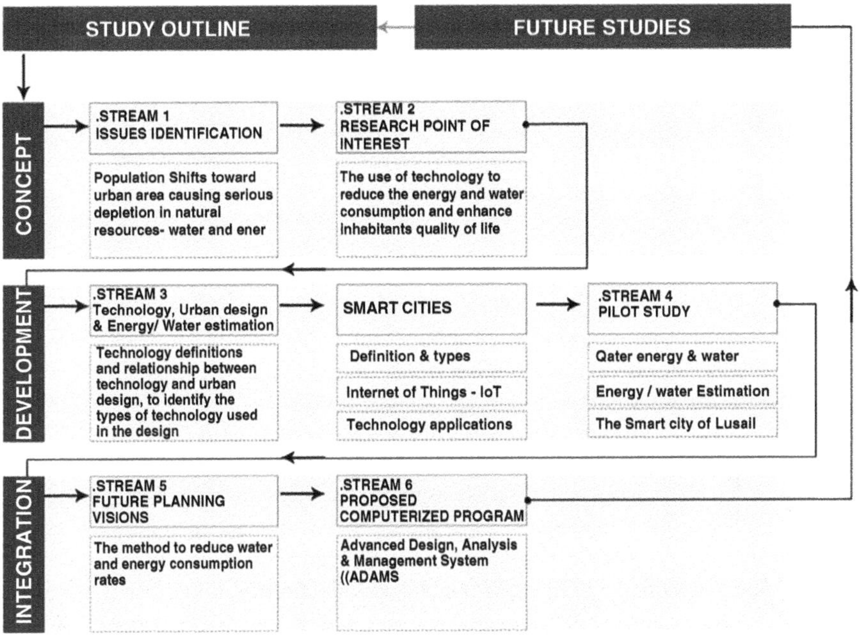

Fig. 6.1 Main stages for the development of ADAMS app

The concept of using intangible methods (theories and studies) to create tangible tools (design and operation programs) is responsible and effective, where the authors suggest that using today's technology – computerized forms of technology, will radically help to decrease the issues and, in some cases, will eliminate the unnecessary usage of such valuable resources.

The main motivation that incited the delivery of this study was started by observing and identifying the issues that are related to the high consumption rates of energy and water. In parallel, the development phase includes the investigation of previous knowledge of the subject that is directly linked to the issues mentioned above. In fact, these investigations have led to formulating a group of recommendations, that directly helps to create computer software that obtains the ability of analyzing, simulating and generates energy and water estimations, this computational tool is referred to as Advanced Design, Analysis and Management System (ADAMS) which works as the tools of resolving the identified issues (Fig. 6.1).

6.3 Concept Development

This section investigates the knowledge related to the use of computational tools and technologies such as CIM applications in the related field of reducing energy and water consumption rates in real-time interactions. In doing so, the authors investigate the current knowledge of urban design and its relationship with technology, as well as the concept of smart cities and the methods of energy and water estimations currently in practice.

6.3.1 Technology and Urban Design

Although, technology is a universal tool that is available and used in every movement of our daily life, yet there are no clear definitions for the term "Technology", that satisfies all scholars, or at least provide mutual common ground for all disciplines. The task of identifying and defining the meaning of technology is complicated and it evolves in time and from a discipline to another (Rooney 1997). The classification of technology involves different typologies like the technology of production, the technology of systems, the technology of power, and the technology of the self-intelligent (Foucault et al. 1988; Rooney 1997). Meanwhile, according to Larry Hickman's point of view, technology is a fundamental analytical process to understand the various outcomes, technology is concerned with the needs of human beings, it expands to include descriptive and normative of the thinking and creating process (Hickman 2001; Innis 2003). This section aims to develop a meaningful terminology for the "technology" to be used for both tangible and intangible processes within the framework of this study.

Technology (machine and ideas) is used in everything surrounding us to facilitate daily tasks. In parallel, urban design is the process of organizing the surrounding environments (built and unbuilt). To sum up; urban design and technology aims to facilitate human needs and enhance the quality of life. The importance of technology comes from its role and ability to merge virtual ideas with factual reality and, therefore reinforces the method to achieve the needs. Hence, technology is directly linked to urban development and its environmental, social and economic dimensions (Stewart 1977). The design process and technology share a unique relationship. Without technology, designs will exist only in our minds and rarely in descriptive documents. The role of technology radically increased in architectural design and urban studies especially during the 2nd industrial revolution, when a combination of artistic design encompassed scientific grounds as part of their practice and education (Emmitt 2009). At a wider scale technology integration in urban design is a must, not only as a support platform, but as a trusted, systematic tool of design, built and operation (DBO) (Fadli et al. 2015).

The focus of this research is on the computerized technology that includes categorization, simulation, analysis, visualization modeling and design tools that facilitate the urban design process, helping to transfer the design decisions from a passive to an interactive state. The idea of using computational technology as a design tools is relatively new. The first partiality intelligent computer program was formulated in the mid-1990s as a coordination tool at the level of a singular building. The program of Building Information Modelling (BIM), has been introduced as the new approach to successful constructions that saves time, effort and reduces the cost of constructions (Eastman et al. 2011).

The cardinal role of technology in design comes from the possibility to anticipate the results and suggest appropriate modification before executing the design process in full (Becerik-Gerber and Kensek 2009) (Becerik-Gerber and Kensek 2009). Similarly, computer programs and related software packages have evolved to obtain the necessary abilities of designs coordination. It also enables the designer to anticipate the patterns and predict any potential problems. They also help track the data of existing construction and serve as the management tool to facilitate data-exchange and interoperability between different environments and platforms.

The powerful integration of City Information Modeling [CIM] technology and urban design formulates the advanced tools for computational programing. This increases creative innovation capabilities of the designer at various stages at all time. It is emphasized at design and operation phases, as well as at operational levels, where the possibility to upgrade the design to consider more variables is higher and important. Figure 6.2 identifies the possible outcomes from the suggested integrations. Outcomes would vary from creating computerized programs to data sharing platforms. It concludes by developing design decision-making systems, leading to direct impact on the quality of life and the users comfort. It indeed, provides powerful tools of resource management, mainly for water and energy management.

6.3.2 *Smart Cities: Between Concepts and Principles*

"Smart city" is a universally used term that usually describes a city having the ability to collect and react towards information's in spatial and interactive dimensions. It is a relatively new concept with two main branches, one related to technology communication and information trends and the other linked to urban areas. A smart city covers

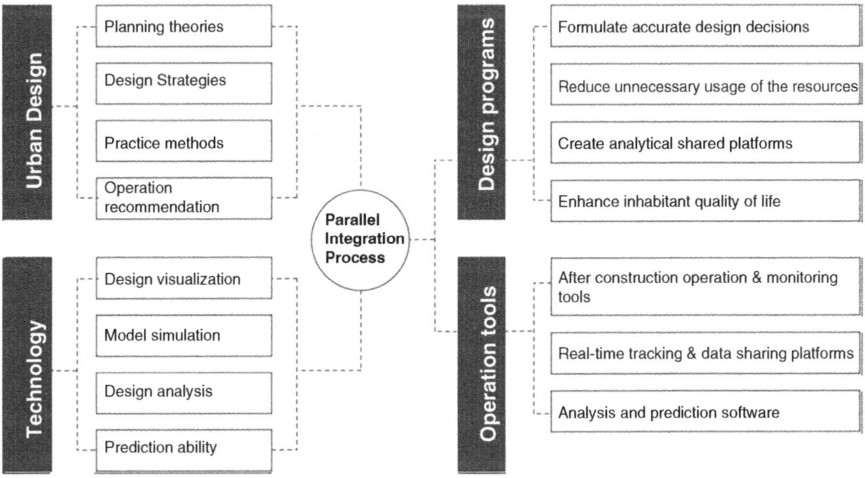

Fig. 6.2 Technology and the integration of Urban Design outcomes

many aspects, including the principles of urban planning, urban design, environment, sustainable development, economic growth, social patterns, technologies with their applications, and so on (Cocchia 2014; Harrison et al. 2010; Hollands 2008; Moutinho 2008). The adjective "smart" includes a wide range of meanings, which are linked to related characteristics and fields of application. Figure 6.3 repertories various types of the smart city components based on objectives and tools classification.

The smart city concept and principles are the results of performance and interaction between the built environment and its users via intelligent physical infrastructure with which it monitors the activities of the independent and self-aware citizens (Giffinger et al. 2007). Meanwhile, according to Caragliu et al. (2011); the combination of a responsible decision with a suitable means of resource management to achieve a high quality of life can be accomplished only by integrating both traditional and modern communication methods with sustainable development, human social patterns, and capital to formulate a sustainable and smart city (Caragliu et al. 2011). The communication and interaction between people, objects, and amenities on one platform through the use of surrounding technologies will radically enhance quality of life, increase logistic performances, decrease energy consumption, streamline resource management, and create what is known as the smart city in the twenty-first century (Dameri 2017). The latter statement refers to Internet of Things and People [IoT&P] (Fadli et al. 2018).

The process of creating a unified definition of the smart city requires us to separate the term into two parts, of which the first, the adjective "smart," means the ability to collect, analyze, and use the following information, which is available from all sensing and monitoring infrastructures and instruments in order to simulate current situations or predict expected scenarios and generate spatial information with the

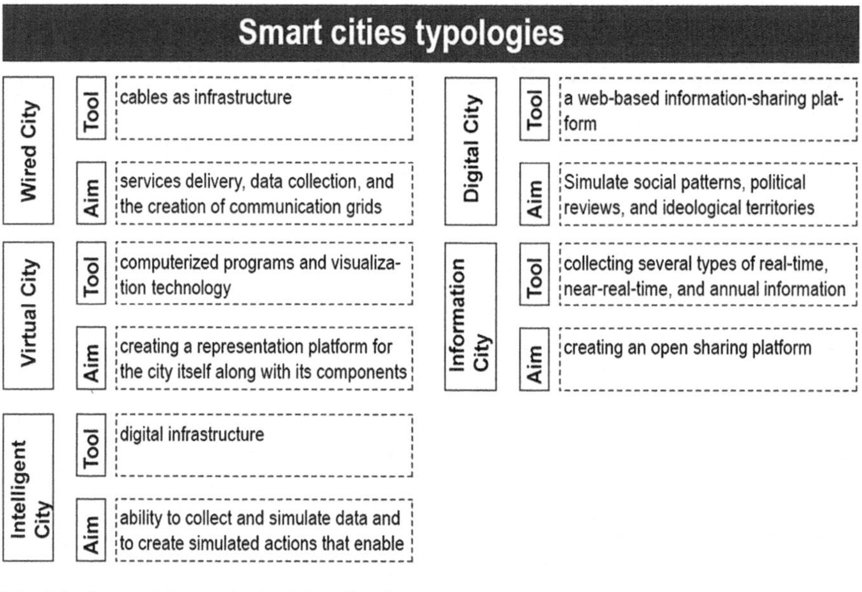

Fig. 6.3 Smart cities typological classification

tabulation of data. Although the level of smartness and intelligence [artificial and human] is usually measured by the capacity of different types of operation to be carried out at the same time. The second part, which is the targeted place "city" from which this information is collected, relates to the data on the physical (transportation, energy and water grids, infrastructure, and so on) and non-physical (social patterns, environmental needs, climatic situation, and so on) components of the city.

The design and creation of smart cities requires both physical (users based operations) and non-physical components (technology base tools) to inter-operate. The inter-operability classification results in the following specifications based on Harrison semantic (Harrison et al. 2010).

Instrumented; in essence, means the ability to collect real-time data from all devices embedded in city fabric. Main aim: to connect the analog and virtual worlds. Designers and users are aware of the benefits of using available soft-infrastructure (all elements and devices that are able to interact with users and collect data). These can be listed as: (1) public CCTV systems, (2) road detectors and sensors, (3) RF identification devices on tunnels and roads, (4) water quality sensors, (5) electrical distribution systems, (6) smart electricity and water meters, (7) telecommunication systems, (8) position reporting systems (GPS), (9) mobile telephone and public networks, and many other tools. This concept is well-explored under the heading "Internet of Things" (Dohr et al. 2010).

Interconnected; the process of collecting the information from soft infrastructure must be followed by a process of integrating these data into systems, organizations, industries, and web-based services, with the aim of the information being available across search engines, social networks, and other logical means of information delivery.

Intelligent; the interconnected data must be used to express facts that affect decisions and required actions that will eventually improve the systemic method of operation and enhance the expected outcomes. Although this will ultimately change (positively) the inhabitants' and users' experience and the city ecosystems, the intelligent process must be in real-time, futuristic, and predictive (Fig. 6.4).

The necessity of creating smart cities comes from its powerful tools and method of operations such as City information Modeling [CIM] technology. Collection of data is considered as the most important phase. Analysis and categorization of the collected data allows users to simulate and select the most suitable decisions to solve several issues such energy and water consumption. Enabling existing cities with soft-infrastructure, which, include monitoring systems, sensing devices and continuous communication systems. These provides real-time data monitoring platforms that enables real-time action plans via effective usage of resources.

6.3.2.1 Internet of Things & People (IoT&P) Concept

Our century has been marked as the century of advance communications methods, the abstract definition of the internet of things and people (IoT&P) concept has been formulated form the facts that 'smart – intelligent' devices are used in everything surrounding us starting from individual smart watches to advanced monitoring

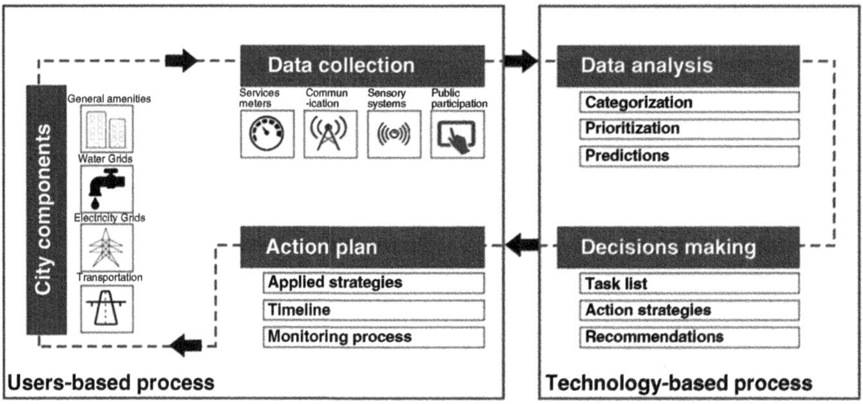

Fig. 6.4 Smart city: from inception to operation

devices that includes ubiquitous communication, pervasive computing and ambient intelligence. The ultimate goal of IoT&P is to provide a constant flow of information that enables continuous users-buildings-machines interaction at all-time using smart devices and integrative systems (Dohr et al. 2010) (AlSaeed and Fadli 2018).

Through this study, we aim to create a shared user-friendly platform connecting buildings, machines and humans. Allowing them to act and interact, identify, locate, sense and connect with each other in real-time. This will lead to novel interactions between people-people, people-things, things-things and things-people (Fig. 6.5). This systematically leads to a significant, accurate and prompt real-time response to unforeseen problems. The novel computational tool and technology aims to enhancing the quality of life, threats emergency-preparedness and responsiveness, and elaborates alternative scenarios for users' needs (Fadli et al. 2015).

Adapting the (IoT and IoT&P) concepts are cardinal to the design and development of smart cities, and interactive built forms with their constant ability to monitor, analyze and manage. Since planting and distributing assigned sensors and monitoring devices around the city is extremely difficult and will consider as unnecessary cost, meanwhile, using the methods of (IoT&P) to collect information and react toward it, using the IoT&P principles provides a more adaptable, user-friendly and affordable application tool to be used in real time by all users of the city, neighborhoods and buildings.

The power of information comes from the ability to make positive changes, where knowledge is the first step towards action, there are so many studies to identify the issues and threats but in most of the cases the solution comes with negative externalities formulated in cost and time, but these concepts can be changed by using passive objects to be interactive, therefore collecting real-time data on specific interest will lead to having better decision making and direct ways to the resolution of the issues.

Meanwhile, collecting the information of energy and water consumption rates leads to formulate data tables identifying the patterns and issues of consumption. It

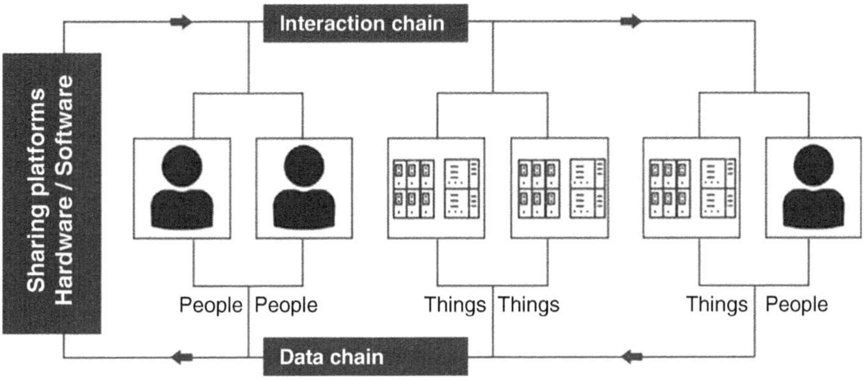

Fig. 6.5 Internet of Things [IoT] operating approach

also identifies the complications leading to establishing a systematic way to the resolution of the high consumption rates. Internet of Things and People [IoT&P] provides the hardware that is required to collect necessary data. The necessity of creating the software is indeed important and can be expanded and adjusted according to users' needs and aspirations within buildings and cities capacities.

6.3.2.2 Smart Urban Design Using CIM and IoT&P Technologies – ADAMS Application-

Conventional Design involves considerable time, effort and expenses. Generating critical assessment information such as cost estimation, energy-use analysis, and operation plan, is costly and timely leading to excessive demand on infrastructure and amenities usage (Hendrickson and Au 1989). Technology integration into design, built and operation (DBO) processes is the next generation of design practice. The ability of simulation, prediction, and consistent monitoring provided by integrated computational tools and technology [CTTs] leads to eliminate the unnecessary usage of the resource through real-time response-interaction.

Today, computer programs and software packages used in design and operation, are well-advanced than the traditional matrix and logarithms. In fact, they have become more intelligent, and have the ability to collect, assess and synthesize data and produce visual displays that are user-friendly and real-time responsive (Jin and Lin 2012). Yet, almost all of the available computer programs try to simulate existing situation or provide tools for new designs, but rarely merge both options (Batty 1997). We therefore, need to understand the variety of existing computer programs and classify typologies, based on well-defined criteria. This will enable the understanding of their role and importance in the process of urban design, in order to reach the ultimate goal of reducing energy and water consumption rates.

The adopted method was based on the scale of design, type of users, level of engagement, accuracy, availability, and operation complexity. These criteria enable the classification of program types into three classes (Fig. 6.6); From singular building design programs, to multi buildings simulation program and further to country planning programs.

However, considering the intelligence level there are two types (***Interactive Programs***; that have the ability to highlight and engage with direct feedback on designs errors such as BIM and, Revit, and ***Command Program***; that only follow user input to produce visual drawings such as Computer Aided Design- AutoCAD), hence, in order for the program to have the intelligent characteristics it must meet several characteristics (Fig. 6.7), such as (1)- digital, (2)- spatial (Ability to generate three-dimensional models), (3)- measurable (the possibility to produce quantity, dimension, query lists), (4)- comprehensive (used to coordinate design intent, monitor building performance, meets construction, operation and finance requirements), (5)- accessible (by all parties involved in the design process), (6)- durable (can be used in all phases of design, built and operation of the facilities) (Kunz and Fischer 2009).

Building Information Modeling (BIM) A design, construction and facility management program, that provides a new method to prepare the designs, and used by all related professionals (architecture, mechanical, electrical and environmental) where the program works on a single building design. The main concepts, method of

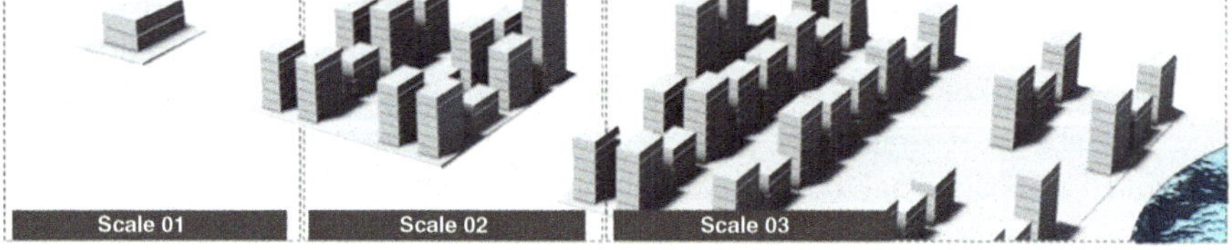

Fig. 6.6 Algorithmic schematic development and program classification

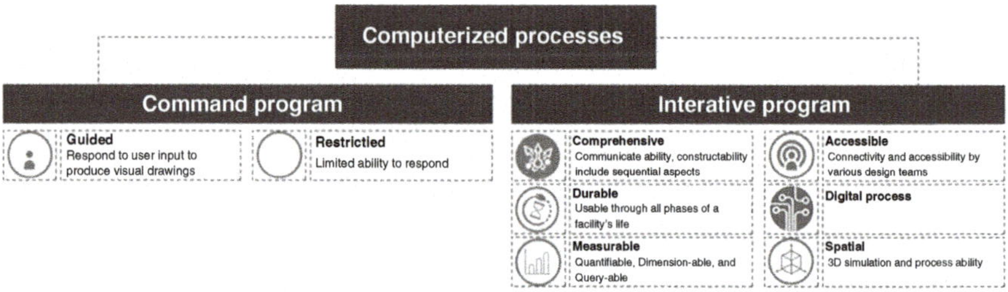

Fig. 6.7 Intelligent simulation: system specifications

operation and process of BIM appeared almost 30 years ago, where the most related term used to describe the process was Building Description System (BDS) (F Fadli et al. 2018). The BDS means the ability to make changes on all design components at once, where all drawings derived from the same source and follow the same arrangement method, all data cooperate with each other at the same time serve the same purpose to meet design and construction requirements (Eastman 1975).

BIM, method of work is based on transferring paper-based modes of coordination and the fragmented design process into an interactive and intelligent process, by overlapping all related sections in one working environment that is accessible and understandable by designers, contractors, managements and owners. BIM is no longer a software or design thing, it's an engineering activity that involves in all construction phases (Eastman et al. 2011). In other words, BIM modeling technology is the process to produce, coordinate, and analyze the building, where the building defined as:

1. **Construction components**; the objects that merge together to formulate the spaces.
2. **Analytical data**: the different types of information that describe the design behavior and the objects purpose and capability,
3. **Coordination data**: the relationships between all component of the building and the connection between the building systems (Birx 2005; Eastman et al. 2011; Maria 2016; McDuffie 2006).

BIM technology provides a multi-task engagement, the benefits of BIM wide and include various scales such as (Fig. 6.8).

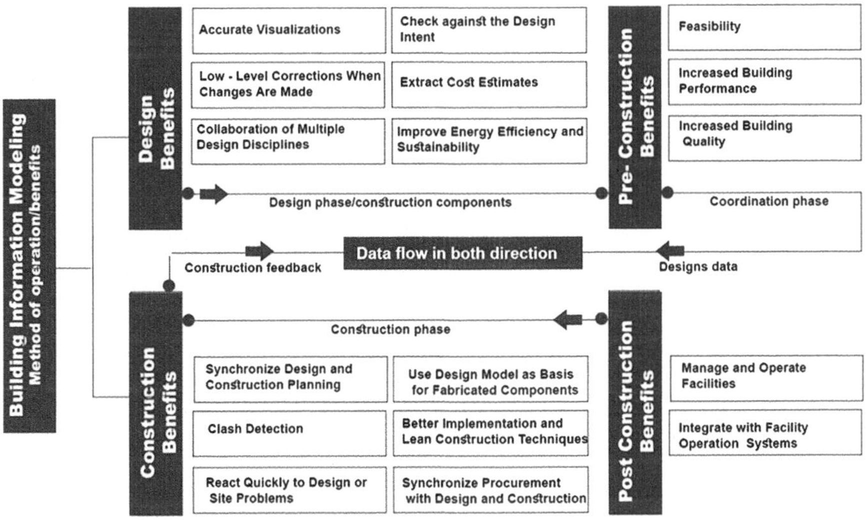

Fig. 6.8 BIM technology benefits. (Adapted from Fadli et al. 2015; Eastman et al. 2011)

Design Benefits include accurate visualization of the building, fast and low effort to make corrections and changes, produce accurate 2D- drawings, multi task and step- by- step coordination between all design disciplines, provide all types of cost estimation and bills of quantities and most importantly create design with sustainability standards to achieve low level of consumption of resource and energy efficiency.

Pre – Construction Benefits comes from the ability to provide clear concepts, feasibility and design option with the aim to increase building performance.

Construction Benefits the program provide a synchronize process between design and construction leading to omit all design errors before it comes to execution sites.

Post Construction Benefits where it helps the management and operation process and integrate various operation programs together, with no doubt this management phase will led to reduce the building consumption of water and energy (Fadli et al. 2014).

City Information Modeling (CIM) Concept Cities are complicated environments, that include not only static models, but also a large quantity of dynamic objects, the normal city vast people, establishments, organization and, infrastructure, a tremendous amount of information is generated in every second. We are now in the age of information explosion, that led to the need to create a classification and extracting method for the useful information to be used (Xu et al. 2014); "Future cities, soft cities and Cyber cities" are the terms used to describe settlements that have the ability to collect, process and, deals with large amount of real time data and information, influenced by building information modeling (BIM), the emerging term City Information Modeling (CIM), came into common use (Beirão et al. 2009); CIM is a cross-disciplinary model of urban design that facilitate the process of generating a spatial data models that used to manage and monitor the various demand for land, infrastructure, and environmental resources, in other words, CIM provides tools to transform urban design from analogue process to digital one (Thompson et al. 2016).

Scholars and developer suggest that CIM is divided into five components that vary in purpose and scale, and all components work to serve the same database that formulate the platform for urban designers to monitor the city and improve its environment, where these components are:

- **Buildings**: In every city, the buildings have their own characteristics, classification and behavior, a rapid digitizing technology must scan all buildings to reach the accurate effective city maps (Goetz 2013).
- **Transportation**: The city exists because its connectivity and transportation availability, the road information such as length, capacity, cost, and situation are very important to monitor how users behave and act toward solving the issues in real-time such as traffic management and services allocating.

- **City furniture**: The quality of life for the city inhabitant is measured with the availability of amenities, the government processes to enhance the services provided must be based on the collected information form several city furniture pieces.
- **Infrastructure**: The mechanical, electrical and water systems are vital to the city life, the process of distributing the infrastructure is very important and it must be carried forth based on the actual needs to serve city lands.
- **Resources**: Natural and manmade resource are the cities backbone, therefore the information generated form such resources must be measured all the time and assessed to create a suitable response system.

CIM method of operation is similar to BIM, yet a bit different, since it deals with data from many sources and it have the ability to track information in real-time, the concept of CIM is based on merging the BIM method of work with Geographical tracking possibility to create this shared platform and information, in which it can be transferred to readable charts, diagrams and tables of information.

The integration of CIM, and BIM technology is a necessity, where the city is composed of several BIM systems, however to comprehend the differences and areas of integration table 01 outlines a comparison between both systems (Table 6.1).

The table of scope and method (Table 02), of operations explains the programs (and concepts of work) method of data input and process in addition it highlights the scope of the program (Table 6.2).

Geographical Information System (GIS) The significance of the program is that it merges the spatial and textual data from several sources into one database, that is accessible and readable for all users. GIS has been used as a tool for urban planning and design since the mid 1980's, where the spatial planning prove its capability and importance in urban design and since GIS works as spatial modelling and analysis tool it has also been used widely (Fig. 6.9) (Han and Kim 1989; Anthony Gar-on Yeh 1991). The program helps significantly in improving mapping for all

Table 6.1 Planning software's comparison

Software	Origin date	Scale of use	Complexity	Type of output
Building Information Modeling (BIM)	Early 1990s	Singular buildings	Complicated: it requires special training and intensive knowledge in design, building and operation.	Drawings 3D models Numeric analysis
City Information Modeling (CIM)[a]	Early 2000s	Group of buildings (neighborhoods)	The concept is based on BIM methods, it requires basic knowledge in urban planning and design, and concentrated knowledge in city modeling and visualization programs	3D models Numeric analysis Data tabulation

[a]CIM is not one computer software, it's a group of software's and sharing platforms that work together to establish the data source (there are several programs that works under CIM concepts such as 'ReCap Pro, InfraWorks, Navisworks Manage, CyberCity 3D, .. etc.)

Table 6.2 BIM and CIM method of operations, scope and benefits

Software	Method of operation	Scope & benefits
Building Information Modeling (BIM)	01- Transfer the designs into spatial form.	Facilitate the coordination of all designs.
	02- Overalls the designs in the same environment and design factors to detect design errors	Transfer design drawings into construction drawings.
	03- Provide visual platform to highlight the designs behavior with each another	Minimize the changes required in case of change in the designs.
		Monitors construction process and facilitate site requirements.
City Information Modeling (CIM)	01- Collect, processes and categorize large amount of data in real-time	Generate real-time information for all city components.
	02- Transfer collected information into spatial visuals	Generate spatial analytical information.
	03- Highlight the predicted issues to be solved and monitored	Formulate a shared platform for information of the city.

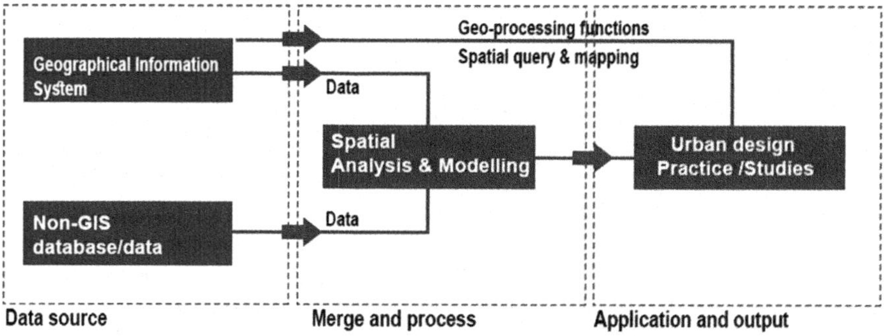

Fig. 6.9 GIS and Urban Planning apps (Adapted from Gar-on Yeh 1991)

city's tangible and intangible components. It fosters the process of data retrieval in a relatively short time, improves the analysis process for existing urban areas, and provides a tool for sustainability analysis (Anthony G-O Yeh 1999).

The role GIS plays, is limited to planning modeling and information presentation and used as a support tool for urban planners and designer at the same time, where planning objectives can be generalized as the determination of planning objectives, resource management and operation, monitoring and analysis of existing situation, modelling and projection, development scenarios, selection of planning methods, result evaluation, and feedback. In other words, GIS can only provide partial data required in the planning process, where other data require a high level of cooperation and coordination between various databases, techniques and models. In the following we discuss the partial role of GIS in the planning process stages.

01 **Resource monitoring**: Integrating the remote sensing data such as satellite images, data readability with geographical information system formulates the source for spatial information that directly leads to continuous monitoring for urban land information (Barnsley and Barr 1996).
02 **Existing situation monitoring**: GIS, helps urban planners to analyze the city's existing situation leading to the avoidance of any conflict with land development and environmental aspects, by creating an overlapping map for all design factors (Anthony Gar-on Yeh 1991).
03 **Modelling and analysis**: The key factor in city planning is the ability to predict future changes and growth requirements (Longley et al. 1994). Therefore, by integrating GIS with existing spatial information's will create modelling platform for city components such as population, economic and, environmental changes.
04 **Development of planning scenarios**: Creating land suitability maps and planning resources is very important in the process of city planning. Integrating GIS into the process can radically help in formulating several planning options that respond to specific threat or needs (Landis 1995; Anthony Gar-On Yeh and Chow 1996) .
05 **Selection of planning scenarios**: Using GIS as an tool of evaluation and multi-criterial decision analysis helps to choose the most effective plans for existing or future city plans (Despotakis et al. 1993; Charles Eastman 1975).
06 **Plans implementation**: GIS used to create multi stages assessment for environmental and economic impacts to minimize the negative impact of planning implementation.
07 **After implementation evaluation and feedback**: Feeding the database with actual land patterns and emerging needs, helps to create an evaluation tool.

GIS is a very powerful tool in urban planning. The use of GIS in city making process has significantly increased in the last decades. Integrating the technology of spatial data with numeric and semantic data lead to creating a visualization platform that can be described as an up to date, accurate and a decision-support system for planning and implementation.

Urban design, technology and smart city associated to BIM-CIM applications, involve the "smart city" as a relatively new concept. A smart city works by integrating tangible and intangible components to create a futuristic vision that uses Artificial Intelligence [AI] technology such as the CIM based-computational platforms. This will support enhancing the quality of life humans-users, and promote a sustained life cycle for the buildings, machines and spaces.

A multitude of computer programs and software packages provide multi-task operations for city design and operation. However, an important shortcoming is noticeable in computational tools and technologies that enables merging all parameters related to water and energy consumption in one package. All existing programs work separately and always focus on the design and construction phases only. There are those, which only aim to monitor (in purpose of management) the

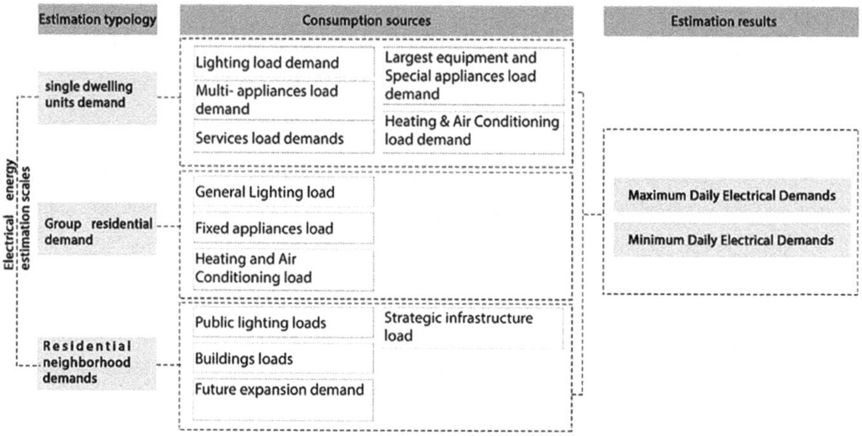

Fig. 6.10 Electrical energy estimation cycle

resources where the intervention is always difficult to eliminate the threat presented by the high rate of water and energy consumption. Therefore, there is a high necessity to harvest the benefits of technology by creating a computational software and information tracking, sharing platforms that aim at first to deal with resource bleeding (water and energy) and reduce the demand on such resources.

6.3.3 Energy and Water Estimation Process

The process of estimating energy and water requirements for the inhabitants of a city is a long and complex procedure that requires the availability of considerable amount of data. Therefore, the estimation process for both energy and water is organized and explained by several international standards and codes of practice that have evolved through time. Recently, the estimation process has started to take suitability into consideration, specifically after the sustainability assessment systems started to form and merge with the design process. This research has identified the main sources of standards and practice code, namely: (a) International Electrotechnical Commission (IEC); (b) National Electric Code (NEC); (c) American Society of Heating, Refrigerating, and Air-Conditioning Engineers (ASHRAE 90.1); (d) American Water Works Association (AWWA); (e) The International Association of Plumbing and Mechanical Officials (IAPMO). These organizations have led the formulation of a theoretical background that has paved the way for an established structured estimation process.

For this purpose, a universal estimation technique has been identified from the investigated practice and theory standards. The energy estimation begins by identifying the source of consumption then applies the consumption factor with its minimum and maximum requirements. Figure 6.10 explains the process and lists the requirements as per the following:

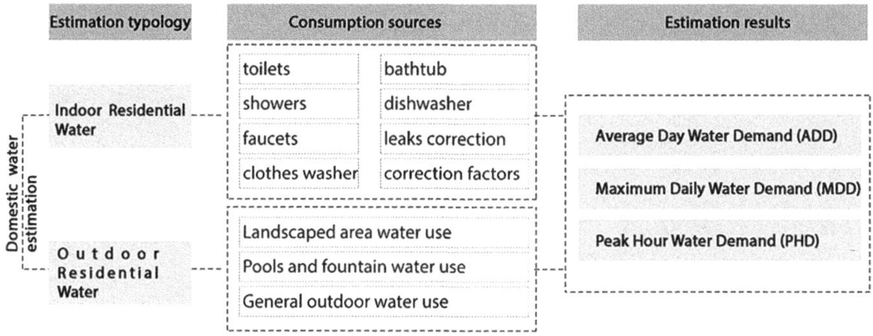

Fig. 6.11 Water estimation cycle

However, the process of estimating water requirements focuses on the number of inhabitants and their rate of consumption, whereas the method followed and recommended by international practice standards classifies water consumption by the type of use (domestic and non-domestic). "Domestic water" refers to the water used indoors to facilitate daily tasks, and "outdoor water" is that which is used for the landscape and other outdoor fixtures. From this, the research has identified and explained the source of consumption as clarified in Fig. 6.11.

Identifying the inputs of energy and water is important. Identifying the source of consumption leads to formulate the adequate estimation tool. The design of the tool is translated from a theory to praxis framework through the integration of estimation guidelines and computational technologies. The estimation method is therefore designed in a systematic automated process that forms the essence of the ADAMS tool.

6.4 Pilot Study

This section of the study explores the concepts of technology, urban design and energy and water issues at specific location, where this study has been carried out in the State of Qatar, first to identify the consumption statistics then after to investigate the City of Lusail as a smart city.

6.4.1 Qatar Energy and Water Statistics

The geographical location of Qatar deprives it of any access to natural resources other than oil and gas, where the underground water is salt and insufficient to fulfil the needs of inhabitants and the lack of sustainable electricity is one of the state largest challenges.

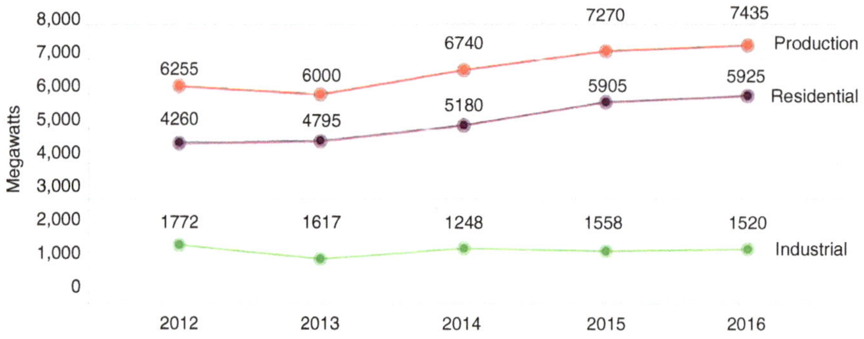

Fig. 6.12 General consumption statistics – electrical. (Source: Kahramaa 2018)

6.4.1.1 Energy Statistics

Aligned with the Qatari government's vision to develop the country in all aspects, and to satisfy the needs of all sectors (industrial, residential and mix use), the total production of electricity has jumped from 4032 MW in 2008 to 10,170 MW in 2017, where the total number of connected meters was 288,903 in 2012, served by 10,000 secondary medium-voltage (MV) and low-voltage (LV) substations. This rose to 344,445 (connected meters) in 2016 with a total of 14,000 substations in the first quarter of 2017. An investigation of the energy indicators reveals a clear increase in the demand for electricity over the last 5 years, as the residential sector alone consumes more that 50% of the total electricity production (Kahramaa 2016b, 2017).

According to Kahramaa (the local services provider), the total demand of the residential sector alone reached 5964 MW in 2016 (Fig. 6.12) and continues to increase radically along with other sectors (industrial and commercial), even though the individual consumption per capita has decreased from 11,100 KW/year in 2012 to 9847 KW/year in 2017 (Fig. 6.12).

The energy statistic is examined to provide a general overview of the total production and consumption, to estimate the efficiency and saving percentage achieved by integrating the system (ADAMS) into the process of design planning and operation.

6.4.1.2 Water Statistics

The water sources in Qatar are classified according to their origin (1) desalination: chemical and electrical process that removes salt from sea water and purifies it to be used as potable water; (2) abstraction of groundwater: natural process that extracts water from under the ground and purifies it using electrical methods and the re-use of treated sewage water; and (3) using chemical processes to clean the water, used for irrigation and agriculture only. Water extraction and production is a rapidly growing sector in the State of Qatar. The total water production in 2012 was estimated at around 437 million m^3/year, which increased to 560 million m^3/year in

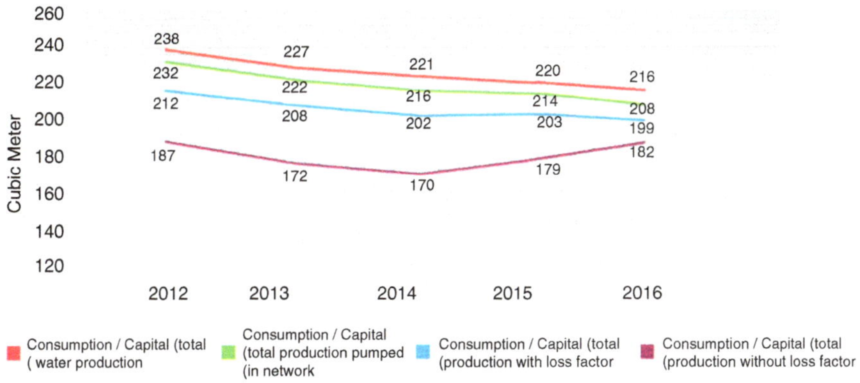

Fig. 6.13 Residential consumption statistics – water. (Source: Kahramaa 2018)

2016 (267 from desalinated sea water and 293 from underground and treated water sources) (Kahramaa 2017).

The latest water master plan reveals that more than 7000 distribution sub networks cover the major cities. However, the total loss due to leakage is estimated to be 7% in 2012 and decreased to 4% in 2012. The aim of QNV 2030 is to reduce the total consumption of water from 238 m^3/year in 2012 to 216 m^3/year in 2016 (Kahramaa 2016a) (Fig. 6.13).

6.4.2 *Energy and Water Estimation Process*

The method for estimating energy and water use followed by practitioners in Doha is a fully manual procedure where there is no unified or comprehensive application that estimates need; however, this research has identified the current method of practice associated with these issues and which in turn leads to identifying the responsible level of intervention by ADAMS:

1. Estimation codes: The codes and standards in Qatar follow international codes, therefore the consideration of Qatari estimation characteristics and consumption factors is limited and considered on a wide scale through the codes and standards prepared by the energy and water general planning authority known as Kahramaa.
2. Estimation cycle: The process of estimation is limited to the authorized designers or consultants, where the consultant prepares and submits for the authority the estimation of the building associated with the calculation, and where the authority's role is to review and match the needs with actual infrastructure capacity.
3. Supervising authority: The estimation result determined by the consultant is sent to the municipality and provided to infrastructure planning agencies to be revised against the service availability, and to make sure that it matches the recommendation of Kahramaa, where the approval of the estimation ensures that the providers are capable of connecting the establishment to the infrastructure.

4. Estimation tool: There are no unified tools to estimate need where the designer uses the international codes and programs that are accepted by the government; the only technological tool that is available is the newly-developed building permit system which organizes the communication between the designer, the authority, and the service providers.

Therefore, this research has identified that the most suitable level of intervention is in the design process, and there must be provided a unified estimation tool that considers local codes and standards at same time as it facilities the designer's accessibility to a shared database. The planning tool also provides a supporting tool for the authority to estimate general requirements and future needs, as well as a management tool that can allow both the householder and the government to monitor consumption rates and resource availability, all with the aim of reducing energy and water consumption rates.

6.4.3 *Lusail: A "Smart" City in Qatar*

Located at the northern porch of Doha city – capital of Qatar, Lusail City is a new city, that aims to create a smart, ambitious, and innovative environment that merges all pillars of sustainable development to fulfil the needs of the inhabitants and establish futuristic sustainable urban fabrics (Tok et al. 2015). Lusail City's urban development extends over 38 square kilometers and includes four elite islands in addition to 19 residential, mixed-use, and services zones. The total population is planned to reach 200,000 inhabitants and almost 170,000 employees, with the total expected population being more than 450,000 people (Scharfenort 2014) (Fig. 6.14).

Information Technology in Lusail being the first city in Qatar to be fully developed with modern concepts of technology in mind, the city provides and uses Information Technology Systems (ITS) at various scales such as smart infrastruc-

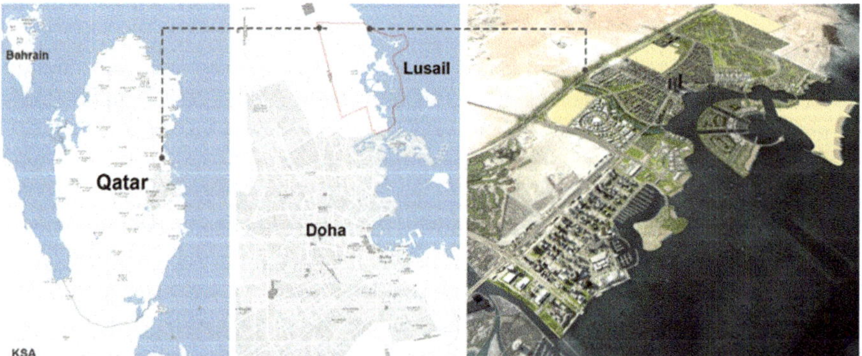

Fig. 6.14 Lusail City in Doha, State of Qatar. (Courtesy of Lusail City Authority, 2018)

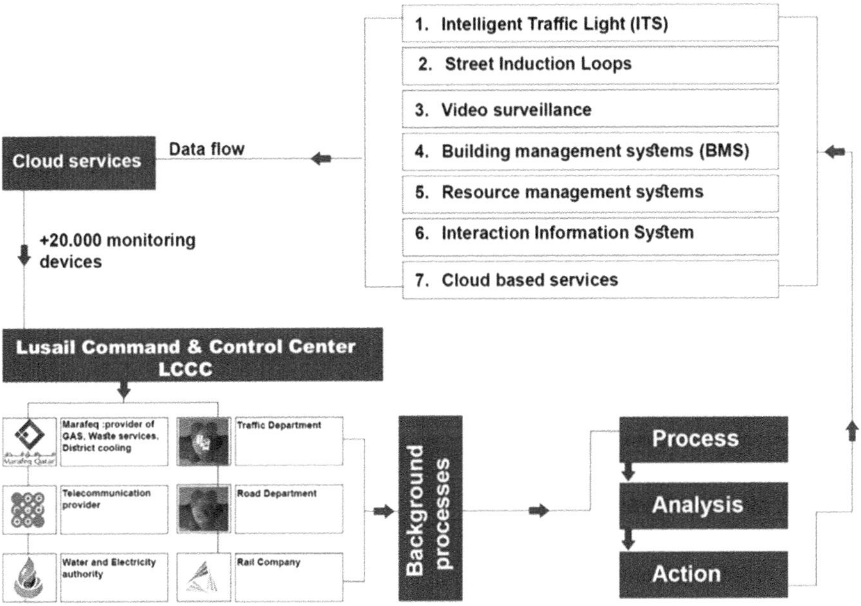

Fig. 6.15 Information Technology Systems [ITS] structure and flow

ture, consistence monitoring, to the individual buildings management systems all of it integrated to Lusail Command & Control Center (LCCC); Lusail (ITS) includes (Fig. 6.15):

1. Intelligent Traffic Light (ITS)
2. Street Induction Loops
3. Video surveillance
4. Building management systems (BMS) which in turn includes (Electricity and Water smart Meters, Cooling management, fiber connection systems)
5. Resource management systems (Smart Irrigation, Smart street light)
6. Interaction Information System (for public use)
7. Cloud based services (all information shared with users by cloud services to mobile devises)

LCCC supervises all actions and processes from the design, construction to the operation phase. The main scope of LCCC is to provide a unique platform for all key authorities and service providers (Marafeq: provider of GAS, Waste services, District cooling- Ooredoo: Telecommunication provider- Water and Electricity authority- Road Department- Rail Company- Traffic Department). This open shared platform enables access and mutual data-analysis in a synchronized manner. This process permits a fast and efficient communication, input, processing and output. This provides a safety system to tackle any environmental, economic and technological threat (LREDC 2015).

Advantages of ITS The integrated process of ITS allows the optimization and analysis of data collected from the smart infrastructure. Data collection occurs in real-time leading to establish fast effective responses. ITS advantages are wide and encompasses several aspects. However, the focus of this study is on water and energy preservation and effective resources management.

1. **Reducing Energy consumption rates**: electricity is vital for all sectors, therefore, the usage and consumption is directly monitored by LCCC. The consumers are divided into buildings, public spaces and transportation systems, where every increase in consumption highlighted by the detection sensors, allowing real time response, resulting in reducing energy demand compared to other location with same parameters to 32% less energy consumption, in addition a group of supporting system is always on operation such as:

(a) *Smart meters*: that provide real-time reading for electricity consumption.
(b) *Intelligent lighting systems*: that respond to weather, day time and actual need for electricity.
(c) *District cooling*: the conventional cooling systems works on providing low temperature air for the buildings, however, ITS system provides the actual need to reach thermal comfort based on time, capacity and location and every unnecessary cooling is removed, where all of cooling capacity is provided by thermal simulation for each building – by integration BMS into the process this will not only reduce energy consumption but cost as well (Fig. 6.16).

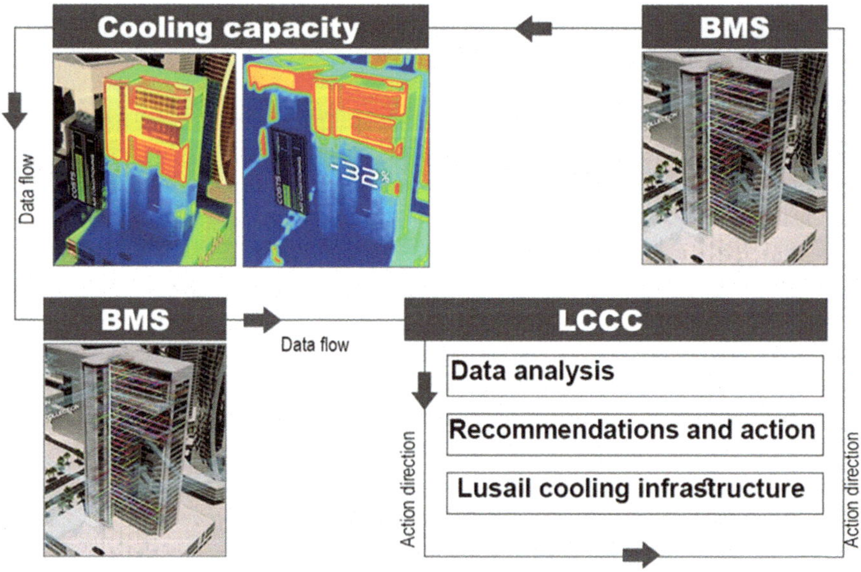

Fig. 6.16 Cooling systems design, development and operation [DDO]

2. **Reducing Water consumption rates**: providing water for inhabitant is very important, the method of delivering the service is conventional, however, the integration of the technology is limited to public spaces, parks and, general amenities, where the LCCC controls the capacity of flow time of operation and required action, where all process are controlled by smart intelligence to estimate the requirements according to weather, time and actual need this result in reducing water consumption to 18% of usual consumption compared to other location with same parameters.

6.5 Future E-Planning Visions

Planning and design with conventional methods is no longer responsible and sufficient to counter environmental, economic and social threats and enhance the inhabitant's quality of life. Urban planning institutions, urban planners, service providers and official authorities must use and develop technological solutions that use and harvest the benefits of applied science of technology, knowing the means of technology and its application is the first step of many toward enabling intelligent planning methods.

Current technology and software packages have proofed their abilities, and applicability to be included in individual design process helping to produce sustainable, affective and responsible designs. Yet, the shortage in current methods is wide and cannot be overlooked due to the limited cooperation abilities where, almost all software work on individual designs, and the possibility to establish coordinates between them is almost absent.

Planning for future cities requires a deep comprehension for the principle of designs and planning as a multi-stage action, therefore technology and its applications shall respond and implemented at all scale of design, planning and operation.

In order to face the increasing demands on energy and water; the computational design-oriented technology must move towards becoming self-sustaining and intelligent. It needs to adopt a wide ability of data collection, simulation and analysis, therefore, to solve the issues the authorities must look into all life cycle of cities (design, built and operation), where the most important action must be in real-time and respond to accurate data.

6.6 Advanced Design, Analysis and Management System (ADAMS)

Aiming to close the gap between theories of urban design, smart cites and technology applications, leads to creating computerized software that is simple and intelligent and focuses on resource maintenance with the ability of consentience monitoring and direct operation. In parallel, the software uses traditional methods of designs interaction (user- computer) allowing it to be a designing tool.

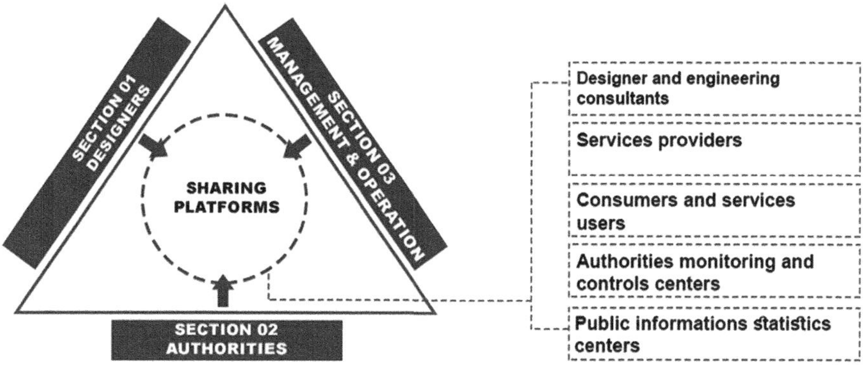

Fig. 6.17 ADAMS main functions and operation

ADAMS is a systematic practical application that provides multiple tools at various scales. Its aim is to close the gap between theories of urban design, smart cities and technology applications, leading to the creation of computerized tools that are simple, self-intelligent and focused on maintaining resources with consistent monitoring and direct operation.

6.6.1 System Function Spectrum

The system functions are divided into three main branches that include (01)- design tools (such as general estimation and simulation), (02)- planning (infrastructure monitoring and services tracking) and (03)- operations management (monitoring and response), each function is composed of several abilities (sub-functions), where all the functions are merged together through a unified sharing platform, to formulate the tools that are required to reduce the energy and water consumption rates.

The proposed method of operation works simultaneously to serve and coordinate the outputs between designers, planners, and building owners' fields of interest. This coordination process is stored and analyzed by sharing platforms that work both directions (as input and source of outputs). The general method of operation is based on the main function provided by ADAMS which includes (Fig. 6.17).

6.6.2 System Configuration

ADAMS proposed method of operation works simultaneously to coordinate the inputs and outputs between designer, users, and authorities, this coordination process aims to generate responsible designs with high ability of coordination prior and after construction, the overall method of operation is based on the main function provided by ADAMS which includes (Fig. 6.18).

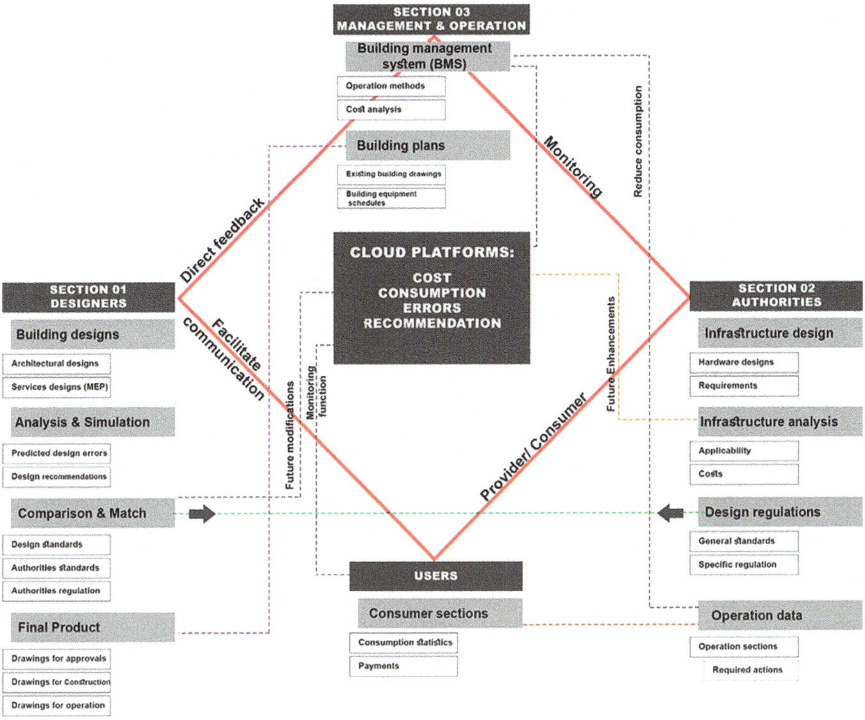

Fig. 6.18 ADAMS operation process

6.6.2.1 Design Tools

As it is the base tool, the aim is to practically develop and computerize the energy and water estimation process. The added values of the tools are the possibility to generate automated estimations (demand calculations) that are compared and matched with international and local standards and regulations with consideration to the efficiency in performance, ensuring that the estimation process is accurate and provides realistic demand estimations. These estimations are as close to the actual needs as much as it could be, which leads to eliminating the waste in energy and water demand on infrastructure and therefore reduces the consumption rates.

Design Function Structure

Divided into three classes that start with inputs, then internal analysis and calculation process, where the result of this phase is reflected through the output screen. Both phase one and three are user-interactive. Meanwhile, the second phase is a fully automated process that operates based on the user inputs in phase one (Fig. 6.19).

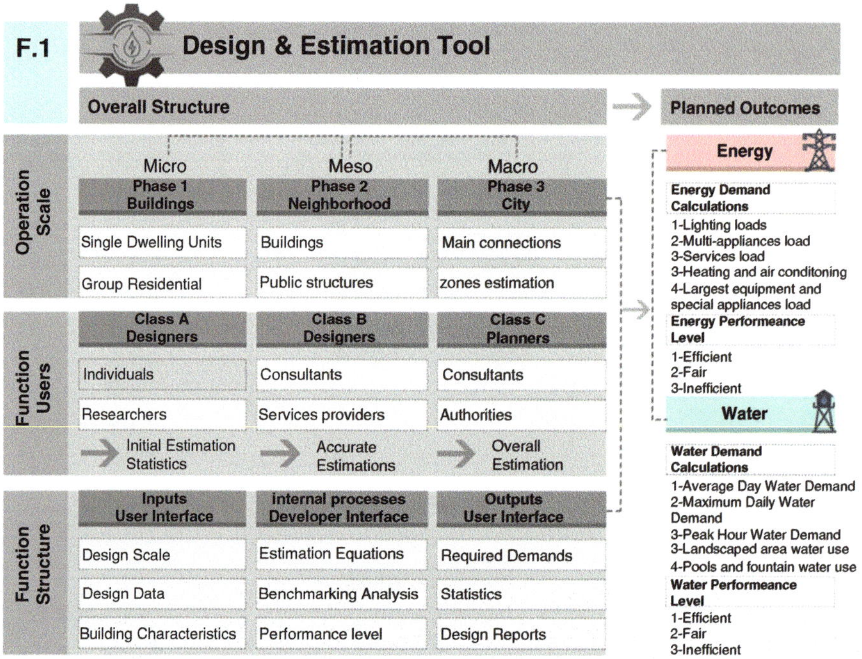

Fig. 6.19 ADAMS system; design and structure

6.6.2.2 Internal Process Chains

The process chain refers to the instruction impeded in the software, which forms the computational algorithm and process matrix. The design function process starts with the input by the user that is identified from energy and water estimation process, then the software applies the pre-set (pre-programed) calculation equations in specific order also identified from the estimation process of energy and water, to finalize the data in the numeric system that displays the result in the user's screen. Aligned with overall assessment value that describe the estimation performance.

The overall process chain is divided into an energy estimation process and a water estimation process, and the mathematical equations used to estimate the energy and water requirements.

The internal process chain represents the intangible aspects of the ADAMS structure, meanwhile the tangible aspect of the design tool is represented in the user-interface (Figs. 6.20 and 6.21), where the command page in the design tool display the required inputs listed in the internal process chain initiating the interaction between user and ADAMS as a system and allowing the system to forms the required sequence of operations.

Authorities Tools this section target the governmental institution that is responsible to provide infrastructures such as (water and electricity grids), the tools generate designs and analysis with users integration, the program can easily generate the

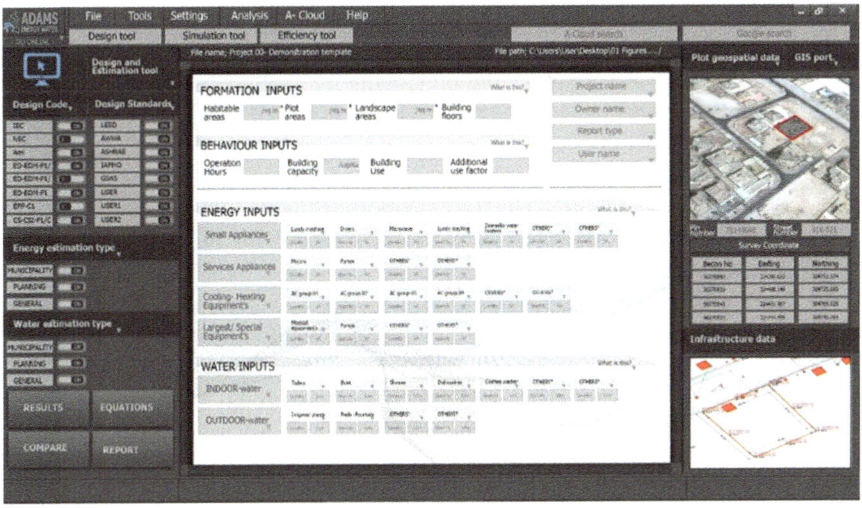

Fig. 6.20 ADAMS user's interface

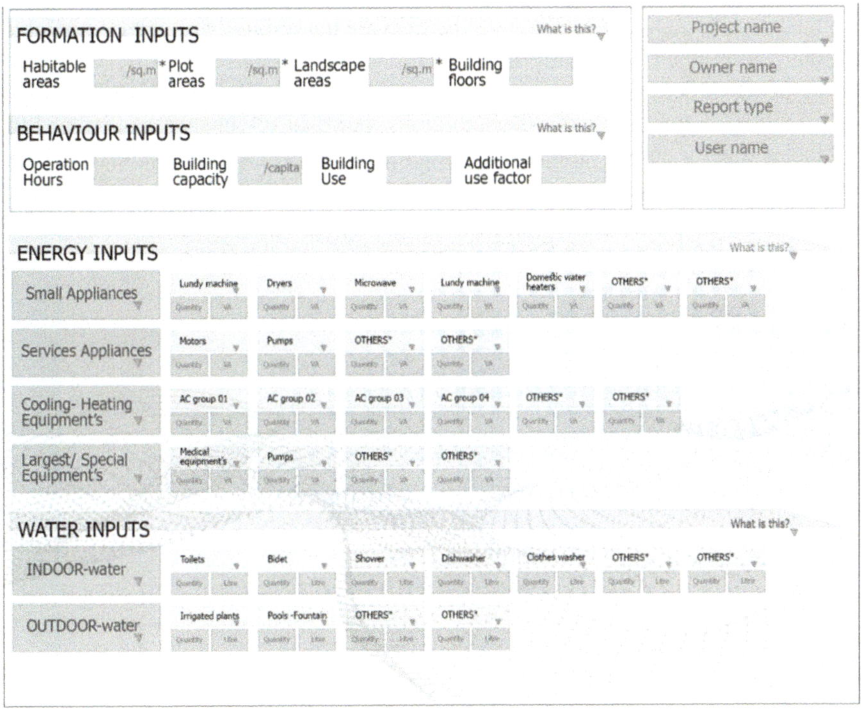

Fig. 6.21 ADAMS input dialogue page (design and structure)

general design standards and the specific regulation for each plot within city limit, in addition the tools is closely integrated with the individual buildings operations, to highlight any issues and propose the most suitable treatments and recommendations, where the collected data and analysis result is shared for future enhancement and current enhancements.

Operation & Management Tools since almost all modern building and designs are using Building Management Systems (BMS), that is the brain of building and the responsible system of building monitoring and operation, the integration of BMS is very important with authorities where the waste in resource will be highlighted and treated in real-time.

Cloud Platforms the advantage of ADAMS is the possibility of sharing information between all design, construction, operation and authorities leading to have real-time data base allowing the responsible parties to monitor and act toward information directly with no delay, leading to channel the attention on the targeted issues and reduce the cost of all operations. In addition, the use of sharing platforms will create accurate data banks that will be used for future studies and design improvements.

Although the aim of ADAMS challenges a complex situation, it provides a smart tool for present and future needs. It adopts a consistent coordination between several disciplines (architectural, electrical, mechanical, management, computer and medical sciences to name just few). It has also the possibility of creating a potential resilient smart open agile platform for the integration of all related disciplines and data types. It is designed in order to directly help in city planning and design to not only reduce energy and water consumptions, but also to enhance quality of life, wellbeing and the design, development and operation of current and future built and planned structures. It will, with no doubt, lead to healthy well designed and managed buildings, neighborhoods and cities in the present and near future.

References

AlSaaed, M., & Fadli, F. (2018). *Computational technology applications in urban design processes; WE-ADAMS an integrated tool to smart energy/water management system.*

Barnsley, M. J., & Barr, S. L. (1996). Inferring urban land use from satellite sensor images using kernel-based spatial reclassification. *Photogrammetric Engineering and Remote Sensing, 62*(8), 949–958.

Batty, M. (1997). Cellular automata and urban form: a primer. *Journal of the American Planning Association, 63*(2), 266–274.

Becerik-Gerber, B., & Kensek, K. (2009). Building information modeling in architecture, engineering, and construction: Emerging research directions and trends. *Journal of Professional Issues in Engineering Education and Practice, 136*(3), 139–147.

Beirão, J. N., Duarte, J. P., Montenegro, N., & Gil, J. (2009). Monitoring urban design through generative design support tools: a generative grammar for Praia. *Paper presented at the Proceedings of the APDR Congress.*

Birx, G. W. (2005). BIM evokes revolutionary changes to architecture practice at Ayers/Saint/Gross. *AIArchitect, 12*, 1–7.
Caragliu, A., Del Bo, C., & Nijkamp, P. (2011). Smart cities in Europe. *Journal of urban technology, 18*(2), 65–82.
Cocchia, A. (2014). *Smart and digital city: A systematic literature review Smart city*. Genoa: Springer.
Council, W. E. (2016). *World energy resources*. London: WECouncil.
Dameri, R. P. (2017). *Smart city definition, goals and performance smart city implementation* (pp. 1–22). Springer.
De Paula, R. (2013). *City spaces and spaces for design. Interactions, 20*(4).
Despotakis, V. K., Giaoutzi, M., & Nijkamp, P. (1993). *Dynamic GIS models for regional sustainable development Geographic Information Systems, Spatial Modelling and Policy Evaluation* (pp. 235–261). Springer.
Dohr, A., Modre-Opsrian, R., Drobics, M., Hayn, D., & Schreier, G. (2010). The internet of things for ambient assisted living. *Paper presented at the Information Technology: New Generations (ITNG), 2010 Seventh International Conference on.*
Eastman, C. (1975). The use of computers instead of drawings in building design. *AIA Journal, 63*(3), 46–50.
Eastman, C., Eastman, C., Teicholz, P., & Sacks, R. (2011). *BIM handbook: A guide to building information modeling for owners, managers, designers, engineers and contractors*. USA & Canada John Wiley & Sons.
EIA (2011). Annual energy review (Reports). *From Energy Information Admission.* https://www.eia.gov/totalenergy/data/annual/index.php#consumption
Emmitt, S. (2009). *Architectural technology; Research & practice*. England: Wiley.
Fadli, F., Sobhey, M., Asadi, R., & Elsarrag, E. (2014). Environmental impact assessment of new district developments. *WIT Transactions on The Built Environment, 142*, 517–528.
Fadli, F., Barki, H., Boguslawski, P., & Mahdjoubi, L. (2015). 3D scene capture: A comprehensive review of techniques and tools for efficient Life Cycle Analysis (LCA) and Emergency Preparedness (EP) applications. *WIT Transactions on The Built Environment, 149*, 85–96.
Fadli, F., Kutty, N., Wang, Z., Zlatanova, S., Mahdjoubi, L., Boguslawski, P., & Zverovich, V. (2018). Extending indoor open street mapping environments to navigable 3D CITYGML building models: Emergency response assessment. *International Archives of the Photogrammetry, Remote Sensing & Spatial Information Sciences, 42*(4), 161–168.
Foucault, M., Martin, L. H., Gutman, H., & Hutton, P. H. (1988). *Technologies of the self: A seminar with Michel Foucault.*
Giffinger, R., Fertner, C., Kramar, H., Kalasek, R., Pichler-Milanović, N., & Meijers, E. (2007). *Smart cities: Ranking of european medium-sized cities. vienna, austria: Centre of regional science (srf), vienna university of technology*. www. smart-cities. eu/download/smart cities final report pdf
Goetz, M. (2013). Towards generating highly detailed 3D CityGML models from OpenStreetMap. *International Journal of Geographical Information Science, 27*(5), 845–865.
Han, S.-Y., & Kim, T. J. (1989). Can expert systems help with planning? *Journal of the American Planning Association, 55*(3), 296–308.
Harrison, C., Eckman, B., Hamilton, R., Hartswick, P., Kalagnanam, J., Paraszczak, J., & Williams, P. (2010). Foundations for smarter cities. *IBM Journal of Research and Development, 54*(4), 1–16.
Hendrickson, C., & Au, T. (1989). Pro*ject management for construction: Fundamental concepts for owners, engineers, architects, and builders*. Chris Hendrickson.
Hickman, L. A. (2001). *Philosophical tools for technological culture: Putting pragmatism to work*. Bloomington: Indiana University Press.
Hoekstra, A. Y., & Chapagain, A. K. (2006). *Water footprints of nations: Water use by people as a function of their consumption pattern Integrated assessment of water resources and global change* (pp. 35–48). Springer.

Hollands, R. G. (2008). Will the real smart city please stand up? Intelligent, progressive or entrepreneurial? *City, 12*(3), 303–320.

IEA. (2016). *Water Energy Nexuse- World Energy Outlook 2016*. From International Energy Agency www.iea.org/t&c/

Innis, R. E. (2003). The meanings of technology. *Techne: Research in Philosophy and Technology, 7*(1), 34–40.

Jadhav, N. Y. (2016). *Green and smart buildings: Advanced technology options* (Vol. 1). Puchong: Springer.

Jin, D., & Lin, S. (2012). *Advances in computer science and information engineering*. Berlin: Springer.

Kahramaa. (2016a). *General statistics report consumption Report (Water section)*. State of Qatar: Qatar General Electricity & Water Corporation.

Kahramaa. (2016b). *General Statistics report consumption report (Electrical Department)*. State of Qatar: Qatar General Electricity & Water Corporation.

Kahramaa. (2017). *Electricity & water statistics report*. State of Qatar: Department of Planning and Quality Assurance.

Kahramaa. (2018). *State of Qatar annual electricity & water statistics report (production and consumption)*. State of Qatar: Department of Planning and Quality Assurance.

Kunz, J., & Fischer, M. (2009). *Virtual design and construction: Themes, case studies and implementation suggestions*. Center for Integrated Facility Engineering (CIFE), Stanford University.

Landis, J. D. (1995). Imagining land use futures: applying the California urban futures model. *Journal of the American Planning Association, 61*(4), 438–457.

Longley, P., Higgs, G., & Martin, D. (1994). The predictive use of GIS to model property valuations. *International Journal of Geographical Information Science, 8*(2), 217–235.

LREDC. (2015). *Lusail City: Sustainability strategies*, from http://www.lusail.com/the-project/sustainability/

Maria, F. M. (2016). *Deriving building information models from legacy paper drawings*.

McDuffie, H. T. (2006). *BIM: Transforming a traditional practice model into technology-enabled integrated practice model*. The Cornerstone, AIA.

Moutinho, J. L. (2008). *Building the information society in Portugal: lessons from the digital cities programm 1998–2000*. Value-added partnering and innovation in a changing world, 215.

Rooney, D. (1997). A contextualising, socio-technical definition of technology: learning from Ancient Greece and Foucault. *Prometheus, 15*(3), 399–407.

Scharfenort, N. (2014). *Off and running: Qatar brands for FIFA World Cup, and life beyond*. Under Construction: Logics of Urbanism in the Gulf Region.

Stewart, F. (1977). Technology and underdevelopment. *Development Policy Review, 10*(1), 92–105.

Thompson, E. M., Greenhalgh, P., Muldoon-Smith, K., Charlton, J., & Dolník, M. (2016). Planners in the future city: Using city information modelling to support planners as market actors. *Urban Planning, 1*(1), 79–94.

Tok, E., Fatemah Al Mohammad, M., & Al Merekhi, M. (2015). *Crafting smart cities in the gulf region: a comparison of Masdar and Lusail Handbook of Research on Digital Media and Creative Technologies* (pp. 448–460). IGI Global.

UN. (2016). *The world's cities in 2016 UN: Department of economic and social affairs, population division*.

Xu, X., Ding, L., Luo, H., & Ma, L. (2014). From building information modeling to city information modeling. *Journal of Information Technology in Construction (ITCon), 19*, 292–307.

Yeh, A. G.-O. (1991). The development and applications of geographic information systems for urban and regional planning in the developing countries. *International Journal of Geographical Information System, 5*(1), 5–27.

Yeh, A. G.-O. (1999). Urban planning and GIS. *Geographical information systems, 2*(877–888), 1.

Yeh, A. G.-O., & Chow, M. H. (1996). An integrated GIS and location-allocation approach to public facilities planning—An example of open space planning. *Computers, Environment and Urban Systems, 20*(4–5), 339–350.

Part III
Urban Health and Wellbeing

Chapter 7
Centenarian Transhumanism Aging in Place

Jennifer Loy

Abstract The rising cost of health care and an aging population are issues that will need to be addressed within a future smart city environment. Digital technology is providing unprecedented opportunities for proactive health strategies to be employed to support healthy aging, including aging in place. However, whilst the technological capabilities supporting this potential are rapidly emerging, the social factors still need further research. This chapter considers the practical and emotional challenges facing people as they age in the twenty-first century context and contributes to discussion on the integration of digital technology into society earlier in life for proactive, healthy aging and to support aging in place for future generations.

Keywords Health · Care · Digital technologies · 3D printing · Data

7.1 Introduction

Actuarial predictions suggest those born this century have a life expectancy of over a 120 years.[1] Debates on the future of work, the nature of retirement and cost of healthcare for an aging population (where the median age increases) raise concerns about how societies can effectively respond. Actuaries argue conventional retirement and superannuation (pensions) with associated government funded, residential aged care will be unable to be facilitated by the working populations of the future, with the Actuaries Institute of Australia, for example, describing the situation as a 'longevity tsunami' (2012), predicting that the percentage of Australians over 65 years of age will grow from 14% to 25% by 2050. Assuming expected birth rates and financial predictions are correct, new thinking is needed as societies address the challenges for sustainable healthy aging. This chapter discusses a proactive approach

[1] http://www.actuaries.asn.au/Library/Events/FSF/2012/FSF2012PaperHowesRafe.pdf

J. Loy (✉)
Deakin University, Geelong, Victoria, Australia
e-mail: Jennifer.loy@deakin.edu.au

N. Biloria (ed.), *Data-driven Multivalence in the Built Environment*, S.M.A.R.T. Environments, https://doi.org/10.1007/978-3-030-12180-8_7

to the design of technology-enabled healthcare within a smart city environment, to support new futures for aging populations. This approach is based on rethinking perceptions of designing for old age by introducing strategies to pre-empt the challenges of physical and cognitive aging. These are possible because of a confluence of emerging digital technologies that support the development of data driven, integrated product systems for personalised health care within smart home and urban environments. Ubiquitous computing, data analytics, digital communication tools and bespoke digital fabrication provide the means for technological change in health care systems for an aging population. However, research into positive human development in a digital era is also needed to provide direction for the essential cultural changes needed to effectively implement such digital solutions.

7.2 Digital Healthcare

An overwhelming desire expressed by individuals on the subject of aged care, is to retain their independence in their own home in the face of diminishing capacity for as long as possible. Staying at home may seem an emotional ideal, but the degeneration of physical and mental acuity that accompanies aging needs mitigation for this to be achieved without increased physical risk (and therefore cost) and social isolation. This applies both to the individual concerned and carers. Healthcare support for older people living at home currently tends to be reactionary, for example in response to physical trauma or recuperation following an illness, with a focus on retrofitting generic, assistive technology, increasing home care visits and finally residential care. Whilst moving into assisted living and residential facilities can provide managed physical support, it can have a negative impact on the emotional well being of the older person because lack of autonomy can undermine a sense of self. As observed by Morgann et al. (2012, p. 130): "There is a level of self-determination that is expected upon becoming an adult. Having control over one's own space – as it relates to who we allow in, how we decorate and furnish it, and what we choose to keep in those private, personal areas – is crucial to the feelings of autonomy and independence. AL (assisted living) necessarily limits how individuals experience their personal spaces as it provides oversight and daily cleaning and ensures safety." As lifespans increase, even with a corresponding extension of capability further into that lifespan, this approach will most likely become too expensive for societies to maintain and in the meantime is not ideal for the individual and carers trying to manage the situation. A radical rethink is arguably needed not only to reduce the cost of aged care, but to more effectively support the desire for independence for future generations choosing to live at home for longer in their old age.

Research into aging in place in a smart cities context explores the potential of digital technologies, such as embedded in the Internet of Things (Rowland et al. 2015), to provide preventative healthcare to support personal empowerment in a technologically-enabled, home-care system (e.g. Ghani 2018, Kalid et al. 2017). Coulter (2011, p. 185) suggests that: "The public has a huge thirst for information about health and healthcare. Healthcare professionals have a responsibility to educate and inform patients and to boost their confidence and skills for making decisions about their health. Often this means a radical change in how medical consultations are conducted, with less emphasis on giving instructions and advice, and more on encouraging patients to determine their own goals and helping them to meet them. Information can have a therapeutic role, improving the patient's ability to cope with illness and enhancing their ability to look after themselves, so clinicians should help patients to access it." According to Farahani et al. (2018), there are four layers of Internet of Things architecture that have implications for the development of e-health systems as part of a smart cities approach: Firstly there is a sensing layer, which integrates the physical with hardware to collect data; then a networking layer, creating connecting systems; a service layer manages services meeting users' needs; and, finally, an overarching interface layer allows for data interaction by users and applications. Greenfield (2006, p. 23) argues that digital technology should be integrated more fully into everyday objects and environments: "These are universals humans have lived with for millennia, elements like walls and roofs, tables and seating, clothing, and, of course, the body itself – our original and our final home. In everyware, all of these present appealing platforms for networked computations." These layers and systems can provide integrated healthcare feedback, as described for example in the Breath project (2015), funded by Ambient Assisted Living program in the UK.[2] However, in addition to monitoring and data driven telemedicine and e-health systems, demonstrated by the European smart homes framework, digital fabrication processes could also be factored in to monitored, digital health systems provide tailored assistive technologies designed to physically empower the user (and carers) at home, provide information on changing physical capabilities and to support mobility. Additive manufacturing has been used to create personalised prosthetics and orthoses, but it is still in its infancy in terms of providing a systems approach to supporting an individual's physical needs. There are, however, examples that are indicators of the emergence of systems practice, such as in the work of Andiamo[3] in the UK. This is a company set up by the parents of Diamo Parvez, whose son had cerebral palsy. They specialise in the use of 3D scanning as the basis for 3D computer models used for the 3D printing of personalised braces for children with cerebral palsy. This system replaces the use of plaster casting which is distressing and slow, with bulky, inflexible results. 3D printing allows for bracing to be designed that can be lightweight, quickly fabricated whilst the measurements are still accurate and adapted on an ongoing basis as the child grows. The monitoring of brace effectiveness on gait in this group is a focus of research (e.g. Smith et al. 2009), relying predominantly on the use of gait lab testing over short distances. Integrating constant feedback systems into a system of evolving braces for a growing child would better inform this type of work.

[2] https://ec.europa.eu/digital-single-market/en/news/breathe-project-privacy-design-ambient-assisted-living

[3] https://andiamo.io/about/

This example illustrates how digital technologies can provide physical bracing, balance and strength, as well as monitoring – an approach which should be directly applicable to the needs of older people. However, for this to be most effective – and realistically accepted into everyday life by older people – the use of adaptive bracing would need to be introduced much earlier in a person's life, fostering a gradual change of thinking about understanding and maintaining the body before old age. Centenarian transhumanism refers to a design-led research approach to rethinking assistive technology and healthcare long-term for the future generations of aging populations, that draws on the opportunities provided by digital technologies to create more integrated cyber-physical systems. This proposition supports a preventative and proactive approach to preparing the population for independence for longer. Essentially, it involves engaging aging individuals with assistive technology at a much earlier stage of life, as well as integrating digital technology systems into daily living with e-health strategies and smart home planning. Currently mechanical aids tend to be brought in to older people's lives in response to specific problems, such as mobility, or practical challenges in the kitchen, e.g. opening cans, turning dials. By building instead interdependent technological relationships between the user and mechanisms in middle age, prior to practical problems arising and before health issues develop, then protective measures can be developed to reduce the risk of critical damage to the body as well as reduce the impact of emotional stress for the person usually brought about by the introduction of assistive technology following a health crisis. By arguably "co-evolving with our technology", (Kelly 2010, p. 37), once health issues do then occur, the patient of the future is used to operating within a technology-enabled support system enhancing their capabilities.

Addressing aging for millennials, rather than for now, it should be possible to build a digitally enabled framework for living with assistive technology integrated into everyday life. From a health insurance and government healthcare system's point of view, this may be long-term, but would be of social and financial benefit for the next generations, for whom it would also be most easily adopted. Researchers, such as Petrova (2014, p. 525) describe those born after the introduction of the Internet as having a "techno-dependency" with related capabilities: "Gen Y have grown up in a world of rapid technological advances affecting the way they learn, their approach to knowledge acquisition and the forms of interaction between themselves… as a result of their techno-dependency and the fact they are accustomed to using computers and Internet to perform any given task, Gen Y has formed unique characteristics and competences."

Establishing this health care approach for a techno-dependent generation potentially effects human evolution in a digital era "the human organism is a paradigmatic case of ontogenetic adaptation: thanks to an enormously flexible cognitive and behavioral repertoire" (Powell 2012, p. 150). As the impact of middle age undermines body function, for example ankle stability, manual dexterity or grip strength – even to a minor degree, it could become standard mitigating practice to integrate digitally-enabled, assistive technology into wearables for everyday life. Devices are becoming more lightweight and affordable with the development of new materials (e.g. Paralympian John Maclean's carbon fibre leg brace[4]), wearables integrating sensors are integrated into healthcare (e.g. body monitoring with photonic textiles: Quandt et al. 2017), aged care use (e.g. Oedema socks by Edema, monitoring the abnormal collection of fluid in legs and ankles: Brown 2018) and advances in digital fabrication technology are supporting customisation (e.g. custom-made foot orthoses, Dombroski et al. 2014). These technologies allow for the development of relatively low-cost, bespoke devices that could be adapted during a person's lifespan, with products such as partial exoskeletons extended over time as needs arose. As arms, legs and backs deteriorated with age, embedded sensors in those exoskeletons could inform incremental adjustments, with devices attuned to compensate. This would empower the individual, protect vulnerable body parts, and so support independent living for longer. If a significant problem then did occur, loss of tendons for example, or neuropathy, or a degree of myelopathy, the user would already be comfortable with a high degree of assistive technology. The change to dependency on technology would not be as emotionally and physically challenging because it would be gradual and proactive, rather than reactive and radical as would occur following a trauma as would be the case under the current system, even if such a degree of personalised assistive technology were readily available.

The idea of creating a process of orthotic adjustment and adaptation is possible because of a confluence of digital technology developments in the twenty-first century, centred on 3D printing (additive manufacturing). 3D printing allows the shift from mass production to customization crucial for bespoke healthcare and has resulted in multiple research initiatives addressing personalised healthcare. For example, the wider adoption of lightweight robotic exoskeletons developed by the Delaware Center for Orthopedics Research[5] was facilitated by 3D printing. The lack of dependence on tooling in additive manufacturing means customised solutions can be incrementally evolved in response to changing experiences and physical needs, based on feedback data at a relatively affordable cost. Tracking monitors and the translation of data into accessible formats could provide users with feedback on the effectiveness of their assistive technology, and the ability to adjust as necessary with a degree of independence. Although less radical, this work relates to the research of Hugh Herr (Markowitz and Herr 2016) whose work includes researching the development of prosthetics that are linked to nerve endings to allow amputees physical feedback from their prosthetics. It also links to the development of hearing aids where users can adjust the sound level, as well as adjust for optimum hearing in different situations, such as in conversation or at a concert hall (e.g. Oticon digital hearing aids[6]). This is significant at this time, as empowering individuals is highlighted in the development of future health care systems (Bridges et al. 2008). Systems integration further into environments, to create a holistic, responsive digital support systems for the aging population, would provide a very different experience of aging for future smart homes and cities.

[4] http://www.johnmaclean.com.au/

[5] http://www1.udel.edu/udaily/2011/nov/dhsa-orthopaedic-research110510.html

[6] https://www.oticon.com/

7.3 Proactive Healthcare

The cost of health care, and in particular residential care for older people, is becoming problematic for society. In addition, there is a growing resistance to moving out of the home to receive a higher level of care in assisted living facilities. Living in the home for longer, termed aging in place, has a level of inherent risk as aging can cause accidents, such as when balance is affected. The basis for the proposal here is the creation of a proactive health care culture that anticipates problems as the body ages before they arise, rather than a responsive one that reacts to problems after a crisis. This approach is based on two pillars:

- The first is providing practical systems to reduce stress and trauma on the body as it ages that causes wearing to the joints, such as knees and ankles, through exoskeletal supports that grow as the challenges to the body grow through aging, physical stress or accident. This also relates to rehabilitative support after an accident. The proposal being that this would become accepted practice culturally and therefore when the person is older and the problems required a more comprehensive, or specialised exoskeleton, they would be used to the practice of wearing it and comfortable working with its idiosyncrasies.
- The second involves creating a responsive, supportive environment based on personal monitoring that adapts to the changing needs of the person as they age to support independence into old age, both physically and cognitively.

Society now has appropriate tools able to address these challenges, and a generation growing up that for the first time could realistically, culturally engage with this proposal, based on their experiences of digital immersion from a young age. The question is whether society is interested in developing systems for future generations or focussed on responding to the current industry-driven challenges without preparing for the future the millennials are inheriting.

7.3.1 Adaptive Support Mechanisms

Transhumanism is the theory that the human race can use science and technology to evolve beyond its current physical and mental limitations: "The human organism is a paradigmatic case of ontogenetic adaptation: thanks to an enormously flexible cognitive and behavioral repertoire, including the ability to acquire and transmit cumulative (intergenerational) cultural adaptations, humans can survive and reproduce across a wide range of otherwise hostile developmental conditions" (Powell 2012, p. 150). If populations continue to age, research into technological healthcare solutions will be needed to help reduce the financial burden of future healthcare in order that is does not overwhelm society. In addition, for the positive mental health of an aging population, the ability to remain active and independent in their own home for longer will be the subject of further research. The current confluence of digital technology is supporting new approaches to addressing healthcare. In addition to sensors, data analytics and communication tools, additive manufacturing provides new ways of responding to bespoke healthcare needs. Additive manufacturing, commonly known as 3D printing, first became commercially available as stereolithography 30 years ago. However, the early machines were only able to provide a prototyping service as the processes and materials were not suitable for functional products. As a result, these systems had little impact on healthcare technology for approximately 20 years beyond as surgical planning tools. In the last decade, research into technologies suitable for end-use product manufacture has come to fruition, providing an ability to create functional products in a wide range of materials, from polymers and ceramics to metals. The reason this is significant in this context, is that whilst there are a wide range of processes within the banner of additive manufacturing, the production approach is based on a 3D computer model of the product and the elimination of tooling. This allows for the customisation of each individual part as required, which is an extremely useful tool for clinicians and designers working in healthcare where the human body provides the ultimate use-case for bespoke manufacturing. Until additive manufacturing, production relied solely on the ability to design products for a mass market to justify the high costs of tooling. Where an individual, customised solution was required, conventional manufacturing was unable to respond. As a result, in situations such as orthopaedic clinics where occupational therapists build splits, the dominant practice is to manipulate these by hand from flat sheets of plastic, informed by the skill and experience of the clinician, to suit the needs of the individual patient. This is a relatively slow, and potentially inaccurate process, without the ability for monitoring and validation of the decisions made by the therapist, or the tracking of patient rehabilitation in response to specific strategies to create a data-base over time. For clinics with long waiting lists, the ability to speed up the process, or remove it from the clinic where possible through the deskilling of the manufacture of the product, allows the clinician to focus on the patient at an expert level and evolve practice based on information gathered over time. Additive manufacturing in the current decade can be used effectively in end-use products, from aerospace to automotive and whilst the range of technologies it encompasses do not compete directly with mass production by printing as scale or speed or cost, they do allow for bespoke manufacturing. The majority of inner-ear hearing aides, for example, are 3D printed based on individual scans and printed en-masse. Orthokids[7] in Australia is a company that uses 3D printing for infant helmets to address medical issues with the development of the skull, based on patient scans. This eliminates the need for plaster moulds, which were problematic when infants were involved. In addition, because of the use of a 3D CAD model as a base for the print, it is possible to reprint a helmet that is damaged, and, if needed, scale the model up as required as the child grows. This iterative development is characteristic of the use of additive manufacturing, with products evolving in response to customer feedback and to changing needs. The accessible

[7] http://www.orthokids.com.au/https://www.youtube.com/watch?v=WoZ2BgPVtA0

adaptability of additive manufacturing provides the opportunity to create products that can be altered by the user themselves or carers.

Additive manufacturing is used in prosthetics, in particular low-cost prosthetics for children. This is because in conventional manufacturing the growth of the child made prosthetics quickly obsolete, as well as heavy and costly and in the majority of cases, children received no prosthetic. 3D printing networks, such as established through the work at e-Nable prosthetics (Schull 2015), mean that prosthetics customised to the child, both in terms of fit and aesthetics, are now achievable. The function of an e-Nable prosthetic is limited, but allow the child to participate more fully in everyday activities. The example of Emma's Magic Arms[8] in 2012 is more relevant to the proposal in this chapter (Webster 2013). Two-year old Emma was born with arthrogryposis multiplex congenita (AMC). This severely limited her movement. Equipment called the Wilmington Robotic Exoskeleton (WREX) was available for children from the age of six to help them control and support their limbs but the equipment was too heavy for a younger child. The head of paediatric engineering and a research designer at the Nemours/Alfred I. duPont hospital scaled the device down and 3D printed it on a Stratasys Dimension to fit the 2-year old. The result was light-weight and low-cost, and the technology accessible which means that as the child grows, replacing parts to allow the mechanisms to grow with her will be possible.

Since that time, there has been considerable development in the use of additive manufacturing to create customised prosthetics. Examples such as the Exo[9] prosthetic by William Root, and the early work of Bespoke Innovations (Sorrel 2010), illustrate the use of the technology to move the product out of the purely functional sphere into the development of relatable product. In this, the example of dancers and athletes, such as Amy Mullins, have helped to change the cultural understanding and acceptance of prosthetics beyond the mirroring of existing limbs (Pullin 2009). Mullins embraced the use of prosthetics to add abilities and projections of character in a conscious way that addresses stigmas attached to prosthetics.

In this proposal, orthoses would become more prevalent and acceptable in the everyday lives of older people. In order for this to be possible, additive manufacturing is needed to create lightweight, personalised products that address specific physical needs. Figure 7.1 shows a scoliosis back brace customised to his personal prescription by the designer, Christopher Miller.[10] By using messo structures of varying thickness, the designer was able to control the amount and direction of movement of the wearer, based on clinical advice. The work of researchers on the development of responsive products that adapt to incoming data, demonstrated in the example of a bicycle helmet that responds to body metrics to open and close vents to optimize the experience for the rider (Novak et al. 2019), illustrate the potential to create a system of integrated monitoring and reactive mechanisms to support health care initiatives in the future. Such digital systems are becoming

[8] https://www.youtube.com/watch?v=WoZ2BgPVtA0

[9] https://www.behance.net/gallery/20696469/Exo-Prosthetic-Leg

[10] https://www.kajewski-miller.com/https://www.lerner.ccf.org/

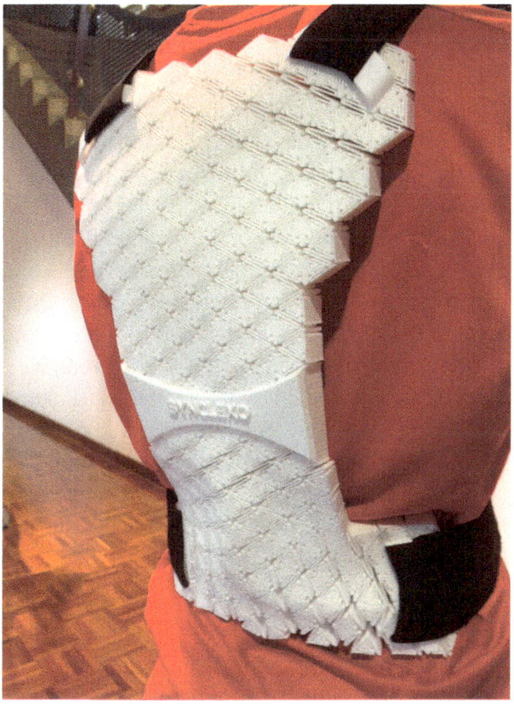

Fig. 7.1 Miller scoliosis back brace 2016

increasingly responsive and complex, providing increasingly complex webs of data. Extending the current aged care monitoring systems to this level of complexity, directly monitoring the human body, and extending into the surrounding environment, provides opportunities for a different level of proactive care. Much as aspects of engineering have shifted through the use of sensors to anticipating structural and material fatigue, allowing the company to replace parts before they fail, reducing downtime, so this approach could create support systems where, for example, a person experiencing difficulties with balance or a hand tremor, even at a level where they are not yet fully aware of it, could be helped before an accident rather than after one.

If exoskeletons were lightweight and developed bespoke to medical needs as the person ages, then they could increasingly support movement and balance. Whereas an older person would be unlikely to be comfortable with wearing one – just as they are frequently resistant to other assistive technology such as walking frames – if they were used to them and if it was commonplace and normal to wear them from a much younger age, then there would be more compliance.

An incentive to begin this process would be to support their integration into sport on the basis of extending the users' involvement with the activity for longer. Either as protection as a preventative as the individual begins to age, becoming more vulnerable to injury, or as a way of continuing to take part in sports as weakness or injury occurs. Individually designed, adaptive braces, supporting ankles or knees for example, could be worn during or between games to reduce the point of everyday wear exacerbated by the particular sport. The customisation of supportive wearables does not have to be limited to rigid components (as illustrated by the work of Bristol University on 3D printing 'soft muscles', Dicker et al. 2017) as increasingly e-textiles are being developed that can alter the performance characteristics of materials for specific use requirements. Whilst sports provide a clear example of where technology can provide physical support, this approach applies to a wide range of quality of life activities, both social and solitary. The ability to continue with hobbies or to develop new hobbies based on technological supports – e.g. supporting arm weaknesses for guitarists, aids to stability for dance or exercise classes and accuracy in sewing, memory aides for lifelong learning – would enhance the quality of life for older people, central to the proactive approach to mental stimulation for older people described by Grotz *et al* (2017) and mental stimulation and emotional well-being discussed by Coulter (2011, p. 256): "A new kind of development is in the offing. A radical plan for the conversion of a long-stay setting into a residential college for older people…now seems much more likely to be adopted by imaginative providers….the new thinking about education, creativity and the quality of life offers promise to us all."

7.3.2 Ubiquitous Computing

Designing products increasingly involves developing systems of online interactions as well as the physical objects. Examples include sporting goods with online community platforms to track data and allow for interactions to compare performance. Specialised sports shoes, such as for professional basketball, can be embedded with sensors that allow tracking for the athlete and coach. Cyclists can race each other over the same stretch of road at different times, with their performance shared online in competition. Mouthguards, such as developed by the Lerner Research Institute[12] and Cleveland Clinic Concussion Centre (Alberts et al. 2017), use digital impression systems for customisation and also track impact data through on-board sensors. The detection systems embedded in the Cleveland Clinic mouthguard record the impacts received to the head by players and measures the factors that can determine if a concussion may have occurred based on whether an impact exceeds a predetermined threshold. The linear and rotational acceleration rates, the location and direction of an impact, are displayed in real time to the training team through a mobile phone app.

Research led by Autodesk research fellow, Mickey McManus, who co-authored the book *Trillions: Thriving in the Emerging Information Ecology* (Lucas et al. 2012), monitored automotive data relating to the performance of the car including impact of exterior forces and environmental conditions on its structure and surfaces over time. However, it also tracked the performance and emotions of the driver, through monitoring systems, for example cloud-based EEG and measuring the pressure of the driver's grip on the steering wheel. This allows the researcher to track the anticipation of the driver to events, as well as reaction times and emotional responses to particular driving situations. In terms of health care for older people living at home, this constant monitoring could be introduced as a preventative. This would provide the individual and their careers with measurable information on the experience of the person throughout the day, allowing them to identify pressure points, times of stress or anxiety, and also their ability to take on levels of personal responsibility and independence. It could also provide the data for the development of a more responsive, integrated environment to support the user in their home interactions, aligned to Greenfield's view of holistic, digital integration (2006, p. 23): "Fifteen years downstream from its tentative beginnings at Olivetti, the idea of the ordinary as a new frontier for computing is finally starting to bear fruit. We're beginning to see the walls and books, sweaters, and tabletops around us reconsidered as sensors, interface objects, or active sites that respond in some way to data they receive from outside. Eventually, we may even come to see them as the articulated parts of a massively distributed computational engine."

In an active-monitoring, enabled environment, mobility for the older person could increase if they could interact with their environment in real time for redirection if they became confused. An activated environment that recognised the individual and provided both reassurances could support greater confidence in venturing out and returning back home. Environment systems, such as for real-time particle monitoring for air quality (Marques et al. 2019), and monitoring systems such as Google Nest,[11] already collect data that builds a database of information about the way a house is used and inform adaptive response of integrated systems to those needs. By creating more responsive environments that learn to attune to stress levels monitored for example by movement or Cloud based EEGs stress could be reduced. This would also be useful in situations where stress can erupt into aggression, for example in accident and emergency departments. Vital signs would be fed from the activated environment into a digital system that fed alerts to staff, similar to those on a hospital bedside monitor. Any warning signs in the waiting patients, such as raised blood pressure, could be responded to before problems arose. An activated environment could track, encourage, facilitate and even respond to the emotional response to individuals. It could also provide reassurance for carers and family.

7.4 Future Generations

"It is essential for humans at this time in our evolution to begin to identify what is being lost through our utter dependence on technology and to determine how it may affect humanity long term. Furthermore, we must not think only of the long-term effects: we must also ask ourselves about the intentions of our actions"(St. Clair 2016, p. 43). The proposal forming the basis of the chapter is that advances in digital technology relating to home care are providing the foundations for a new

[11] https://nest.com/au/

cyber-physicality, that could support aging in place, by demonstrating their ability to enable greater independence and a changed relationship between the person, their support team and their environment. The culture around health care and assistive technology is changing, as illustrated by the prosthetics and orthoses discourse, where increasingly extrovert extensions to the human body are accepted and celebrated in society, for example in the artistic designs for Viktoria Modesta within The Alternative Limb Project.[12]

For the already digitally immersed, millennial generation, it is arguably possible to take this to a level where digitally enhanced healthcare is integral to their lives, potentially reducing health care costs in the future and allowing more people to live at home for longer. The time is right for a rethink of healthcare for the coming generations. There is an unprecedented acceptance of data monitoring, gathering, sharing, analysing and applying to problem solving that the millennial generation onwards will be immersed more comfortably immersed within. According to Greenfield (2006, p. 11): "In this context, "ubiquitous" meant not merely "in every place," but also "in everything." Ordinary objects, from coffee cups to raincoats to the paint on the walls, would be reconsidered as sites for the sensing and processing of information and would wind up endowed with surprising new properties. Best of all, people would interact with these systems fluently and naturally, barely noticing the powerful informatics they were engaging. The innumerable hassles presented by personal computing would fade into history." Electronics have dropped in price with production expanding exponentially since the turn of the century. According to the McKinsey Global Institute, the economic impact of connected products and IoT applications could be from $3.9 trillion to $11.1 trillion per year by 2025 (Manyika & Chui 2015). ARM[15], one of the largest microprocessor IP companies in the world, had an annual production in excess of three billion per year in 2008. In 2018, they are aiming to support the seamless management of trillions rather than billions of connected devices. Data analytics is at a level where it is driving decision making on the stock exchange, too fast for humans. Machine learning is developing rapidly, according to McManus, who described, during the RAPID manufacturing conference keynote (2017), *Networked Matter and the Nature of Things*, microprocessors that learn 'like a child'. Machine learning in robotics has advanced, both in terms of creating increasingly human-like robots but also in respect to online avatars that can respond to queries previously addressed in a call centre, to distributed robotics where levels of automation and robotics are embedded into structures and environments to create an integrated system.

In the future that the younger generations will be growing up into, the physical and virtual environments will most likely be far more integrated, with augmented or cross reality creating more overlaps on a daily basis. Narototzky (2016, p. 157) states "In the early twenty-first century, it is becoming increasingly clear that the new digital era heralds much more than a simple improvement of existing capabilities." It could be that in the future going out without lightweight glasses fitted with augmented reality (AR) capability will not be possible, as road signs and directions

[12] http://www.thealternativelimbproject.com/

are provided by AR, allowing for change from a central location on demand. Vehicles and people will be tracked, much as they already are by BMW to create a massive, flowing data base analysed at a meta level as well as monitored at a micro level (Marr 2017). In the twenty-first century, the younger generations are brought up in societies where pop-culture references challenge ideas of uniformity. Instead they support the shift to personal control over projected appearance and character. This is illustrated in the 2018 film *Ready Player One,*[13] set in a post-apocalyptic world where humans have given up trying to repair the damage to the planet inflicted through war and environmental destruction, and instead live as much as possible in a virtual world where they can choose their own avatars, socialise and even work within the system. There has also been a rise in body-hacking. This is both in relation to adding aesthetic prosthetics to the body, for example skull horns, and in respect to electronics, for example embedding passes under the skin. On the surface of the skin, there have been developments in the applications of temporary tattoos 3D printed onto the body with conductive inks, for example to alert soldiers to chemical attacks or spills and the 3D printing of electronics is gaining traction. Research funded by the US Defence Advanced Research Project Agency carried out by the U.C. Berkeley's Human Engineering and Robotics Laboratory resulted in a lightweight exoskeleton called the Berkeley Lower Extremity Exoskeleton (BLEEX), that allows an individual to essentially pilot a heavy payload rather than directly carry it themselves. At the same time, Lockhead Martin and Berkeley Bionics research has focussed on the development of the Human Universal Load Carrier aimed at augmenting performance whilst reducing metabolic cost. Whilst these developments are targeted at specific functions required for Defence Force requirements, this research, alongside products designed to support specific industry workers, such as the Eksovest[14] in the construction industry, which supports the arms much as in the Emma's Magic Arms project, are providing increasing numbers of examples of products that demonstrate human physical augmentation relevant to the proposals for supporting healthy aging in this chapter, both for the older person and for the physical challenges facing carers described by Briane and Wray (2016, p. 98): "The effects of caregiving on physical health have received less attention than the effects on psychological health. Yet the evidence suggests that caregiving can have a deleterious effect on the physical well-being of caregivers because caregiving often involves some level of physical effort. This physical work may include providing a wide variety of assistance with activities of daily living, including bathing, toileting, dressing, lifting, moving and transferring, and doing additional physical chores." In addition to physical, practical considerations, artistic works, such Anouk Wipprecht's digitally enhanced wearables[15], illustrate how the personalisation of product through the use of digital technologies can extend to emotional interactions and responses in the future. Wipprecht's work includes the Spider Dress, which is fitted with sensors that an individual can set to mark their personal

[13] https://en.wikipedia.org/wiki/Ready_Player_One_(film)

[14] https://eksobionics.com/

[15] http://www.anoukwipprecht.nl/

space, with the dress reacting to entry past that barrier. Her most recent dress for BMW provides reactive mood lighting based on biometrics. Whilst this research is expressive and provocative, its implications for enabling greater, potentially more nuanced, and certainly more inclusive, levels of communication are evident. A research focus on the practical mechanics of creating support systems, both in relation to e-health and physical assistive technologies, is understandable. However, the human element of designing for a cultural acceptance by individuals and social groups needs to be central for compliance. Design for ability has changed the discussion of supportive technology from medical device to wearable (Pullin 2009). Terminology is changing, and the relationship between an individual and assistive technology is becoming more personal (illustrated in the work of the Alternative Limb company) and more empowered. The historically paternalistic view of medical health, in terms of access to records, specialist referrals and test results, as well as the functional aesthetics constraints of medical devices of the twentieth century is being increasingly challenged in the twenty-first. The cultural acceptance of digital technology-enabled or constructed devices needs to be built alongside their mechanical performance. Haptic devices to ensure the physical and digital remain connected and together are human centred and a collaboration between the engineering and scientific community and the arts and humanities to ensure that the positive aspects of digital technology as empowering the individual are not overwhelmed by a disconnect from the human experience that fosters quality of life and reduces isolation. Maybe, too, by creating a virtual life with more depth and longevity than current social media provides, the individual could reconcile the digital and physical space into a more integrated view of the world as shared between the two. As Lipson and Kurman (2013, p. 13) suggest: "The end of the 20th Century was about information becoming digital. The 21st Century is going to be about bringing the virtual world into closer alignment with the physical one."

7.5 Conclusion

Designed smart environments have been an inevitable development of the expansion of computing across platforms. Supporting healthcare is a positive application of integrated technologies. However, where people are involved, the transition to systems thinking in this context needs to be managed over time. It is essentially a change in mindset that needs to be fostered by design. New cultural practices need to evolve that respond to a digitally integrated approach. As the twenty-first century brings digitally immersion, the change in mindset should be possible for the next generation if it is addressed sensitively now. It may be too, that those in middle age, who have demonstrated a willingness to work with digital technology for activities such as sport and weight-loss, would be open to a new approach to preparing for their older years if it led to the possibility of staying at home for longer. Personal and community empowerment and financial sustainability is the aim, with lifelong life enabled by technology as a conscious, proactive healthcare goal.

Glossary

Transhumanism The belief or theory that the human race can evolve beyond its current physical and mental limitations, especially by means of science and technology.

Centenarian A person who is 100 years or older.

Internet of Things Objects that are fitted with microchips and connected to the internet in a network that allows them to interact with each other and to be controlled remotely as a system.

References

Actuaries Institute of Australia (2012). *Australia's longevity Tsunami: What should we do?* Actuaries Institute White Paper.

Alberts, J., Linder, S., Russman, A., Figler, R., Cruickshank, J., et al. (2017). Utilisation of an electronic incident report to document injury-related demographics and medical triage in youth, high school and college athletes. *British Journal of Sports Medicine London, 51*(11), A12. https://doi.org/10.1136/bjsports-2016-097270.29.

Briane, M., & Wray, J. (2016). *Supporting families & carers: A nursing perspective*. Boca Raton: CRC Press Tailor & Francis Group.

Bridges, J., Loukanova, S., & Carrera, P. (2008). Patient empowerment in health care. In Heggenhougen, H. (Ed.), *International encyclopedia of public health* (pp. 17–28). Elsevier, Science Direct.

Brown, P. (2018). *The future of healthcare may reside in your smart clothes*. Mouser Electronics: https://au.mouser.com/applications/healthcare-may-reside-in-smart-clothing/

Coulter, A. (2011). *Engaging patients in healthcare*. Maidenhead/Berkshire: McGraw Hill.

Dicker, M. Baker, A., Iredale, R., Nacify, S., Bond, I., Faul, C. Rossiter, J., SPinks, G., & Weaver, P. (2017). *Light-triggered soft artificial muscles: Molecular-level amplification of actuation control signals, nature scientific reports*. Published: 23 August 2017. Nature.com/scientific reports.

Dombroski, C., Balsdon, M., & Froats, A. (2014). *The use of a low cost 3D scanning and printing tool in the manufacture of custom-made foot orthoses: A preliminary study*. BMC Research Notes 2014, 7:443. http://www.biomedcentral.com/1756-0500/7/443

Farahani, B., Fizouzi, F., Chang, V., Badaroglu, M., Constant, N., & Mankodiya, K. (2018). Towards fog-driven IoT eHealth: Promises and challenges of IoT in medicine and healthcare. *Future Generation Computer Systems, 78*, 659–676. Elsevier, Science Direct.

Ghani, A. (2018). Healthcare electronics – A step closer to future smart cities. *Information & Communication Technology Express*. Elsevier. https://doi.org/10.1016/j.icte.2018.01.009

Greenfield, A. (2006). *Everyware: The dawning age of ubiquitous computing*. Berkeley: New Riders. AIGA.

Kalid, N., Zaidan, A., Zaidan, B. Salman, O., Hashim, M., & Muzammil, H. (2017). Based real time remote health monitoring systems: A review on patients prioritization and related "Big Data" using body sensors information and communication technology. Journal of Medical Systems, (2018) 42: 30. https://doi.org/10.1007/s10916-017-0883-4

Kelly, K. (2010). *What technology wants* (p. 37). New York: Penguin Group.

Lipson, H., & Kurman, M. (2013). *Fabricated*. Indianapolis: Wiley.

Lucas, P., Bailey, J., & McManus, M. (2012). *Trillions: thriving in the emerging information ecology*. Hoboken: Wiley.

Manyika, J., & Chui, M. (2015). By 2025, Internet of Things applications could have $11 trillion impact. *Fortune*, July 22.
Markowitz, J., & Herr, H. (2016). Human leg model predicts muscle forces, states, and energetics during walking. *PLOS Computational Biology*, 1–30. https://doi.org/10.1371/journal.pcbi.1004912.
Marr, B. (2017). How BMW uses artificial intelligence and big data to design and build cars of tomorrow. *Forbes*, August 1.
Marques, G., Roque Ferreira, C., & Pitarma, R. (2019). Indoor air quality assessment using a CO_2 monitoring system based on Internet of Things. *Journal of Medical Systems*. https://doi.org/10.1007/s10916-019-1184-x
Morgann, L., Frankowski, A., Roth, E., Keimig, L., Zimmerman, S., & Eckert, J. (2012). *Quality assisted living: Informing practice through research*. New York: Springer.
Narototzky, V. (2016). Beyond perfection. In P. Sparke & F. Fisher (Eds.), *The Routledge companion to design studies* (pp. 156–168). Abingdon on Thames: Routledge.
Novak, J., Burton, D. & Crouch, T. (2019). Aerodynamic test results of bicycle helmets in different configurations: Towards a responsive design. *Journal of Sports Engineering and Technology*. https://doi.org/10.1177%2F1754337118822613.
Petrova, R. (2014). *Educating designers from generation Y: Challenges and alternatives*. In DS E&PDE14 proceedings, Design Education and Human Technology Relations, New York, NY, p. 525.
Powell, R. (2012). The future of human evolution. *The British Journal for the Philosophy of Science, 63*(1), 145–175.
Pullin, G. (2009). *Design meets disability*. Boston: MIT Press.
Quandt, B., Braun, F., Ferrario, D., Rossi, R., Scheel-Sailer, A., Wolf, M., Bona, G., Hufenus, R., Scherer, L., & Bosele, L. (2017). Body-monitoring with photonic textiles: A reflective heartbeat sensor based on polymer optical fibres. *Journal of the Royal Society Interface, 14*, 20170060. https://doi.org/10.1098/rsif.2017.0060.
Rowland, C., Goodman, E., Charlier, M., Light, A., & Lui, A. (2015). *Designing connected products: UX for the consumer Internet of Things*. Sebastopol: O'Reilly Media.
Schull, J. (2015). Enabling the future: Crowdsourced 3D-printed prosthetics as a model for open source assistive technology, innovation and mutual aid. In *Proceedings of the 17th International ACM SIGACCESS conference on computers & accessibility*, 26 October (pp. 1–1). https://doi.org/10.1145/2700648.2809870
Smith, P., Sahar, H., Graf, A., Flanagan, A., Reiners, K., Kuo, K., Roh, J., & HArros, G. (2009). Brace evaluation in children with dipelgic cerebral palsy with a jump gait pattern. *Journal of Bone and Joint Surgery, 91*(2), 356. https://doi.org/10.2106/JBJS.G.01369.
Sorrel, C. (2010). *Bespoke designs makes beautiful custom prosthetic legs, wired*. https://www.wired.com/2010/12/bespoke-designs-makes-beautiful-custom-prosthetic-legs/
St. Clair, A. (2016). Critical thinking, wisdom and paying homage to the human experience. *Voices, 42*(1/2), 41–43.
Webster, S. (2013). Additive manufacturing: A custom solution for the medical industry. *Manufacturing Engineering, Dearborn, 150*(4), 87–91.

Chapter 8
Grey Smart Societies: Supporting the Social Inclusion of Older Adults by Smart Spatial Design

Nienke Moor and Masi Mohammadi

Abstract In this chapter, we explore the possibility to use the living environment (of inpatient and outpatient care settings) for facilitating and encouraging the social inclusion of older adults in an increasingly smart society. We therefore pay attention to the spatial and smart design of emerging housing typologies for older adults in the Netherlands in which social activities and encounters take place.

Our first explorative research question reads: To what extent can the social inclusion of older adults with physical and/or mental disabilities contribute to their well-being? Based on (sociological) theories and existing knowledge from the literature, we can conclude that there are sufficient indications that the social inclusion of senior citizens in society have positive effects on their well-being, by strengthening social resources, in the case of intimate ties, and by stimulating public familiarity and random encounters. Moreover, it can be argued that encounters between elderly people with (either physical or mental) disabilities and healthy others can have a positive influence on the social acceptance of the former.

Following on the above, our second research question examines which spatial and smart interventions in and around inpatient and outpatient care settings can stimulate social inclusion. In this light, we discussed two new housing typologies in the Netherlands that can positively affect the inclusion of senior citizens in society: Farm sharing, which is particularly suitable for vital older adults who want to live independently for as long as possible, and the Care Estate, that seems to be a suitable form of living for vulnerable elderly people with physical and mental comorbidity, such as dementia. These housing typologies demonstrate the existence of an

N. Moor
Kivi Chair Architecture in Health, HAN University of Applied Sciences,
Arnhem, The Netherlands
e-mail: Nienke.Moor@han.nl

M. Mohammadi (✉)
Chair Smart Architectural Technologies, Eindhoven University of Technology,
Eindhoven, The Netherlands

Kivi Chair Architecture in Health, HAN University of Applied Sciences,
Arnhem, The Netherlands
e-mail: m.mohammadi@tue.nl

N. Biloria (ed.), *Data-driven Multivalence in the Built Environment*, S.M.A.R.T. Environments, https://doi.org/10.1007/978-3-030-12180-8_8

interplay between spatial design and smart technologies, in the sense that these factors can make each other superfluous or can provide added value.

In order to be able to optimize the well-being and health status of their residents, housing typologies must meet the needs of (vulnerable) older adults with regard to care, and social interaction, autonomy as much as possible. The art of designing new suitable housing typologies for older adults therefore should be based on linking different layers of people's living environment: the care environment, the socio-spatial environment, and the digital environment. The two examples of housing typologies that we cover in this chapter, demonstrate how these different layers can be interconnected in order to design a new suitable housing concept.

Keywords Emerging housing typologies · Older adults · Social inclusion · Smart homes · Smart neighbourhoods

8.1 Introduction

Nowadays, housing and care in many countries all over the world are facing a number of significant challenges, such as double ageing, the reducing number of caregivers, the growing number of one-person households (among older adults), urbanization and adjusting to the digital era. As a result, the existing housing and care models have to be adapted. The current sectoral and hierarchical structures in the Netherlands are gradually making way for new ways of thinking that are based on customer-driven demand, informal community systems, integrated network-based collaboration, co-creation and trust. These social and technological changes require a renewed view from all stakeholders, with the focus shifted from being a 'producer' to 'becoming a service provider'. The user is the main part of this ongoing, multi-sectoral approach.

This chapter is written for experts who (want to) actively participate in the field of smart living (care) environments. Over the past decade, many experimental housing typologies in the field of smart technologies and care have been developed. This chapter provides insight into the current situation of housing for a rapidly ageing population residing in rural areas in the Netherlands, and explains how architecture is becoming a service provider by applying concepts like care estate and farm sharing. It also provides a basis for identifying factors that could influence implementation of smart technology in these housing typologies.

8.1.1 Social Inclusion in Health Care

Community participation is considered to be an important element of human functioning (Young et al. 2004; Verdonschot et al. 2009), because it may contribute to living a meaningful life, being comfortable and feeling at home. Especially in old age, when a person occupies less and less space (Oswald et al. 2005; Wiles 2005). The strength of (self-organized) civic society in the Netherlands forms a good basis for flourishing communities. In order to create an age-friendly community, the design of the living environment should be adapted to the physical and mental disabilities that older adults often face, and should support them in their daily routine and social activities (Lui et al. 2009).

In developed countries, a major change in the health care system in recent decades is the transition from social exclusion to social inclusion of (older) people with physical and mental disabilities (Tonkens and Weijers 1999; Leff and Warner 2006). As a reaction to ageing society, older adults are encouraged to live independently for as long as possible. Older adults who require care nowadays live less frequently in (segregated care) facilities, but live relatively independently, with the necessary support, in a residential area (Van Alphen et al. 2010; Verplanke et al. 2010). Who needs care, receives support from formal care providers, but for an increasing share they are dependent on support provided by informal care providers (Van Houtven and Norton 2004). For receiving affection and support, older adults therefore become increasingly dependent on their own social network. Moreover, the way in which their social contacts are organized becomes increasingly important, because these often do not take place in an organized context and in designated areas, as is often the case in inpatient care settings.

Also, in inpatient settings, when older adults can no longer live independently, the emphasis is increasingly on promoting social integration and participation. Although in many of these facilities there is a strong focus on social activities, this does not automatically lead to the social inclusion of the residents, as the activities do not always meet their needs (Knight and Mellor 2007). Moreover, the organized social activities are often focused on stimulating social interaction with fellow residents and not so much on stimulating social interaction with the outside world.

In this article, we explore the possibility to use the living environment (of inpatient and outpatient care settings) for facilitating and stimulating the social inclusion of older adults in an increasingly smart society. We therefore pay attention to the spatial and smart design of emerging housing typologies for older adults in the Netherlands in which social activities and encounters take place.

8.1.2 Residential Care Facilities as Communities and Social Institutions

Policy makers emphasize that older adults (with physical and mental disabilities) are part of society and must remain in contact with people from outside their own community. Social inclusion of this target group is expected to be important, as it contributes to their dignity and autonomy and reduces the likelihood of social isolation (Guest and Wierzbicki 1999). However, Cummins and Lau (2003) argue that community integration is not the same as community exposure. In order for community integration to be beneficial for people (with disabilities), a 'sense of community' needs to be created. Cummins and Lau doubt whether this sense of community can be created in the general community, or only in the community of people with disabilities. Although there are some indications that social interaction is beneficial for the well-being of older adults (with disabilities) (Moyle et al. 2011; Huxhold et al. 2013; Shankar et al. 2015), it remains unclear under which conditions these positive effects occur.

In this chapter we will discuss the living environment of inpatient and outpatient care settings as a potential meeting place, both from a sociological and a built environment perspective. Based on theoretical considerations, we hypothesize about the impact of social inclusion and random encounters on the well-being of people. Subsequently, we discuss recent developments in spatial and smart design of inpatient and outpatient care settings that can promote random encounters and social inclusion, and new housing typologies that follow from this. To illustrate these developments in the domain of housing, we describe two new housing concepts for older adults that are currently under development. First, we discuss farm sharing; a new housing concept in which people live in a small community on a (former) farmyard. This concept can be of interest for multiple target groups, but is especially interesting for older adults who want to live independently for as long as possible, and who want to be prepared for a future in which they may have to deal with health problems. Secondly, we want to discuss the care estate, a new housing concept in the Netherlands that can facilitate or even stimulate random encounters with people from nearby villages. As it concerns an inpatient care facility, we will focus here on the target group of elderly people with dementia. After all, this rapidly growing group in society sets certain strict conditions for housing and the living environment.

Our research questions therefore read: To what extent can the social inclusion of older adults with physical and mental disabilities in society contribute to their well-being? Which spatial and smart interventions in and around inpatient and outpatient care settings can stimulate social inclusion?

8.2 Open Communities and the Social Environment

The realization of open care communities, in which older adults with a care demand can continue to be part of society, presupposes a certain level of social inclusion. After all, older adults with disabilities who live in open in- or outpatient residential care facilities make use of the same living environment as other people do. This raises the question why social inclusion is desirable for older adults with physical or mental disabilities, and for what reasons social interaction with healthy others should be stimulated.

8.2.1 Brief Encounters in the Neighbourhood

From the resources perspective (Hobfoll 1989; Diener and Fujita 1995), it can be argued that social resources are part of basic human needs, as they provide people with affection, social support and social integration, and can in a way protect people against negative life events (Jang et al. 2002; Moor et al. 2013). In his work 'Bowling alone', Putnam (2001) argues that social capital is important in maintaining a healthy and safe society. He distinguishes between bonding and bridging social capital. Bonding social capital refers to connections between people of equal status, whereas bridging social capital refers to connections between people who have very little in common. Therefore, bridging social capital is assumed to be an important precondition for the acceptance of minority groups and special target groups, such as older adults with physical or mental disabilities.

The question remains unanswered to what extent social connections can have a positive impact on creating a healthy and safe environment when they are not intimate. The assumption that social resources are important for people's mental well-being is after all based on the idea that people develop intimate relationships with people who are close to them. In the living environment surrounding inpatient and outpatient care settings, however, encounters between older adults and people from the nearby community will often be brief, superficial and accidental in nature. Can they still provide bonding and bridging social capital?

8.2.2 Public Familiarity

In this regard, Blokland (2003, 2008) comes with the concept of public familiarity. She points out that brief encounters in the public space in most cases do not automatically lead to social cohesion, but can be important for the liveability of the neighbourhood. Random encounters can evoke positive feelings among people without serving a specific purpose. They can positively affect people's feelings of safety and security and make them feel at ease in their home environment (Bouwman and Mohammadi 2013). Moreover, it can be argued that public familiarity is important in bridging gaps between groups of people (Cattell et al. 2008), in our case between residents of inpatient and outpatient care settings and (healthy) others. Encounters in the public space can lead to public familiarity in two ways: by facilitating simultaneous use of the public space and by facilitating social interaction through observation (Van Eijk and Engbersen 2011).

Thus, social fabrics are related to place and its design, at least by their shared relationship to chance encounters. From this perspective, place and its smart design can manipulate the occurrence of (random) encounters between people, and the level of social inclusion of older adults (with physical and mental disabilities) in the wider community.

8.3 Open Communities and the Emerging Housing Typologies

8.3.1 Shift from a Medical Model to a Social Model

In the past 20 years, the importance of the physical and social environment in supporting older adults became increasingly stressed (Davis et al. 2009; Yen et al. 2009). The living environment must meet the needs of senior citizens; for the group of vital older adults who are preparing for a future in which they may become vulnerable, and for the group of elderly people who have to deal with physical or mental disabilities. This was put in motion with the arrival of the social model of disability as an alternative to the medical model of disability. According to the medical model, disability is a medical condition that should be fixed in order to provide disabled people with a normal life of good quality. In contrast, the social model of disability states that societal forces are the most important factor in putting people with a disability in a disadvantaged position in society, irrespective of their medical condition. Physical, psychological and intellectual impairments can only lead to 'disability', when society fails to include people with these limitations in its midst. Although the social model of disability received a lot of criticism (Shakespeare 2006), the de-medicalisation of disability is steadily considered to be important. External factors, including the built environment and spatial design, are supposed to support older adults with impairments and to help them integrate in society.

To determine the sense of well-being, we should consider factors beyond the aging body (Tiernan et al. 2013). There is a manifest shift towards preventive concepts that address healthy lifestyles and cities. Accumulated evidences suggest that the integration of the physical and social environment will lead to higher levels of well-being. Literature stresses the importance of such a living environment for an independent, long, vital, and social life. To encourage healthy behaviour, the design of both place and space should be taken into consideration. Place, as the setting which is experienced by residents, and that outlines community engagement, and space, as the need to meet the requirements of users on various domains, like of housing, social participation, health care, and leisure. The design of new housing typologies for older adults and the surrounding living environment should include aspects like sound infrastructure, safety, nature, future-proofness and age-friendliness.

8.3.2 Inclusive Neighbourhoods

As most older adults with mild to moderate impairments remain living at home as long as possible, it is not very surprising that research on the design of outdoor environments in health care focused on the design of public spaces, such as neighbourhoods. However, also in the case of inpatient care facilities, the design of the neighbourhood receives more attention lately, as it often forms part of the living environment in which residential care facilities are situated.

There is increasing recognition for the fact that people with physical and mental disabilities should not live in segregated environments, but in their own environments that should meet the needs of people with and without disabilities (Brorsson et al. 2011). However, in order to allow older adults with physical or mental disabilities to stay and live at home, the neighbourhood has to be designed in such way that it helps people to navigate, to stimulate them to go outside, and to minimize any possible hindrance. When the requirements of people with dementia are not met by the design of the neighbourhood, they run the risk of becoming homebound and socially isolated (Mitchell and Burton 2006).

Mitchell and Burton conclude that outdoor environments in more general, and dementia-friendly neighbourhoods more specific, should be places that are familiar, legible, distinctive, accessible, comfortable and safe (2010, p. 16). The outdoor spaces in neighbourhoods do not only offer opportunities for physical activity and sensory stimulation, but also for social interaction. Therefore, the neighbourhood should not only be understood as a physical space, but also as a social place in which weak and strong links between people can develop and are maintained (Gardner 2011; Keady et al. 2012). The home and direct living environment of older adults play a key role in their social life, as their social recourses are increasingly connected with social life in the neighbourhood (Guest and Wierzbicki 1999). Conversely, a neighbourhood that is not supportive regarding older adults, can make them feel out of place, which can eventually lead to social disconnectedness and even isolation (Burns et al. 2012).

8.3.3 Empathic Technologies and the Democratization of the Living Environment

The spread of ICT into all aspects of our daily lives appears to have radically increased the scale, range, and the manner of social interaction. Game-changing technologies like IoT, social media, Visual and Augmented Reality can improve the connection between people's needs and their living environment, and connect the indoor life to life outdoors, as well. On the one hand, an age-friendly environment, according to a large number of researchers (e.g. Skouby et al. 2014), needs to be smart. On the other hand, smart technology also means that older people need to know how they have to handle the technology and how they have to cope with the demands that the smart environment places upon them. This makes the (home-based) technology both an opportunity and a challenge, enabling and disabling at the same time. Getting old in our 'hypercognitive society', as Post (2000) states, where assumptions about cognitive ability are implicit, seems to increasingly become a challenge for a large number of older adults. Though, in order to create an age-friendly community with open care, the living environment must be more than just smart and become empathic (Mohammadi 2017). Mohammadi advocates for the total integration of the physical, social and digital environment. Living environments that fully anticipate and adapt to habits and daily patterns of users.

By this we also mean that the living environment must meet the needs of all target groups who are part of the community. This is especially challenging when some target groups, such as older adults with disabilities, make specific demands on the design of their home and neighbourhood. A supportive living environment in which social activities of older adults are facilitated or even encouraged is an important precondition for an empathic neighbourhood. It applies a multidisciplinary focus to the relation between older persons and their socio-spatial surroundings. From this perspective, smart technologies can contribute to the 'democratization' of the living environment (von Hippel 2005), in the sense that its empathetic design meets both implicit and explicit needs of the different target groups in society. For older adults, especially with disabilities, this is an important step forward in creating socially inclusive communities.

8.4 Organized Independency: Shared Spaces, Shared Lives?

Various studies (e.g. Mens and Wagenaar 2009) show that housing for older adults has become more dynamic over time and increasingly new typologies have been established. Three factors have mainly determined the development of the housing for this target group: (1) the societal transformations including the changing position of older people in society, (2) the policies and regulations dealing with the organization of care, and (3) emerging technologies. The older adults are becoming a highly heterogeneous target group with a dynamic need pattern.

It seems as if they are simultaneously becoming more individualistic and more socially engaged; whilst the individualization trend continues, developments such as community-forming are manifesting themselves. 'Social sharing', also amongst the older adults, has even become an economy.

One can state that older citizens have been organizing their own independent future (Mohammadi et al. 2018). Recent phenomena such as the participation society, the principle of self-governance and innovative living and care cooperation, are raising a demand for new housing typologies, but are also sources of new creative initiatives.

In this case, the discussion about architecture mainly focuses on how the space can contribute to positive health and social interaction among residents. Architecture is seen as an enabler for both the individual and the community. The so-called 'Architecture of Place' creates the optimal interaction between space and social structure and stimulates activities. An example of a new housing typology in this perspective is farm sharing, which focuses on the importance of social participation and (re)activation in housing for older adults.

8.4.1 Farm Sharing as an Example

An example of a new housing concept in the Netherlands in which 'sharing spaces' is central, is farm sharing. This housing concept situated in rural areas is a possible answer to the demand for new housing typologies for older adults who want to continue living independently for as long as possible. It also can be considered a reaction to current and future societal and demographic challenges, such as population ageing, inpatient to outpatient care transitions, and rural depopulation.

In addition to the fact that liveability in rural areas has come under pressure, another important development is taking place within the agricultural sector: farmland abandonment. It is expected that in the coming years many farmers will quit their business. As a consequence, a considerable part of the agricultural real estate will lose its function and become vacant. This development leads to the extensive task of demolishing or renovating agricultural buildings and stables in such a way that it will not damage, or even improve, the quality of the living environment. In this light, in several municipalities in the Netherlands, local regulations exist that encourage (former) farmers to demolish the agricultural buildings on their farmyard. The general idea is that when (former) agricultural buildings are demolished, owners are compensated by being granted construction rights. For example, a new home can be built on the property. These local regulations offer room for creative thinking about innovative solutions for both renovation and demolition of agricultural real estate.

In the light of the above-mentioned local regulations, the new housing concept of farm sharing seems to be a promising bottom-up initiative. This housing concept is situated on a (former) farmyard on which several houses have been built. The (former) farm can serve as the main house, in which space can also be designed for shared use. The concept of farm sharing focuses on small-scale living in a green and rural environment and facilitates and even stimulates social interaction and solidarity between its residents. Farm sharing can also be part of rural development, as it provides a destination to former agricultural real estate, in such a way that the rural and agricultural identity of the living environment is not harmed.

Although farm sharing could be attractive for several target groups, in particular it seems to be a positive initiative in the context of population ageing and increasing loneliness among older adults. This housing concept offers people the possibility to establish several generations on one farmyard, thereby facilitating social interaction and informal care. The concept also offers the possibility to offer housing to a group of seniors who, whether or not in advance, choose to grow old together in a rural environment and want to share facilities with each other.

8.4.1.1 Smart Design in Farm Sharing

Mohammadi (2014) examined the implementation of 75 Dutch home automation projects, realized in more than 8000 homes, between 2002 and 2013. She concludes that creating a smart living environment for older adults can help them live independently longer, while maintaining quality of life. However, the use of home automation in elderly homes is not implemented on a large-scale yet.

Home automation applied in homes for older adults can have different functions, such as increasing comfort, establishing contact between residents and (professional) caretakers, creating a safe and secure living environment, and registering people's health status. However, this study demonstrates that there is an import difference in the use of smart technologies in inpatient and outpatient care settings. In inpatient care facilities, in addition to increasing comfort, home automation is mainly used to guarantee people's safety, such as monitoring people's health status and preventing them from harm. In contrast, the focus in outpatient care settings is much more on increasing people's (feelings of) security, such as having camera surveillance and to be able to contact directly with family members and health care professionals.

In the housing concept of farm sharing, the focus is on living together in a small community and sharing common spaces. Social contact with fellow residents is facilitated and even stimulated by this new housing concept. Therefore, home automation directed at improving people's sense of security seems to be less applicable. After all, the residents within the social community pay attention to each other and can reach each other in case of emergency. The design of this housing concept, so to speak, incorporates the underlying social structure of farm sharing.

8.5 Emerging Typologies for Inpatient Facilities: Redesigning Dementia Care

As a result of demographic and societal challenges, people not only impose different demands on outpatient facilities, but also on inpatient facilities. As people are encouraged to stay at home as long as possible, the group of people for whom this is not possible and who live in inpatient facilities has changed its composition. People who live in inpatient settings have become more vulnerable and have a greater demand for care than was the case at first. Within this target group, the group of dementia patients is increasing rapidly (Prince et al. 2015). Therefore, when developing new typologies for inpatient care facilities, special consideration should be given to the connection of the living environment to the special needs of this target group. When 'democratizing' the living environment, the group of people with dementia is perhaps one of the biggest challenges.

8.5.1 Possible Consequences for Dementia Patients

8.5.1.1 Social Engagement

When we talk about social interaction, public familiarity, and bonding and bridging social capital, the question arises how these concepts apply to people with dementia. To what extent are people with dementia capable of social interaction, do they get the chance to meet people from outside their care community, and do these encounters have a positive impact on their well-being? In the literature, there is much attention for the possibility that participation in social and leisure activities later in life may reduce the risk of dementia (Wang et al. 2002; Fratiglioni et al. 2004). However, less attention is paid to the importance of social engagement and participation in the life of dementia patients.

With the progression of the disease, people with dementia often experience a decline in social functioning, due to problems with memory abilities, verbal fluency, word-finding, and social cognition (Sabat and Lee 2011). However, research findings indicate that people with dementia are still capable of verbal and nonverbal communication, and meaningful social interaction (Sabat and Gladstone 2010; Ward et al. 2008). People with dementia attending an adult day centre used verbal and nonverbal communication with each other and demonstrated a mutual emotional understanding and support (Sabat and Lee 2011). Also, when people with dementia are not able to express themselves verbally, they meaningfully use nonverbal communication to express themselves and make clear to others what they mean or what they want (Hubbard et al. 2002). Although dementia has a negative impact on social relations and dementia patients lose many friendships during the course of the disease, some (long-term) friendships remain (Harris 2013).

Sabat and Lee (2011) argue that the decline in social functioning in people with dementia is not only caused by brain injury, but also by the way these people are treated by healthy others. The behaviour of people with dementia is often misinterpreted and wrongly attributed to the disease, rather than to external factors. This misinterpretation, called 'labelling', can result in the depersonalization of people with dementia: characteristics of the individual are overruled by characteristics of the disease. Although people with dementia in a moderate stage of the disease are able to engage in social behaviour, efforts to communicate are often misunderstood or even ignored. This treatment of dementia patients can compromise their self-esteem and can increase the risk of social exclusion.

On a regular base, dementia patients are treated by others if they are socially dead and are not entitled to full citizenship (Brannelly 2011; Sweeting and Gilhooly 1997). This runs counter to the concept of social inclusion, or the idea that the participation of all people in society must be guaranteed. Therefore, in dealing with people with dementia, the focus should be on their personhood: viewing dementia patients as persons, and the disease as only a part of their lives (Kitwood and Bredin 1992; Kitwood 1997). The personhood of people with dementia for a large part is based on their relationships with others. Depersonalizing people with dementia has a negative effect on their personhood, whereas treating them as valued individuals will nurture personhood (Smebye and Kirkevold 2013). From this perspective, it can be expected that participation in meaningful social activities can make an important positive contribution to people's personhood and thus to their well-being. Indeed, there is some empirical support for the assumption that positive and enjoyable engagement in activities is associated with a higher level of well-being of people with dementia in long-term care settings (Cadieux et al. 2013; Chung 2004; Hill and Kürüm 2010).

8.5.1.2 The Acceptance of Dementia Patients by Healthy Others

Apart from the expected positive impact on the well-being of people with dementia, we argue that encounters between dementia patients and healthy others can have a positive influence on the social acceptance of the former. The understanding the general public has of dementia is based on scientific and medical information combined with assumptions based on individual experiences, the experiences of others, and information from the media (Mc Parland 2014). This mix of information often leads to a stigmatizing response from the general public towards people with dementia, which can be labelled dementiaism (Brooker 2003). Dementia is directly related to old age and is considered to be a symbol of unsuccessful ageing. Although people in general feel sympathy for dementia patients, they also regard dementia with fear, as it presents a frightening part of ageing. People do not want to be reminded of the possibility that a similar fate can await them when they reach old age. Dementiaism for a large part is based on fear (Mc Parland 2014).

The contact hypothesis argues that when people come into contact with each other in a positive and neutral context, stigmatization and prejudices can be diminished (Allport 1954). Until now, this hypothesis is mainly used as a possible tool for theorizing about ethnic and racial prejudices and interethnic conflict. However, nowadays the contact hypothesis is also being applied to other stigmatized groups in society, such as people with mental disabilities. The hypothesis assumes that when healthy others come into contact with people with dementia, stigmatization will be reduced and hence the fear to interact with them (Corrigan and Penn 1999). From the different strategies that exist to reduce psychiatric stigma, promoting contact can be considered the most successful one (Couture and Penn 2003). People's experiences with dementia patients are not always consistent with their prejudices, and as a result they have to change the way they think about this marginalized group in society.

From this point of view, brief and random encounters in and around residential care facilities can provide people with bridging social capital. In the public space of residential care facilities, people from within and outside the care community can meet and observe each other, even when they participate in different activities. This could potentially contribute to a greater acceptance of the residents by people from outside the care community.

8.5.2 Redesigning Dementia Care

When we assume that social engagement can be beneficial for the well-being of people with dementia, the question arises how this concept should be incorporated in the spatial and smart design of the dementia care environment, both indoors and outdoors.

As there is no cure for dementia, the social care aspect is even more important when treating people with dementia. External factors, such as the spatial and smart design of the living environment, can help people with dementia to maintain a life of adequate quality as long as possible. Therefore, the treatment of people with dementia is mainly directed at improving people's quality of life and not so much on medical treatment. According to a report by the Organisation for Economic Co-operation and Development (Moise et al. 2004), policies in OECD countries are aimed at delaying institutionalisation and keeping people with dementia at home as long as possible. When institutional care is needed, it should be as home-like as possible.

8.5.3 Design Principles for Dementia Care

As it is noted that the physical and social environment play an important part in improving the lives of people with dementia, more attention is paid to designing environments suitable for people with dementia, both in the home environment and in institutional settings. The design of a dementia friendly environment needs to support the remaining abilities of people with dementia and needs to compensate for their disabilities (Davis et al. 2009) and support them in developing and maintaining social relationships (Wiersma and Pedlar 2008). According to Davis et al. (2009), a dementia friendly environment can be defined as "a cohesive system of support that recognises the experiences of the person with dementia and best provides assistance for the person to remain engaged in everyday life in a meaningful way" (p. 187). Innes et al. (2011) emphasize the complexity of dementia care design, as it should consider not only the needs and wishes of people with dementia, but also that of family members who visit and the staff of the care facilities.

A growing number of studies examines the relationship between the built environment and the quality of life of people with dementia. Amongst others, it was found that design features that strongly prioritise safety and health can have negative effects on people's quality of life, whereas design features that prioritise engagement in social and domestic activities, focus on living experiences and encourage curiosity have positive effects (Chalfont and Rodiek 2005; Torrington 2007). Despite these new insights in building design and recent developments in models of dementia care, practical applications in designing care environments often lag behind (Davis et al. 2009).

8.5.3.1 Facility Layout and Design in Relation to Social Interaction

In the redesign of dementia care, the early work of some pioneers, such as Marshall (1998), resulted in key design principles for dementia care facilities. During the last decades, these principles where discussed, criticized, examined and modified (Davis et al. 2009; Fleming and Purandare 2010; Fleming et al. 2015). One of these design principles states that the design of dementia care facilities should be welcoming for relatives and the local community. Dementia care homes should provide spaces where people can be alone and have some privacy and spaces where people can meet with others from within and outside their care facility.

It is assumed that by creating a homelike atmosphere in the care facility people are encouraged to participate in activities of daily living and, as a result engage with others (Verbeek et al. 2009). Especially the involvement with family members are considered to be important, as they know the residents well and are the primary contacts of the residents outside the care community. Therefore, it is important that the design of dementia friendly environments is also inviting and welcoming to family and friends. A homelike environment that offers (private) spaces where family members can be involved in everyday activities with residents is recommended (Davis et al. 2009). Although there is some evidence for this relationship between the principle of home likeness and participation in activities, it is very difficult to disentangle the effects of the physical environment from that of staff encouragement and support (Fleming and Purandare 2010).

Due to its institutional character and the stigmatization of people with dementia, dementia care facilities are often not considered to be a welcoming or inviting place for outsiders. However, this does not mean that it is not important to encourage a healthy relationship between the residents and people from the local community. The inclusion of the care facility as part of the local community can be beneficial, as it can improve the quality of life of the residents and lead to a better understanding of people with dementia (Davis et al. 2009). Although encouraging and strengthening community links are often part of the social program of care facilities, for example by organizing activities in the nearby village, it is not incorporated in the architectural design of care environments. According to Davis et al., the main obstacle in taking into account community connections into the design of care facilities is a lack of imagination (2009, p. 195). They emphasize the possibility of establishing facilities in the care facility, such as a restaurant or a childcare centre.

8.5.4 The Outdoor Environment as an Enabler for Community Connectedness

In the design principles for dementia-friendly care environments, the provision of a safe and stimulating outdoor environment is often included. Nonetheless, there is no clear guidance in designing the outdoor environment in institutional settings and in the home environment (Mitchell et al. 2003). Despite the increase in the number of studies focusing on the relationship between the design of outdoor spaces and the quality of life of people with dementia, there is an underuse of outdoor areas and resources in dementia care facilities (Chalfont and Rodiek 2005; Edwards et al. 2013). The outdoor environment can be important in dementia care, as is can stimulate people to be physically active and stimulate their senses. However, it remains unclear to what extent the outdoor environment can also be useful in stimulating social interaction and social inclusion in the wider community. It is suggested, for example, that outdoor spaces can stimulate participation in social activities and for that reason have a positive impact on the quality of life of people with dementia (Fleming and Purandare 2010).

8.5.4.1 The Outdoor Environment in an Institutional Setting

Although nowadays there is more recognition for designing dementia-friendly and inclusive neighbourhoods where people with dementia can remain socially active, less attention is paid to the inclusive design of the outdoor environment in an institutional setting. In recent years, healing and sensory gardens are more frequently used in the treatment of people with dementia (Gonzalez and Kirkevold 2014). Apart from the direct effect of being connected to nature, healing and sensory gardens are expected to have a beneficial effect on reducing challenging behaviour, delaying cognitive decline and promoting well-being of people with dementia, by stimulating physical activity and offering multisensory stimulation (Edwards et al. 2013; Whear et al. 2014). It is even suggested that socializing can be seen as an advantage of using the outdoor environment of residential care facilities. Social contact and communication can increase, at least on the short term, by participating in (gardening) activities in the outdoor environment (Gonzalez and Kirkevold 2015). However, this finding relates to contact and communication within the care community; fellow residents, visitors and staff. Gardens and outdoor spaces of residential care facilities can only create opportunities for social interaction between residents and people from the wider community when they are made accessible for others.

8.5.5 The Care Estate as an Example

The care estate is a new housing concept in the Netherlands for care recipients with dementia. Unique to this type of housing is the scale of the property in combination with its special target group. The care estate offers a green environment on which facilities can be created to promote encounters between residents with dementia and people from neighbouring villages. The inclusion of dementia patients in the wider community therefore plays an important role in the development of this new housing concept.

Care estates are a relatively new phenomenon in the Netherlands. Therefore, little is known about this new type of housing and the consequences of living on the estate for the residents (with dementia) and professional care givers. The care estate is believed to be a healing environment where the residents can enjoy nature and participate in outdoor activities that stimulate them both physically and mentally (Hassink et al. 2007). A distinctive feature of the care estate is the outdoor space that is available to the residents and for a large part accessible to the public. This outdoor space offers the residents the opportunity to meet people from outside the care community and facilitates spontaneous encounters. This raises the question how we should arrange the outdoor space of a care estate, so that encounters between residents and people from neighbouring villages are not only facilitated, but also stimulated.

Explorative research on this topic (Moor et al. 2015) shows that by organizing (horticultural) activities in the outdoor space of the care estate brief encounters between people from inside and outside the care community can be stimulated. In the inviting setting of the care estate people from inside and outside the care community can meet each other when they participate in different outdoor activities. Careful consideration must be given to the question how these outdoor activities should be situated in the outdoor space. From this perspective, the research findings identified three zones to locate the outdoor activities: the care house or private zone, the encounter zone, and the context-related or welcoming zone (as can be seen in Fig. 8.1). In the context-related zone outdoor activities should be situated that attract people from the nearby villages to visit the estate, whereas in the encounter area

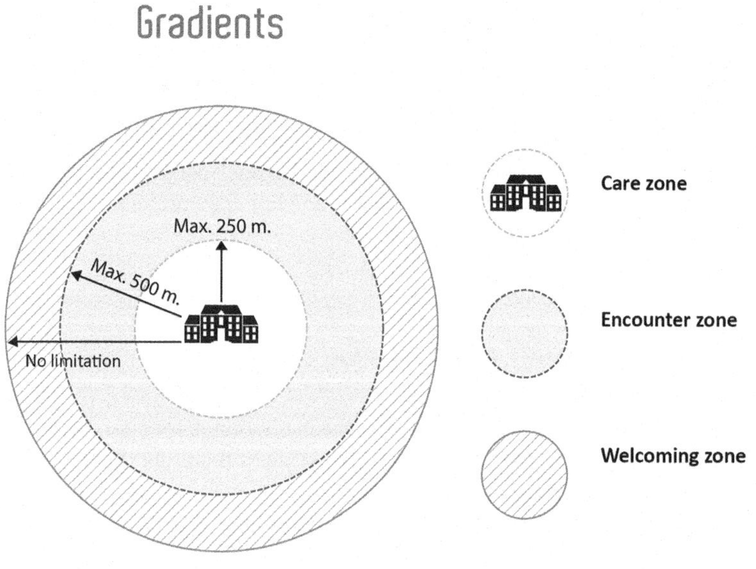

Fig. 8.1 Three zones to transform a care estate into a place that facilitates spontaneous encounters between residents and people from neighbourhood

activities should be situated that are suitable for both the residents (with dementia) and the visitors. Additionally, the selection of activities must be made in such a way that the supply of activities and facilities on the care estate is *complementary* to the existing supply in the surrounding villages. In this way, inhabitants from these villages can be persuaded to visit the care estate and meet its residents. By offering complementary facilities and activities in the outdoor environment of residential care facilities, not only social opportunities arise (for encounter), but also economic opportunities (employment).

8.5.5.1 The Care Estate as a Smart Living Facility

Creating opportunities for encounter on the care estate makes certain demands on the outdoor environment. To stimulate encounters with people from outside the care community, residents with dementia a) should be given some freedom of movement, and b) must be guided through their environment when using the space. With the help of smart technology, a good balance can be sought between guaranteeing safety for the residents with dementia, and offering freedom of movement and guidance to these residents in order to facilitate and stimulate (passive and active) social interaction.

The residents can only meet people from outside the care community if they are given the chance to wander in the outdoor environment directly surrounding the residential care facility. Residents with dementia can be offered digital freedom, by using remote monitoring, which can enhance mobility, wayfinding and access. People can be monitored in such a way that caregivers are aware of their location and their health status, while, at the same time, ensure as much freedom of movement and independence as possible (Thielke et al. 2012).

The outdoor environment of the care estate can, for example, be made more accessible to residents with dementia by transforming into a 'guiding environment' (Mohammadi 2017). According to Mohammadi, the guiding environment should give a sensory impulse at the right time to elderly people (with dementia), in order to perform general daily activities in such a way that it enables them to live independently for a longer time. Nonetheless, the concept of the guiding environment can also be applied to inpatient care settings. Using smart sensor technologies, the interactive environment acts as a memory aid for a resident with incipient dementia. By using smart sensor technologies, the interactive design of both the indoor and outdoor environment of the care estate can assist residents in walking across the estate, in directing them to safe and interesting locations, and in stimulating them to participate in (horticultural) activities. This smart environment also keeps an eye on things and encourages the resident to move or eat sufficiently.

8.6 Conclusion & Discussion

The mission of architecture in the twenty-first century, in our opinion, goes beyond the aesthetic desirability or making architecture. It is about shaping socio-spatial systems and services that boost a future that respects diversity and encourages inclusion.

A higher sense of awareness and more support has emerged in relation to the necessity of technological renewal in both the construction industry and healthcare sector. Better connections between scientific work and health care and building practices are established. The time has come and the paradigm is aimed at steady advances in the future.

There is increasing recognition for the belief that senior citizens should not live in segregated environments but should remain part of society as they get older and face physical and mental limitations. We are social creatures. The frequency and quality of social interaction with significant others is one of the key determinants of our well-being. In Dutch ageing society, the majority of senior citizens can be considered relatively vital and healthy. This group of older adults can be part of society without any problems but are not sure of this in the future. Although these vital senior citizens make no special demands on their living environment, they may want to anticipate a future in which they will get (mobility) problems and health complaints.

A smaller group of older adults, however, can be classified as vulnerable, since they suffer from comorbidity, and several chronic physical or mental conditions. In order for this group to be involved in society, the living environment of these people should be adapted in such a way that the daily activities can be supported.

Our first research question was whether the social inclusion of senior citizens (with physical and mental disabilities) in society can contribute to their well-being. Based on current (sociological) theories and existing knowledge from the literature, we can conclude that there are sufficient indications that the social inclusion of senior citizens in society can have positive effects on their well-being. Social resources can positively affect people's well-being, and, in a way, can protect people against negative life events. This is the case, however, when it comes to intimate relationships with, for example, family members and close friends. Although neighbours can also be good friends, many contacts that people have in their neighbourhood are not intimate in nature. Nonetheless, brief and random encounters in the neighbourhood can also have a positive effect on people's well-being, as it can result in public familiarity. Encounters in the public space can evoke feelings of safety and security among people, and make them feel at ease in their living environment.

Apart from the expected positive impact on the well-being of older adults, it can be argued that encounters between elderly people with physical or mental disabilities and healthy others can have a positive influence on the social acceptance of the former. Based on the contact hypothesis, it can be argued that when elderly people with disabilities come into contact with healthy others in a positive and neutral context, stigmatization and prejudices can be diminished.

Our second research question is whether smart interventions in and around inpatient and outpatient care settings can stimulate social inclusion of senior citizens. In order to create an inclusive and age-friendly society, housing typologies for senior citizens and the direct living environment should directly connect to the needs of both vital and vulnerable older adults. The design of housing and the living environment must offer vital senior citizens the certainty that they can continue to live there in the future, while supporting frail elderly people in their daily activities indoors and outdoors. Smart technologies can contribute to the social inclusiveness of the living environment, by bridging the gap between the needs of older adults and what the living environment has to offer them. In inpatient housing typologies for senior citizens, smart technologies often are used to guarantee's people's safety, whereas in outpatient housing typologies, smart technologies are used more often for increasing security.

In this chapter, we discussed two new housing typologies in the Netherlands that may positively affect the inclusion of senior citizens in society: farm sharing and the care estate. First, we discussed farm sharing, an increasingly becoming popular housing concept that can be particularly suitable for vital older adults who want to live independently for as long as possible, whether or not in a family context. This housing concept is situated on a (former) farmyard on which several houses have been built. The people on the farmyard live together in a small community, have their own homes, but also share common spaces. As the social structure of togetherness in this housing concept has been incorporated in its design, smart technologies to some extent seem to be superfluous in providing security to its residents.

Secondly, we discussed the housing concept of the care estate, that seems to be a suitable form of living for vulnerable elderly people with physical and mental comorbidity, such as dementia, who can no longer live independently. The care estate offers a nature-based housing solution: a green environment on which facilities can be created to promote encounters between residents with dementia and people from neighbouring villages. The inclusion of dementia patients in society is therefore supported by this housing concept. Smart technologies can play an important role in this housing concept in bridging the gap between the needs of the residents with dementia and the risks that the design of the outdoor environment entails. With the help of smart (tracking) technology, the residents with dementia can be given some freedom of movement, while their safety is not compromised. The outdoor environment can also be transformed into a smart 'guiding environment', in which the residents are assisted in walking across the care estate. In this case, the smart environment can even be considered an important precondition for social inclusion, as it allows residents to use the outdoor spaces surrounding the care facility while at the same time avoiding unnecessary risks, such as wandering.

Figure 8.2 shows a set of housing typologies for older adults, which is arranged according to the degree of (in)dependence of the potential residents. At the beginning of this set outpatient housing typologies can be placed that are suitable for senior citizens who live independently, but who are anticipating potential problems

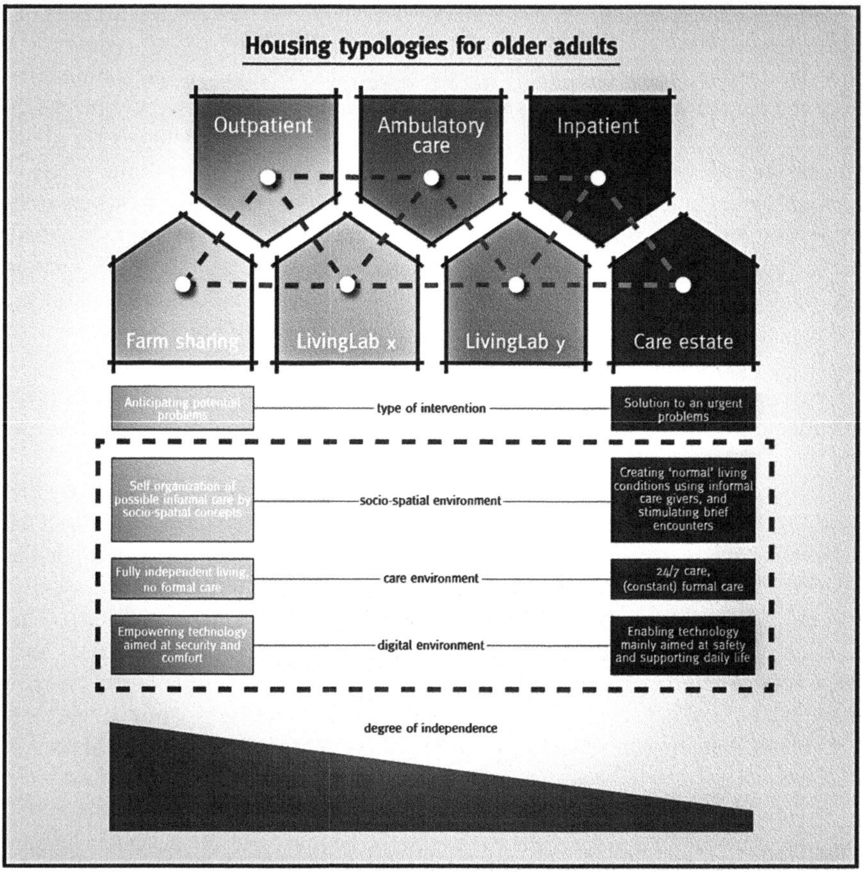

Fig. 8.2 A set of housing typologies for older adults, which is arranged according to the degree of (in)dependence of the potential residents

in the (nearby) future. At the end of the set, inpatient housing typologies can be placed that are suitable for elderly people who have a great need for care and can no longer live independently. Farm sharing and the care estate, the two examples of new housing typologies that we have just discussed, can be placed on both ends of this range. Other new housing typologies can also be placed on this set, depending on the target group they are focussing on.

The fact that new housing typologies for older adults have to meet the needs of their residents regarding "different layers of living" is also clearly reflected in Fig. 8.2. In order to be able to optimize the well-being and health status of their residents, housing typologies must meet the needs of (vulnerable) older adults with regard to care, social interaction, and autonomy as much as possible. The art of designing new suitable housing typologies for older adults therefore should be based on linking different layers of people's living environment: the care environment, the socio-spatial environment, and the digital environment. In the two examples of housing typologies that we have covered in this chapter, these different layers have been cleverly linked with each other in order to design a new housing concept.

A recommendation to designers and policy makers for that reason is to assess new housing typologies for older adults, often starting as bottom-up initiatives in society, on the basis of their combination of the "different layers of living". The impact of each layer on the well-being and health status of older adults can then be tested in different living labs around upcoming bottom-up initiatives.

References

Allport, G. W. (1954). *The nature of prejudice*. Reading: Addison-Wesley.

Blokland, T. (2003). *Urban bonds. Social relationships in an inner-city neighbourhood.* Cambridge: Polity Press.

Blokland, T. (2008). *Ontmoeten doet ertoe*. Rotterdam: Vetia.

Bouwman, M., & Mohammadi, M. (2013) On the relation of spatial design and social fabrics: Relating place and spatial design to social fabrics through chance encounters, *Abstract for the Fourth International and Interdisciplinary Conference on Emotional Geographies*. Groningen, The Netherlands, 1–3 July 2013.

Brannelly, T. (2011). Sustaining citizenship: People with dementia and the phenomenon of social death. *Nursing Ethics, 18*(5), 662–671.

Brooker, D. (2003). What is person-centred care in dementia? *Reviews in Clinical Gerontology, 13*(3), 215–222.

Brorsson, A., Öhman, A., Lundberg, S., & Nygård, L. (2011). Accessibility in public space as perceived by people with Alzheimer's disease. *Dementia, 10*(4), 587–602.

Burns, V. F., Lavoie, J. P., & Rose, D. (2012). Revisiting the role of neighbourhood change in social exclusion and inclusion of older people. *Journal of Aging Research, 2012, 1–12.*

Cadieux, M. A., Garcia, L. J., & Patrick, J. (2013). Needs of people with dementia in long-term care a systematic review. *American Journal of Alzheimer's Disease and Other Dementias, 28*(8), 723–733.

Cattell, V., Dines, N., Gesler, W., & Curtis, S. (2008). Mingling, observing, and lingering: Everyday public spaces and their implications for well-being and social relations. *Health & Place, 14*(3), 544–561.

Chalfont, G. E., & Rodiek, S. (2005). Building edge: An ecological approach to research and design of environments for people with dementia. *Alzheimer's Care Today, 6*(4), 341–348.

Chung, J. C. (2004). Activity participation and well-being of people with dementia in long-term—Care settings. *OTJR: Occupation, Participation and Health, 24*(1), 22–31.

Corrigan, P. W., & Penn, D. L. (1999). Lessons from social psychology on discrediting psychiatric stigma. *American Psychologist, 54*(9), 765–776.

Couture, S., & Penn, D. (2003). Interpersonal contact and the stigma of mental illness: A review of the literature. *Journal of Mental Health, 12*(3), 291–305.

Cummins, R. A., & Lau, A. L. D. (2003). Community integration or community exposure? A review and discussion in relation to people with an intellectual disability. *Journal of Applied Research in Intellectual Disabilities, 16*, 145–157.

Davis, S., Byers, S., Nay, R., & Koch, S. (2009). Guiding design of dementia friendly environments in residential care settings: Considering the living experiences. *Dementia, 8*(2), 185–203.

Diener, E., & Fujita, F. (1995). Resources, personal strivings, and subjective well-being: A nomothetic and idiographic approach. *Journal of Personality and Social Psychology, 68*(5), 926–935.

Edwards, C. A., McDonnell, C., & Merl, H. (2013). An evaluation of a therapeutic garden's influence on the quality of life of aged care residents with dementia. *Dementia, 12*(4), 494–510.

Fleming, R., & Purandare, N. (2010). Long-term care for people with dementia: Environmental design guidelines. *International Psychogeriatrics, 22*(7), 1084–1096.

Fleming, R., Kelly, F., & Stillfried, G. (2015). I want to feel at home': Establishing what aspects of environmental design are important to people with dementia nearing the end of life. *BMC Palliative Care, 14*(1), 26.

Fratiglioni, L., Paillard-Borg, S., & Winblad, B. (2004). An active and socially integrated lifestyle in late life might protect against dementia. *The Lancet Neurology, 3*(6), 343–353.

Gardner, P. J. (2011). Natural neighborhood networks—Important social networks in the lives of older adults aging in place. *Journal of Aging Studies, 25*(3), 263–271.

Gonzalez, M. T., & Kirkevold, M. (2014). Benefits of sensory garden and horticultural activities in dementia care: A modified scoping review. *Journal of Clinical Nursing, 23*(19–20), 2698–2715.

Gonzalez, M. T., & Kirkevold, M. (2015). Clinical use of sensory gardens and outdoor environments in norwegian nursing homes: A cross-sectional e-mail survey. *Issues in Mental Health Nursing, 36*(1), 35–43.

Guest, A. M., & Wierzbicki, S. K. (1999). Social ties at the neighborhood level: Two decades of GSS evidence. *Urban Affairs Review, 35*(1), 92–111.

Harris, P. B. (2013). Dementia and friendship: The quality and nature of the relationships that remain. *The International Journal of Aging and Human Development, 76*(2), 141–164.

Hassink, J., Elings, M., & Steenstra, F. A. (2007). *Kwaliteiten van zorglandgoederen* (No. 136, p. 34). Plant Research International.

Hill, N. L., & Kürüm, E. (2010). Agreeableness and activity engagement in nursing home residents with dementia. *Journal of Gerontological Nursing, 36*(9), 45–52.

Hobfoll, S. E. (1989). Conservation of resources: A new attempt at conceptualizing stress. *American Psychologist, 44*(3), 513–524.

Hubbard, G., Cook, A., Tester, S., & Downs, M. (2002). Beyond words: Older people with dementia using and interpreting nonverbal behaviour. *Journal of Aging Studies, 16*(2), 155–167.

Huxhold, O., Miche, M., & Schüz, B. (2013). Benefits of having friends in older ages: Differential effects of informal social activities on well-being in middle-aged and older adults. *Journals of Gerontology Series B: Psychological Sciences and Social Sciences, 69*(3), 366–375.

Innes, A., Kelly, F., & Dincarslan, O. (2011). Care home design for people with dementia: What do people with dementia and their family carers value? *Aging & Mental Health, 15*(5), 548–556.

Jang, Y., Haley, W. E., Small, B. J., & Mortimer, J. A. (2002). The role of mastery and social resources in the associations between disability and depression in later life. *The Gerontologist, 42*(6), 807–813.

Keady, J., Campbell, S., Barnes, H., Ward, R., Li, X., Swarbrick, C., et al. (2012). Neighbourhoods and dementia in the health and social care context: A realist review of the literature and implications for UK policy development. *Reviews in Clinical Gerontology, 22*(02), 150–163.

Kitwood, T. (1997). *Dementia reconsidered: The person comes first.* Buckingham: Open University Press.

Kitwood, T., & Bredin, K. (1992). Towards a theory of dementia care: Personhood and well-being. *Ageing and Society, 12*(03), 269–287.

Knight, T., & Mellor, D. (2007). Social inclusion of older adults in care: Is it just a question of providing activities? *International Journal of Qualitative Studies on Health and Well-being, 2*(2), 76–85.

Leff, J., & Warner, R. (2006). *Social inclusion of people with mental illness*. Cambridge University Press.

Lui, C. W., Everingham, J. A., Warburton, J., Cuthill, M., & Bartlett, H. (2009). What makes a community age-friendly: A review of international literature. *Australasian Journal of Ageing, 28*(3), 116–121.

Marshall, M. (1998). Therapeutic buildings for people with dementia. In S. Judd, M. Marshall, & P. Phippen (Eds.), *Design for dementia* (pp. 11–14). London: Hawker Publications.
Mc Parland, P. (2014). *Dementia: What comes to mind? An exploration into how the general public understands and responds to dementia*. University of Stirling, thesis.
Mens, N., & Wagenaar, C. (2009). *De architectuur van de ouderenhuisvesting: bouwen voor wonen en zorg* (p. NAi010). Rotterdam.
Mitchell, L., & Burton, E. (2006). Neighbourhoods for life: Designing dementia-friendly outdoor environments. *Quality in ageing and older adults, 7*(1), 26–33.
Mitchell, L., & Burton, E. (2010). Designing dementia-friendly neighbourhoods: Helping people with dementia to get out and about. *Journal of Integrated Care, 18*(6), 11–19.
Mitchell, L., Burton, E., Raman, S., Blackman, T., Jenks, M., & Williams, K. (2003). Making the outside world dementia-friendly: Design issues and considerations. *Environment and Planning B: Planning and Design, 30*(4), 605–632.
Mohammadi, M. (2014). *Domoticakompas: Inzichten uit een decennium slimme zorgprojecten in Nederland*. Eindhoven: Van Litsenburg B.V.
Mohammadi, M. (2017). *Empathische woonomgeving*. Eindhoven: Technische Universiteit Eindhoven.
Mohammadi, M., van Buuren, L. P. G., Hammink, J. H. W., Dominicus, M. M. T., Hamers, K., & Yegenoglu, H. H. (2018). The evolution of housing typologies for older adults in the Netherlands from 1945–2016: An analysis in the context of policy, societal and technological developments. *Journal of Housing for the Elderly*, 1–22.
Moise, P., Schwarzinger, M., & Um, M.Y. (2004). *Dementia care in 9 OECD countries*.
Moor, N., de Graaf, P. M., & Komter, A. (2013). Family, welfare state generosity and the vulnerability of older adults: A cross-national study. *Journal of Aging Studies, 27*(4), 347–357.
Moor, N., Mohammadi, M., & Curulli, I. G. (2015). Designing encounters: Care estate as an enabler to support the social fabric of dementia patients. *Advances in Social and Behavioral Sciences, 10*, 105–110.
Moyle, W., Venturto, L., Griffiths, S., Grimbeek, P., McAllister, M., Oxlade, D., & Murfield, J. (2011). Factors influencing quality of life for people with dementia: A qualitative perspective. *Aging & Mental Health, 15*(8), 970–977.
Oswald, F., Hieber, A., Wahl, H. W., & Mollenkopf, H. (2005). Ageing and person–environment fit in different urban neighbourhoods. *European Journal of Ageing, 2*(2), 88–97.
Post, S. G. (2000). The concept of Alzheimer disease in a hypercognitive society. In *Concepts of Alzheimer disease: Biological, clinical and cultural perspectives* (pp. 245–256). Baltimore: Johns Hopkins University Press.
Prince, M., Wimo, A., Guerchet, M., Ali, G. C., Wu, Y. T., & Prina, M. (2015). *World Alzheimer report 2015. The global impact of Dementia. Alzheimer's Disease International*. London: Alzheimer's Disease International (ADI).
Putnam, R. D. (2001). *Bowling alone: The collapse and revival of American community*. New York: Simon and Schuster.
Sabat, S. R., & Gladstone, C. M. (2010). What intact social cognition and social behavior reveal about cognition in the moderate stage of Alzheimer's disease a case study. *Dementia, 9*(1), 61–78.
Sabat, S. R., & Lee, J. M. (2011). Relatedness among people diagnosed with dementia: Social cognition and the possibility of friendship. *Dementia, 0*(0), 1–13.
Shakespeare, T. (2006). The social model of disability. *The disability studies reader*, 2, pp. 197–204. New York: Routledge.
Shankar, A., Rafnsson, S. B., & Steptoe, A. (2015). Longitudinal associations between social connections and subjective wellbeing in the English longitudinal study of ageing. *Psychology & Health, 30*(6), 686–698.
Skouby, K. E., Kivimäki, A., Haukiputo, L., Lynggaard, P., & Windekilde, I. M. (2014). Smart cities and the ageing population. In: *Proceedings of the 32nd Meeting of WWRF*, Marrakech, Morocco, 20–22 May 2014.

Smebye, K. L., & Kirkevold, M. (2013). The influence of relationships on personhood in dementia care: A qualitative, hermeneutic study. *BMC Nursing, 12*(1), 29.
Sweeting, H., & Gilhooly, M. (1997). Dementia and the phenomenon of social death. *Sociology of Health and Illness, 19*(1), 93–117.
Thielke, S., Harniss, M., Thompson, H., Patel, S., Demiris, G., & Johnson, K. (2012). Maslow's hierarchy of human needs and the adoption of health-related technologies for older adults. *Ageing International, 37*(4), 470–488.
Tiernan, C., Lysack, C., Neufeld, S., & Lichtenberg, P. A. (2013). Community engagement: An essential component of well-being in older African-American adults. *The International Journal of Aging and Human Development, 77*(3), 233–257.
Tonkens, E., & Weijers, I. (1999). Autonomy, solidarity, and self-realization: Policy views of Dutch service providers. *Mental Retardation, 37*(6), 468–476.
Torrington, J. (2007). Evaluating quality of life in residential care buildings. *Building Research & Information, 35*(5), 514–528.
Van Alphen, L. M., Dijker, A. J., van den Borne, B. H., & Curfs, L. M. (2010). People with intellectual disability as neighbours: Towards understanding the mundane aspects of social integration. *Journal of Community & Applied Social Psychology, 20*(5), 347–362.
Van Eijk, G., & Engbersen, R. (2011). Facilitating 'light' social interactions in public space: A collaborative study in a Dutch urban renewal neighbourhood. *Journal of Urban Regeneration & Renewal, 5*(1), 35–50.
Van Houtven, C. H., & Norton, E. C. (2004). Informal care and health care use of older adults. *Journal of Health Economics, 23*(6), 1159–1180.
Verbeek, H., van Rossum, E., Zwakhalen, S. M., Kempen, G. I., & Hamers, J. P. (2009). Small, homelike care environments for older people with dementia: A literature review. *International Psychogeriatrics, 21*(2), 252–264.
Verdonschot, M. M., De Witte, L. P., Reichrath, E., Buntinx, W. H. E., & Curfs, L. M. (2009). Community participation of people with an intellectual disability: A review of empirical findings. *Journal of Intellectual Disability Research, 53*(4), 303–318.
Verplanke, L., Verplanke, L. H., Duyvendak, J. W., Duyvendak, W. G. J., & Groenendijk, J. (2010). *Onder de mensen?: Over het zelfstandig wonen van psychiatrische patiënten en mensen met een verstandelijke beperking*. Amsterdam: Amsterdam University Press.
von Hippel, E. (2005). *Democratizing innovation*. Boston: MIT Press.
Wang, H. X., Karp, A., Winblad, B., & Fratiglioni, L. (2002). Late-life engagement in social and leisure activities is associated with a decreased risk of dementia: A longitudinal study from the Kungsholmen project. *American Journal of Epidemiology, 155*(12), 1081–1087.
Ward, R., Vass, A. A., Aggarwal, N., Garfield, C., & Cybyk, B. (2008). A different story: Exploring patterns of communication in residential dementia care. *Ageing and Society, 28*(05), 629–651.
Whear, R., Coon, J. T., Bethel, A., Abbott, R., Stein, K., & Garside, R. (2014). What is the impact of using outdoor spaces such as gardens on the physical and mental well-being of those with dementia? A systematic review of quantitative and qualitative evidence. *Journal of the American Medical Directors Association, 15*(10), 697–705.
Wiersma, E. C., & Pedlar, A. (2008). The nature of relationships in alternative dementia care environments. *Canadian Journal on Aging/La Revue canadienne du vieillissement, 27*(1), 101–108.
Wiles, J. (2005). Conceptualizing place in the care of older people: The contributions of geographical gerontology. *Journal of Clinical Nursing, 14*, 100–108.
Yen, I. H., Michael, Y. L., & Perdue, L. (2009). Neighborhood environment in studies of health of older adults: A systematic review. *American Journal of Preventive Medicine, 37*(5), 455–463.
Young, A. F., Russell, A., & Powers, J. R. (2004). The sense of belonging to a neighbourhood: Can it be measured and is it related to health and well-being in older women? *Social Science & Medicine, 59*(12), 2627–2637.

Chapter 9
Real-Time Interactive Multimodal Systems for Physiological and Emotional Wellbeing

Nimish Biloria and Dimitra Dritsa

Abstract There has been lately significant progress in the design of clinically assistive technologies for physiological and emotional wellbeing, driven by developments in Human Computer Interaction, Virtual Reality systems for rehabilitation and social interaction and Rehabilitation Robotics. The clinical, task-driven nature of such systems though often affects negatively the user acceptance of technology, resulting in lesser interactions with the user. At the same time, interactive environments which are not constructed for strictly medical applications, can also instigate interaction dialogues which generate physiological and emotional benefits for the user, while also incorporating a more playful dimension. As there is currently lack of communication channels between Clinically Assistive technologies and Socially Interactive Design Systems, the chapter attempts to merge these domains by identifying parameters related to physiological and emotional wellbeing that could inform the design of interactive systems for health and wellbeing at variable scales. These parameters are presented as a set of guidelines for Interaction design for healthcare and wellbeing, and the chapter elaborates on their practical application through three case studies: RoboZoo, Textrinium and Reflectego. All the presented case studies operate as public indoor or outdoor installations and have been tested in different contextual conditions, in Netherlands, Spain and France.

Keywords Architecture · Real-time interaction · Robotics · User behaviour · Tangible interaction

9.1 Introduction

Over the last two decades, an increasing interest has been demonstrated in designing technologies for physiological and emotional wellbeing. The domain of Human Computer Interaction has made significant progress in addressing user needs of the

N. Biloria (✉) · D. Dritsa
Faculty of Design Architecture Building, University of Technology Sydney, Ultimo, Australia
e-mail: nimish.biloria@uts.edu.au; Dimitra.dritsa@uts.edu.nl

N. Biloria (ed.), *Data-driven Multivalence in the Built Environment*, S.M.A.R.T. Environments, https://doi.org/10.1007/978-3-030-12180-8_9

elderly, children and users with a need for physiotherapeutic treatment, social interaction training and emotional support. Current studies on the development of assistive technologies are focused either on addressing functional or social aspects. For instance, Virtual Reality (VR) systems for healthcare and Rehabilitation Robotics have shown potential in treating motor impairments for lower, upper and full body extremities in the context of post-stroke rehabilitation (Luo et al. 2005; Yakub et al. 2014), while the social dimension is explored in Virtual and Augmented Reality systems for social interaction training settings (Lahiri et al. 2011) and within Social Robotics, with applications such as social interactive robots that act as pet companions (Kidd et al. 2006; Wada and Shibata 2007) for the elderly.

Such applications of a medical nature mostly operate at a product scale, while socio-technical interactive systems of a larger scale, also referred to as interactive environments (Bullivant 2007) or interactivated spaces (Harris and Bongers 2002) are mostly situated in either urban open public spaces, or public buildings such as galleries and museums, and operate on the borders of art and science. Such systems have very similar sensing and actuation protocols with the aforementioned clinical applications, and while the primary intent of such real-time interactive systems is to entertain the visitor, their embedded interaction dialogues can also be interpreted from a health and wellbeing perspective. For instance, an interactive floor with real-time location tracking and embedded behavioral modes for attracting and engaging visitors (such as that of Delbrück et al. 2007) indirectly results in the increased movement of the users within the space, as an unintended consequence of the interactive game like structure which the floor perpetuates.

When comparing such interactive installations with clinical assistive technologies for addressing similar health and wellbeing issues, the disadvantage of the former is that interactive installations for public spaces are designed for the average user, without considering specific physical or cognitive impairments of the users, while assistive technologies operate within a well-defined set of constraints, driven by the physical condition and the profile of the user. On the other hand, the enjoyment and pleasure that a user feels in more experimental open-ended scenarios have been consistently appearing as a critical factor that positively affects user acceptance of technology, in the discourse on user interaction with social robots, computers and information systems (Heerink et al. 2010; Sun and Zhang 2006; Heijden 2004). In the case of assistive technologies that lack this playful dimension and are strictly associated with medical use, users tend to feel that their interaction with such clinical objects can bring stigmatization in their social circle, and therefore end up using them to a lesser degree than what is medically suggested (Hirsch et al. 2000; Steele et al. 2009).

It is thus deemed to be of value, to start establishing communication channels between Clinically Assistive Technologies, and Socially Interactive Design Systems of a more experimental nature, in order to shape user-centered experiences that are tailored towards the advancement of the health and wellbeing of the target user, but are not task-driven to an extent that tunes down the open-ended and affective aspects of the interaction. The chapter serves as a report on creative attempts to merge these two domains by identifying parameters related to physiological and emotional well-being that could inform the design of interactive systems for health and wellbeing at variable scales. In this context, the paper aims to establish a set of guidelines for the design of interactive environments for health and wellbeing. These have been tested via three research driven design case studies, conducted under the author's guidance at the Technical University of Delft, The Netherlands. Two of these projects were conducted as research experiments under a European Union Culture Grant called METABODY and the third project is a professional project commissioned by one of Netherlands most prestigious Science Museums: NEMO.

The guidelines proposed in Sect. 9.3 are not expressly intended to serve as a new definitive framework; rather, they build upon relevant research subjects in the field of interaction design, such as the Sensoric or Cognitive aspects of the interaction and the design of Movement (Harris and Bongers 2002; Bilda et al. 2007) or the Spatial Dimension (Harris and Bongers 2002; Oosterhuis 2002; Taysheng 2005), and work more as an extension of extracted themes. The Chapter thus first examines in Sect. 9.2 existing frameworks that formulate the basis for this research, Sect. 9.3 introduces the broad themes to be taken into consideration in the context of interaction design for enhancing wellbeing, Sect. 9.4 elaborates on these themes through three case studies, and Sect. 9.5 reflects on the presented topics and concludes by shaping the directions for future research.

9.2 Interaction Design and the Design of Technologies for Healthcare and Wellbeing

Designing interactive systems for enhancement of physiological and emotional wellbeing requires an intertwining of movement instigating design tailored to specific settings of physical rehabilitation coupled with spatial aspects as well as with the impact that these factors have on increasing the quality of the social interaction between the users and the interactive system. In researches that study the application of models such as the Unified Theory of Acceptance and Use of Technology in the context of assistive technologies, factors such as the age, the self-efficacy and the anxiety of the user have been identified as parameters of direct or indirect influence in the interaction between the user and respective assistive technologies. (Heerink et al. 2010) Such parameters, as well as the vast differences that the users can have in terms of physiological condition and social needs, should be included in the set of user requirements and design parameters and constraints. In this context, this section discusses interaction design in relation to social interaction, cognition and bodily movement, and briefly explores subtopics such as materiality, haptic interaction, bodily positioning and spatial relations, which are all themes that will be later reinterpreted or expanded in the context of wellbeing. The discussed approaches do not by any means aim to cover the extensive body of research that has been conducted in the overall field, but instead act as a representative sample for the demonstration of how components from different interaction design frameworks and guidelines can be positioned together and further extended in the context of enhancing wellbeing.

Social interaction was put in the center of interaction design by Hornecker and Buur (2006), which is noteworthy as a shift from the prevalent designing for task effectiveness norm. Their approach provides a set of design guidelines built around four themes: Tangible manipulation, spatial interaction, embodied facilitation and expressive representation. Within the theme Tangible manipulation, materials and their properties related to tangible interaction are briefly discussed in relation to the sensory feedback that comes from the interaction; spatial interaction situates bodily movement within space, and raises questions such as if the whole body is used, and what is the spatial relation between the body and the interactive object; embodied facilitation discusses spatial configurations and their ability to instigate social interaction within a group setting.

In adjacent fields, such as rehabilitation robotics, the relationship between the user and the interactive object has been often explored with a focus on functional aspects rather than social. Such is the case in the development of physical therapy robots (Yakub et al. 2014). In Social Robotics or certain applications of Virtual Reality for healthcare and wellbeing, social interaction becomes the core objective; in this case, the relation between spatial configurations and social interaction in individual or group settings that Hornecker and Buur explore (2006) acquires an additional layer of complexity in conditions which cause an impairment of social communication skills, such as autism spectrum disorder (ASD). In such cases, social interaction with objects and organisms is preferred due to their more predictable and easily decipherable behavior (Lahiri et al. 2011; Yakub et al. 2014). The number and the duration of the interactions in an individual or group setting and in relation to the age of the user is also a challenge that has been pinpointed in the field of Social Robotics, since it can affect the familiarization between the user and the interactive object (Leite et al. 2013). It would be of value to take aspects such as the social and psychological aspects of the relationship between the user and the interactive object also in rehabilitation scenarios that are currently only exploring the functional aspect; while the body of research on this topic is not so extensive, it has been proven that social interaction within the context of rehabilitation therapy can raise the patient's motivation and encouragement. Parameters such as the intensity and rhythm of the encouraging sound effects during the exercise, or the physical presence of a social agent that provides guidance and support, instead of a video recording or a simulation, have been identified here as elements of importance (Matarić et al. 2007).

The evaluation of interactive art experiences as a cognitive experience was a layer added by the approach of Bilda et al. (2007) who analyzed the presence of Body, Thought and Feedback as three interrelated components that are dominant in varying percentages in interactive experiences. The first component refers to the part of the interaction where the participant becomes aware that their body causes a change in the system; the second component, Thought, refers to mental processes reported during the interactive experience, related to the understanding of the causal relationship between bodily movement and interactive system output. This part plays a crucial role in the interactive experience, as it represents the moment that the user starts consciously using their body or thoughts as an instrument of the interaction. The third component, Feedback, refers to the observation of visual or auditory changes in the interactive environment, resulting from the participant's input.

This identification of distinct components within the interactive experience, and the analysis of the duration and sequence of each component, as well as the moments of their juxtaposition, shapes a highly useful tool for identifying their interrelations and plan their sequence and concurrences in future experiments. In order to plan an interactive experience tailored to the specific needs of the user, the performative decline in terms of hearing and vision could be an issue to be considered here in the case of aging individuals, as it has been discussed in the field of Health game design (Been-Lirn Duh et al. 2010) and Rehabilitation Robotics (Yakub et al. 2014); in the context of interaction design, auditory and color sensitivity can render a range of colors and sounds imperceptible, or affect negatively the emotional state of the user. The difference in response speed in users with declining cognitive and locomotor skills should therefore be considered in order to ensure that the interactive experience will affect positively the user.

Bodily movement has also been a topic of investigation in the context of interactive design, with the most influential approach being that of Harris and Bongers (2002) who explore the nuances of bodily positioning in relation to each of the sensors and actuators that compose the system. Bodily movement is described in terms of axial positioning (described as Degrees of Freedom along X,Y,Z axes) and the association between the body and the sensor is described as Range of the sensor, referring to three potential scales: the 'Intimate scale', where the sensor is within hand reach; the arm range or the bodysphere, and the 'Architectural or Spatial Body Movement', where the sensor is within 0–10 m. For rehabilitation robotics, which involve a wide range of exercises specific to the impairment of different body parts, such as training of upper or lower limbs (Brewer et al. 2007; Fasoli et al. 2003), gait training (Pennycott et al. 2012; Patton et al. 2008), rehabilitation of hand and fingers for the treatment of grasp pathologies (Polygerinos et al. 2015) and wrist rehabilitation (Krebs et al. 2007; Gupta et al. 2008), the categorization of the experiments in terms of allowed degrees of bodily positioning, rotation and movement, is certainly of value.

9.3 Guidelines for Interaction Design for Healthcare and Wellbeing

The proposed guidelines are divided into two categories: *Design* and *Interaction*. The explored themes within this research chapter related to *Design* are *Scale* and *Materiality*; themes related to *Interaction* are parameters related to movement and its nuances, such as *Range of movement, Spatial relations, Rhythm and Predictability of responses* (Fig. 9.1). The guidelines have been developed after reflecting on

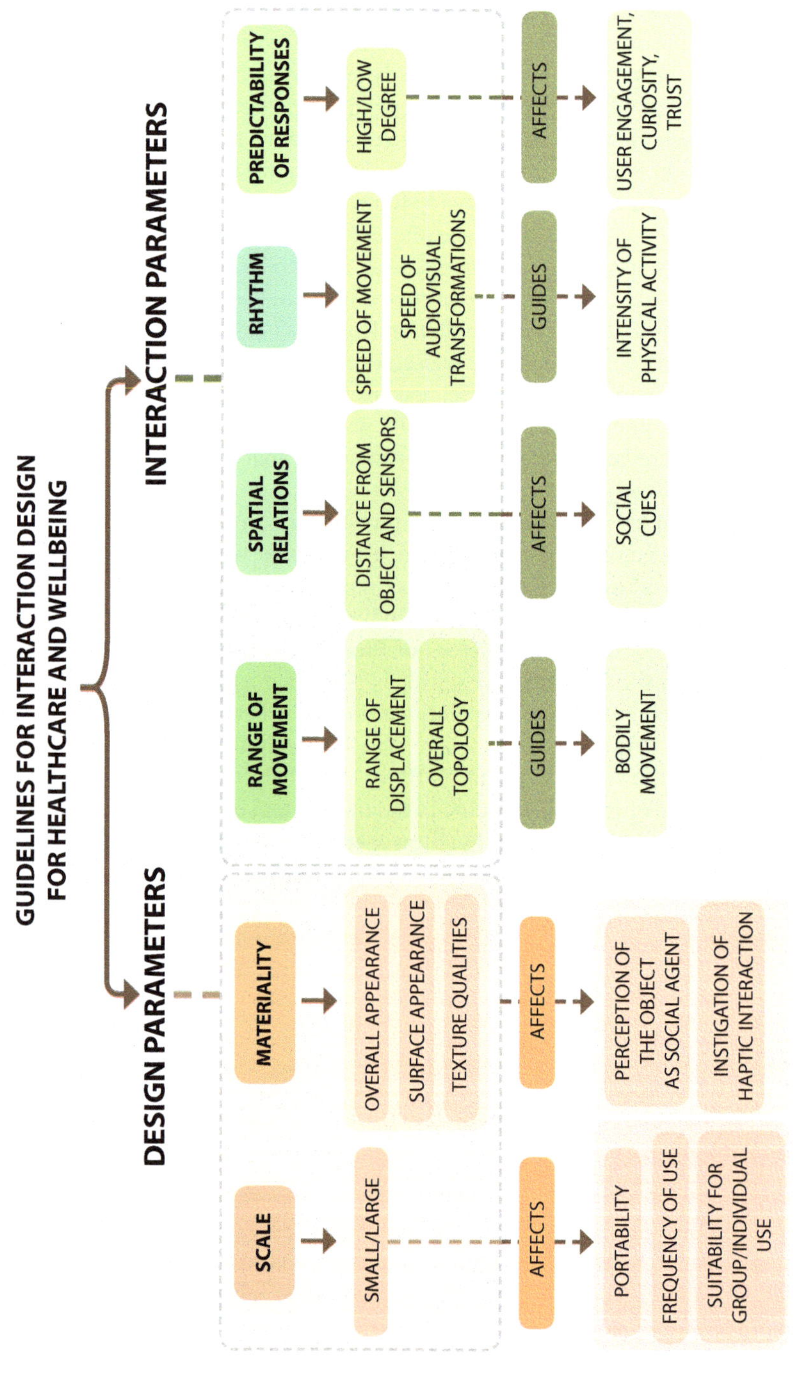

Fig. 9.1 Guidelines for interaction design for healthcare and wellbeing

accomplished and tested physical experiments with real-time interactive environments and social robotics. Three of these are presented in the form of case studies which are presented in the next section. The following three scenarios were considered as the possible application settings, as they reflect some of the most frequently encountered themes in HCI for healthcare and wellbeing:

(a) The enhancement of physical activity, which is expressed as increased daily walkability, or increased movement within a specific spatial setting
(b) The enhancement of physiological wellbeing in a rehabilitation setting
(c) The enhancement of emotional wellbeing related to supporting users with social withdrawal and isolation, training users with impairments of social communication skills, and increasing social interaction.

A short elaboration is given below on each of the categories and the subthemes, while later studies will expand on each theme and also cater to specific needs of different case studies.

A1. Scale

Two scales are examined in this category: the small (or product) scale, and the medium/large scale, which can be an architectural installation in the form of an architectonic element such as a ceiling or a floor. Along with Scale, as the primary parameter, the following factors are considered as secondary set of parameters associated with it:

(a) *Degree of mobility of the interactive systems*
(b) *Distribution and interdependence of the interactive components*
(c) *Number of users*

Interactive systems which have a high degree of mobility can be more easily transported and do not require overt installations, thus allowing their usage in multiple places; large-scale interactive systems, which adhere to/attached to building elements such as floors or roofs, tend to constrain the interaction to one space. Characteristics related to portability, such as easy transportation, light weight and freedom of movement and relocation, are useful features in the case of interactive objects designed for rehabilitation settings, which may not require extensive supervision. Frequent repetition of exercises is critical for the improvement of the condition of the targeted body member (Yakub et al. 2014), therefore allowing the user to perform exercises anytime of the day, without constraining them to a specific rehabilitation space, would be a highly desirable property. For the enhancement of emotional wellbeing, these features are essential in cases where the object also acts as a social companion. Freedom of movement would also be of importance in the case of enhancing daily physical activity, floor movement or walkability, by using one or more interactive components that can move independently, akin to a walking partner or a pet that triggers the user to follow them around.

Medium and large-scale interactive systems are deemed more suitable within controlled settings, where the physical activity or rehabilitation exercises can be supervised and are usually constrained to the movement of specific body parts. In this case, the scale of the interactive system constraints the space and time of interaction, since the user has to be in the place where the system is anchored. Such interactive systems however, promote other benefits such as emergent social cohesion and interaction patterns, self-promoted gaming, competitive attitude generation and social engagement at a larger scale. Attributes of emotional wellbeing, implicit companionships and physiological movement can be triggered via such a large-scale interactive system. The architectural space can also gain affective qualities operating as a living organism which can assist the user in cases of social isolation or emotional dysfunction by triggering emotional responses from the user and engaging in social interplay.

As for the spatial arrangement or distribution of the components, the design of the spatial arrangement could become a tool to instigate customized social interaction. This could also result in unplanned and proactive interactions with users. Componential independence would be important in this case, in order to allow switching between all these scenarios and selectively reconfiguring the scale of the intervention and opening it to the public.

Finally, additional parameters, such as the *number of users, the scope of the intervention and the usage patterns* of the intervention space, are also important in determining the choice between a large or small-scale system: In the case of physiological wellbeing, for instance, an interactive floor or roof that triggers physical activity via multimodal interaction would be more suitable for a larger group, while an interactive walking partner, with the capability to be personalized to understand one's emotional state would be more fitting for an individual.

A2. Materiality

Material qualities are important factors in determining how the user perceives the interactive object or system and interacts with it (Fernaeus and Sundström 2012; Hirsch et al. 2000). The parameters of materiality discussed here are:

(a) *The overall appearance*
(b) *Parameters related to the surface appearance, such as the exposure of electronics*
(c) *Textural qualities such as the degree of softness*

Regarding the overall appearance of the system, in cases that focus on social interaction, objects with anthropomorphic or zoomorphic elements incorporated in the design tend to be more easily accepted as partners in social interplay and instigate caring behavior (Leite et al. 2013) which would be important for treating social isolation. The exposure of electronics also has to be considered here (Fernaeus and Sundström 2012), since the interactive object or system might not seem friendly and inviting if the hardware and the wiring are visible.

For cases where the touching or stroking the object is an important part of the interaction, texture qualities such as softness become a critical aspect of the design. This happens especially in cases of enhancing emotional wellbeing, where social interaction is at the core of the objectives, and haptic interaction becomes integral for creating a bond with the interactive object. Finally, the degree of texture softness would also be important for rehabilitation settings which incorporate strongly haptic interaction, such as a medicine ball squeezed by the fingers of the users for testing and increasing finger dexterity.

B1. Range of Movement

In the case of enhancing physical activity, as well as in rehabilitation settings, there is a set of medical guidelines regarding the range of movement that the body parts of the user that are more active in the specific exercise should either conform to, or try to achieve. The need to constrain bodily movement within this specific range means that the components of the interactive system should have a built-in ability to guide the user towards satisfying this requirement. The parameters discussed here are:

(a) the *range of displacement of the whole body of the object,*
(b) *the overall topology of the object*
(c) *the range of movement of components.*

In the context of enhancing walkability, for objects that fit in the small-scale category and have the ability to move freely, the objective is to increase the overall time of floor movement (the overall physical activity of the day) which can be translated to a specific range of movement for the whole body of the interactive object, or a distance that the object is encouraged to cover.

In the context of rehabilitation, involving medium- or large-scale interactive systems, one or more components of the interactive system can be physically transformed, akin to the guiding movement of a physiotherapist which the user is mimicking. The overall structure and topological characteristics of the interactive system can also guide the movement of the user, influencing the way that the user positions and moves their body to interact with the system. Two factors are therefore of importance: the ability of the overall design (topology) of the system, as well as the ability of specific components of the system to trigger a movement within the desired range as a response from the user.

A focus on the overall topology would be more suitable in cases where the whole body is participating in the rehabilitation exercise; the focus on the movement range of independent components, on the other hand, would.

be fitting in a scenario where the focus is on specific body parts, such as the arm movement.

B2. Spatial Relations

This parameter refers to the distance of the user from the sensor and the components of the interactive system. Proxemic behavior is an important part of social presence, and has been a topic of interest for the field of Human Robot Interaction, in the effort to increase the perception of a machinic object as a counterpart that can participate in verbal or non-verbal dialogue in a social setting (Fiore et al. 2013). This factor becomes crucial in settings where enhancing social interaction is a part of the objective; the minimum and maximum distance between the interactive object/system and the user, and the manner in which this distance alters throughout the interaction dialogue, can be interpreted as a series of social cues which significantly influence social qualities to the interactive object.

The distance becomes minimum in rehabilitation sessions where the use of haptics is a part of increasing neuromuscular activity (Turolla et al. 2013), but also in cases where tactile interaction in the context of emotional wellbeing it is a part of the objectives. When the interactive system/object plays the role of a social companion, tactile contact is crucial for the formation of social bonds between the user and the object (Lee et al. 2006) In such cases, the embodiment of sensors that track haptic interaction, such as conductive wire or pressure-sensitive pads in the surface material of the system, adds another layer of electronics in the surface material, the exposure of which needs to be considered as discussed in the section A2.

B3. Rhythm: Speed of Movement or Physical/Audiovisual Transformation

This parameter refers to the time needed for a component of the interactive system to change from state A to state B. This change can be physical, audiovisual transformation or both; rhythm, therefore, refers here to the speed of this transformation.

When the enhancement of physical activity is the goal, the rhythm, or speed of movement can be related to the intensity of the physical activity. Parameters related to the specific profile of the user, such as age and potential disabilities, have to be considered here. In rehabilitation settings for neuromuscular recovery, the rhythm is again of importance, as the speed with which the user is instructed to move the body part that is the focus of the exercise needs to be controlled, to prevent muscle tension. These medical guidelines could be translated to a suggested speed of movement (or change in light and sound) of the component which will guide the movement of the user.

In all cases, the cognitive capacity of the individual, as well as the speed of response to audiovisual stimuli has to be considered in order to program a speed and range of movement which will be perceptible by the user, tuned with the rhythm of their movement, and also easily decipherable in terms of social cues in social interaction training settings.

B4. Predictability of Responses

This section refers to the degree to which the user can foresee the actions of the interactive system. Relevant research on human-robot interaction has shown that a higher degree of unpredictability can raise the curiosity and engagement of the user. These characteristics would be sought in scenarios that target the enhancement of physical activity, where a higher degree of animosity of the interactive system could act motivationally towards more intense physical activity of the user. High levels of curiosity and user engagement could also assist in the provision of sufficient motivation to use the interactive object or system in the first place, which is critical for seniors that tend to have a lesser degree of familiarity with technology (Been-Lirn Duh et al. 2010) and is an issue also discussed within Rehabilitation Robotics (Yakub et al. 2014).

In rehabilitation scenarios, repetition of the same set of exercises is essential, so the part of the system that constrains or guides the bodily movement during the exercise would need to be programmed with higher predictability in its actions. This could change in the case that the interactive system has also agents or components that play a more social and motivational role; the levels of unpredictability need to be considered carefully though, since unforeseeable behavior can also result in lower levels of trust (Law et al. 2017). High levels of predictability should be programmed in cases such as therapeutic environments for autism spectrum disorder, where structure and predictability are critical factors (Javed et al. 2015).

9.4 Exploration of the Presented Themes Through Three Case Studies

The following section shall elaborate upon three case studies conducted under the guidance of the author (Dr. Nimsh Biloria) which were built on the thematic presented in Sect. 9.3. Each experiment deals with a different degree of scale, materiality, range of movement, spatial relationship and rhythm, while addressing different modes of social, mental and physiological engagement at both individual and group level. The experiments were conducted as an exhaustive body of work on real-time interactive environments as part of a European Union Culture grant project titled METABODY under the leadership of Dr. Biloria. The experiments are specifically chosen owing to their multi-modal interaction nature and the manner in which they address the issue of wellbeing at variable scales. Non-verbal communication and exploration of socio-spatial and socio-technical interdependencies became a major feature of these projects. The three projects: RoboZoo, Textrinium and Reflectego elaborated upon in this section shall thus specifically outline the specificities in addressing the aforementioned themes.

4a. Robozoo

RoboZoo, was conceived as an experiment in social robotics consisting of an ecology of small scale robotic-bots which operate on the premise that motion/movement and non-verbal communication can be understood as interfaces of emotional interaction and cognition. The installation aimed at critically examining and assessing the manner in which the divide between humans and machines can be blurred to an extent where aspects of empathy and shared emotional agency become emergent consequences of interactions between the two. Instigating a healthier community engagement, as a critical aspect of wellbeing in urban public spaces via actively merging human and machinic agencies, wherein ambiguity and diffused affordances take center stage, thus provoking pro-active engagements for creating new social structures became a primary objective of Robozoo. (Fig. 9.2).

The project was conceived to operate in two ways for enhancing both physiological and emotional wellbeing. Firstly, it can be deployed in large public spaces including venues such as museums, rehabilitation centers, public squares etc. Here, the interaction motives are focused on enhancing group-based social cohesion and chance encounters. Secondly, RoboZoo can also be used at an individual level wherein it acquires the dimension of a customized pet/companion and thus aids in

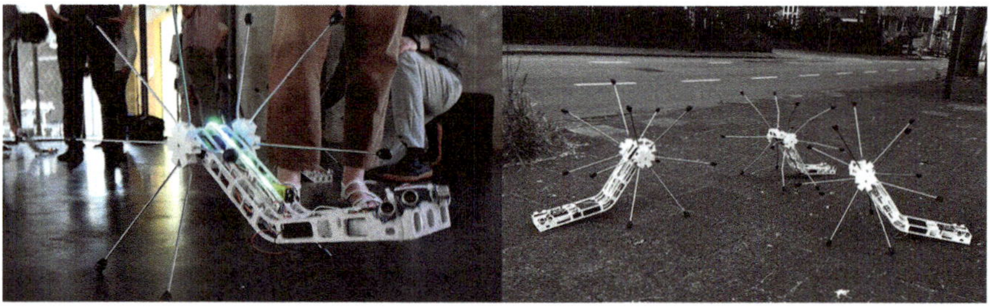

Fig. 9.2 RoboZoo: an ecology of small scale robotic bots. (Image courtesy Dr. Nimish Biloria)

social isolation at an individual scale. This companionship can be facilitated at both indoor and outdoor environments. Robozoo, as an interactive swarm of robots was thus conceived as small-scale bots, which, operate on the basis of a multi-agent swarm computing model. Each bot operates as an individual agent, with embedded proximity sensors, micro-controllers and servo motors, powered by a battery pack. Each agent is further programmed with control rules (akin to a swarm) which enables it to sense its context (people and obstacles), sense the speed of movement/ approach of people as well as other agents towards it and thus propel itself towards people (based on how they approach: gentle movement equates to a friendly approach vs sudden and rapid movement equates to an unfriendly, imposing approach), while maintaining contact with other agents in its vicinity. The bots and humans inter-activate each other in order to create novel social patterns and in the process constantly redefine space via establishing unspoken ecological dependencies.

Scale RoboZoo is conceived at a Product/Object scale as an interactive small-scale swarm of robots, which, operate on the basis of a multi-agent swarm computing model. Each bot operates as an individual agent, with embedded proximity sensors, micro-controllers and servo motors, powered by a battery pack. The bots and humans inter-activate each other in order to create novel social patterns and in the process constantly redefine space via establishing unspoken ecological dependencies. In terms of movement, the bots are completely mobile and are thus free to move in the x and y dimensions via wheel like arrangement of steel spokes with rubberized endings for added safety and grip over different terrain. The embedded sensing ability of the bots and the ability to communicate amongst each other with respect to their geo-location allows them to interact with both group and individual users. The bots can thus be seen as a part of a bigger socio-technical ecology while each one of the bots acts as an individual component with context driven customized behavior.

Materiality RoboZoo, specifically departs from a typical humanoid expression and acquires an abstract zoomorphic appearance. The bots are built of simple kit of parts easy to assemble parts which can be laser cut out of flat sheet material, which in the case of the prototypes was chosen as plastic for the entire body and stainless

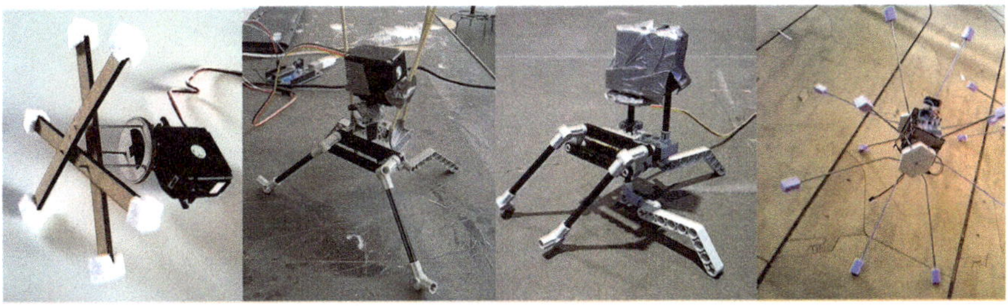

Fig. 9.3 Exploration of the materiality of RoboZoo according to user feedback. (Image courtesy Dr. Nimish Biloria)

steel spoked as wheels. The bot thus gives the appearance of an animate being which is not over imposing and non-threatening. The plastic body acted as a casing for all the electronic hardware, which in the case of RoboZoo was fully exposed to the users. Despite this exposure of its hardware, the overall appearance of the bots even without any facial (human) gesture-based clues was embraced very warmly by children and the elderly alike. Overall, the materiality, which was essentially hard and rough in its texture contradicted the overall user embracing socially outgoing nature of the bots. (Fig. 9.3).

Range of Movement Each bot is programmed with basic control rules (akin to a swarm) which enables it to sense its context (people and obstacles), sense the speed of movement/approach of people as well as other bots towards it and thus propels itself towards people (based on how they approach: gentle movement equates to a friendly approach vs sudden and rapid movement equates to an unfriendly, imposing approach, while maintaining contact with other bots in its vicinity. This allowed for bots at an individual level to showcase customized behavior while making sure that the overall population of bots did not stray away and stayed within determined boundaries. The large range of movement and the explorative nature of the bots resulted in enhancing the overall physical activity of the users, as they developed the tendency to mentally connect and care for the bots and instinctively follow their movements.

Spatial Relations Spatially, apart from self-maintaining boundary conditions, the bots would make physical contact with the users either by actively seeking proximity to individuals within a space or by unexpected interactions with users who would go out of their way to help bots which were physically stuck and were expressing the need to be helped via their physical movement patterns. While tactile interaction was not a part of the designed behaviors, the tendency of the bots to come within close proximity was interpreted by the users as a social cue to caress the bot as a pet, thus forming an emergent social bond. These unexpected user interactions coupled with the ability of such machinic behavior to create novel social engagements created varied socio-spatial relations. (Fig. 9.4).

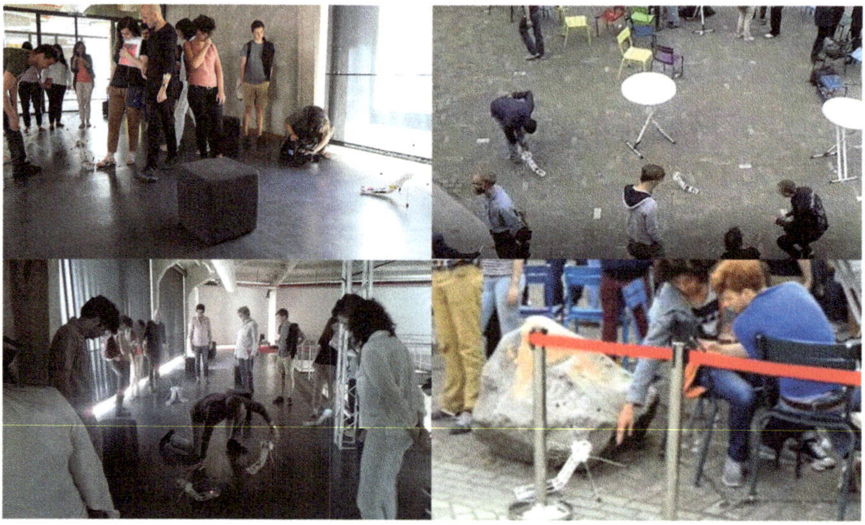

Fig. 9.4 Interactions with RoboZoo during an open to public science event in Delft: upper right and bottom right image and an exhibition at the Media Lab Prado, Madrid, Spain: upper left and bottom left image. (Image courtesy Dr. Nimish Biloria)

Rhythm RoboZoo's rhythms ranged from seemingly erratic behavior to deliberate behavior traits such as following, seeking, approaching etc. These emergent patterns of rhythm constantly occupied the user in a dynamic relationship with otherwise sterile robotic interactions and allowed a sense of inter-connectedness between the user and the machine. This also kept the users mentally engaged and physiologically active while at the same time developing an emotional engagement with the bots (a behavior specifically observed in the elderly, who wanted to name the bots and carry them home).

4b. Textrinium

Textrinium is a smart textile based interactive structure for promoting full-body interaction based physiological wellbeing (Fig. 9.5). The main appearance of the structure is based on the mathematical embedded minimal surface discovered in 1982 by Celso José da Costa. The topology is created by puncturing a compact surface, therefore becoming a finite topology. The current design is a topologically thrice-punctured torus which is deformed until the planer end becomes catenoidal. The name of the project is Textrinium based on the interweaving of different components within the textile, architecture and mathematical geometry. Textrinium interacts with its surroundings via physical movement, change in the color of its textile by differentiating in resistance and integrated sensors like ultrasonic sensors and conductive wire. All the used components are part of the same knitted fabric. (Fig. 9.6).

The structure is supported by an internal glass-fiber flexible skeleton. Extensive research in material systems, topology optimization, stress and deformation simulation within fabrics, weaving patterns and fiber directionality, integrating (knitting)

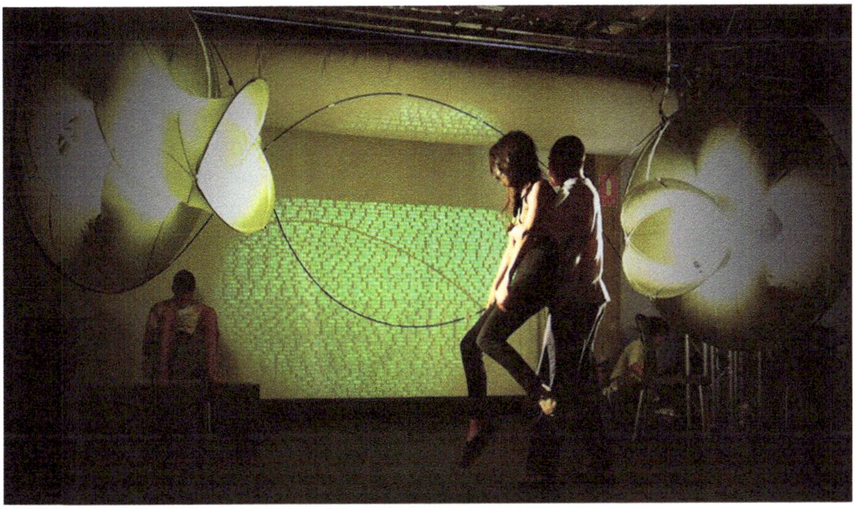

Fig. 9.5 Textrinium: a smart textile based interactive structure. (Image courtesy Dr. Nimish Biloria)

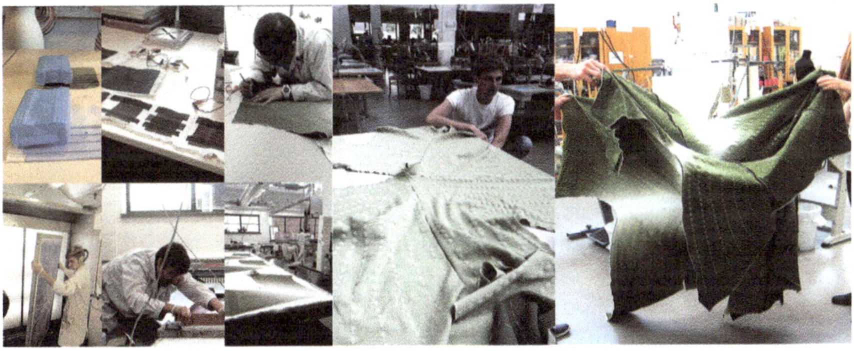

Fig. 9.6 Different phases of the construction of Textrinium, including testing the conductive wire, printing the thermochromic paint on the fabric and assembling the different components. (Image courtesy Dr. Nimish Biloria and Dimitra Dritsa)

sensing, sewing techniques exploration, actuation and control systems within the textiles, thermo-chromic textile-based applications, phosphorescence applications and computation numerically controlled fabrication went behind the making of Textrinium.

Scale Textrinium was a Large scale real-time interactive installation, composed of 2 inter-communicating components made of a flexible glass-fiber skeletal system wrapped with a smart textile with embedded sensing and actuation systems. The two components promote full physical body interaction and are anchored/positioned within a designated spatial zone resulting in limiting the interactions with only the users who visit the installation space. The installation's behavioral affordance was based on interaction with single users per component and a data communication protocol from one component to the other was evolved from studying such interactions. This resulted in the development of competitive behavior between the two components resulting in a surge for attracting potential users towards each other via physical movement, light and sound pattern generation and color gradient transitions. The shape of the components was specifically developed to be highly inviting to the users and produced behaviors of physical immersion into the two components.

Materiality Textrinium, as a therapeutic installation involves physical contact and tactile feedback between the user and the two components. This determined a soft fabric material as the material of choice to become the external face of the two components. The fabric in itself is a smart fabric which is specifically developed for the installation and is developed from a thermochromic material with embedded heat emitting fibers woven in as a part of the knit. This allowed for traces of human touching and stroking in the form of bright outlines of the palms, fingers etc. to be left behind, creating visual feedback. Besides this the embedded conductive wires allowed for automated emission of heat in order to produce emergent patterns for attracting visitors. Fabric speakers, made out of conductive coils and small magnets woven within the smart fabric were also activated by the frequency of the touch. The electronics were fully embedded within the make-up of the Smart Textile and were hardly noticeable to the naked eye, thus creating the impression of a softer, more inviting structure which could be easily touched (Fig. 9.7).

Range of Movement The range of movement of the components was programmed at two levels: Firstly, Physical x, y and z axis (within a spatial boundary) displacement using motorized manipulation of specific structural points per component accompanied with the turning on/off of embedded lights in order to attract users. The component getting lesser attention (detected via lesser number of touching and stroking by users) will produce rapid movement and light patterns in an attempt to attract more attention. Secondly, once the users have been isolated the movements

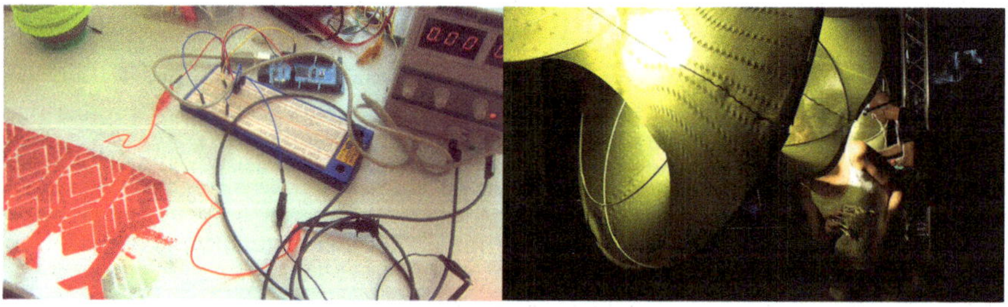

Fig. 9.7 Left: Testing the conductive wire embedded in the fabric. Right: Interaction of the users with Textrinium at the Media Lab Prado, Madrid, Spain. (Image courtesy Dr. Nimish Biloria and Dimitra Dritsa)

become subtler and allow for users to immerse themselves (Torso upwards) into the components themselves. The topology of the components reflects this immersive intent. (Fig. 9.7).

Spatial Relations Textrinium deploys two kinds of sensing mechanisms: proximity sensing and comparative touch indexing. This implies that the components independently can compare the distance of people from them and can compare the amount of attention each one is getting by comparing the amount of times they have been touched individually. These trigger respective movement patterns in order to foster specific social interplay to capture the attention of the passer-by. Haptic interaction which binds the user's touch with emergent sound patterns and color changes establish a deeper relationship with the user wherein spatial boundaries are dissolved via corresponding physiological gestures by both counterparts to display acquired familiarity with each other. Once immersed within the component, the user can further embrace, touch, stroke and intimately hear novel sonic patterns from the embedded speakers (Fig. 9.8).

Rhythm Textrinium thus presents two different rhythms for different levels of engagement: a fast paced, three-dimensional displacement and a slow-paced transformation of sound, color and light accompanied with slower pulsating tactile feedback. Apart from a slow initiation of inter-personal contact via the installations rhythmic character, the installation, once engaged with the users predominantly acquires a softer and submissive dimension to avoid abrupt neuromuscular contractions while promoting upper body movement and mental stimulation.

4c. Reflectego

Reflectego was conceived as an interactive art installation to enhance physiological wellbeing by attracting a large number of people to interact with it within a public setting. The design derives from a kaleidoscopic composition of faceted mirrors, aimed specifically at distorting perception. In the project, the user literally becomes the physical object inside a kaleidoscope in which he sees his image scattered and recomposed as a result of his movement patterns. The structure consists of a suspended faceted mirror-surface with embedded proximity sensors, which hovers and physically changes the inclination and directions of its facets in real-time based on the people it can sense below it. The user is thus visually displaced, since his perceptual affinity of seeing him/herself in a mirrored surface is suddenly challenged. The installation is suitable for a group level interaction wherein emergent social patterns would emerge in a dynamic fashion (Fig. 9.9).

Scale Reflectego is a Large-scale installation which operates akin to an animated architectural roof surface. It is thus anchored in place and requires the consideration of various security protocols. While the installation is being restricted in space, owing to its large dimension and its being installed within catchment areas (entrance lobbies, courtyards etc.) of large-scale public buildings such as Museums, Shopping malls etc., it benefits from the thoroughfare of large number of people. The installa-

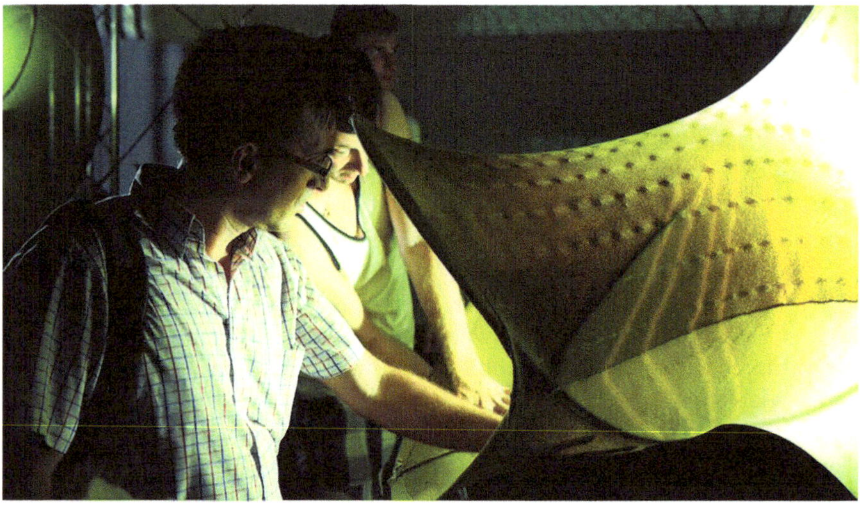

Fig. 9.8 Users interacting with Textrinium by actuating the conductive wire with their touch. (Image courtesy Dr. Nimish Biloria)

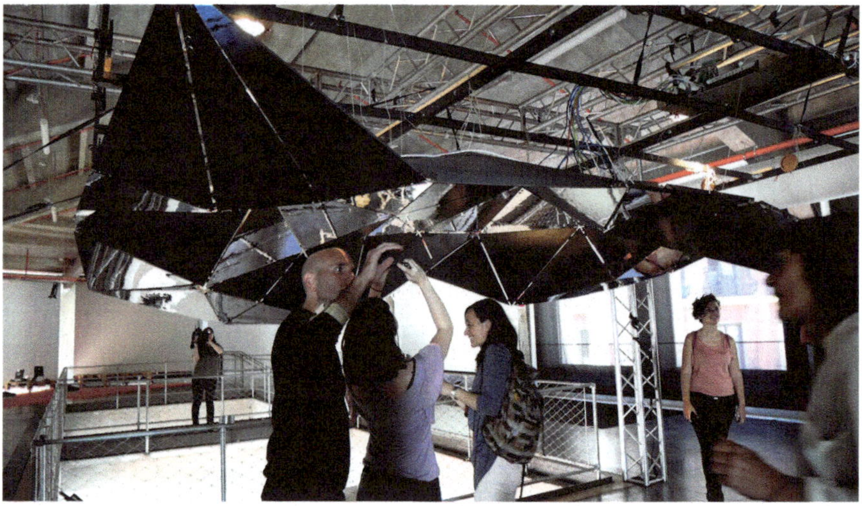

Fig. 9.9 Reflectego: an interactive roof surface. (Image courtesy Dr. Nimish Biloria)

tion is conceived as a collection of components with a low level of individuality. They are self-similar in nature and are able to produce a defined behavior upon actuation.

Materiality Reflectego is conceived as a hard textured, highly geometric, singular patterned tessellation bearing installation with embedded electronics (Figs. 9.9 and 9.10). The surface facing the user (after being suspended) is highly reflective and

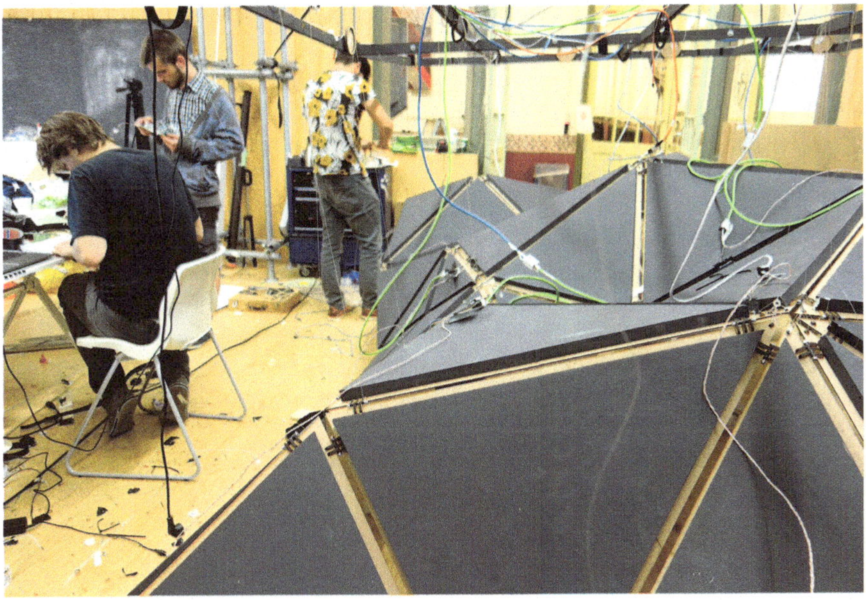

Fig. 9.10 The embedded electronics, hidden on top of the interactive components. (Image courtesy Dr. Nimish Biloria)

glossy in order to discourage tactile interaction and capture the reflections of the passers-by. The installation in itself is made out of light weight material in order to avoid any existing surface/spatial element that it is anchored to. The installation required a rigid wood frame structure which harnesses external motors and a series of proximity sensors embedded at regular intervals throughout the installation.

Range of Movement The installation acquired a tessellated physical form in order to make a seemingly flat surface actuate and expose its reflective tessellations three dimensionally. The actuations (in the form of strings being pulled by a motorized pulley attached at the intersections of the tessellated surfaces) were local in nature and were only initiated when the presence of an individual was detected below the surface. The movement of the entire surface, though operating on a simple and singular rule of pulling strategic vertices transformed the otherwise flat roof/surface to a fluid, highly interactive surface. As the users constantly moved in multiple directions, immersed in the observation of their scattered reflection patterns, the angular transformations of the installation resulted in the activation of a much larger floor-space area than the footprint of the roof, thus increasing the overall floor movement time of the users.

Spatial Relations The interactive object was not meant to be touched in this case, but to be perceived as an organism which engages in social interplay by constantly reconfiguring its distance from the user (see proxemics as explained above). A predefined distance was kept on purpose as a buffer between the object and the user, to enhance this effect. The interactions and associations which people made with the installation were also very local in nature, with people specifically immersed in interacting with the surface area on top of them. Gestures ranged from extending the body towards the surface, extension of arms, Jumping, redirection arm movement underneath the surface to actuate other parts etc.

Rhythm The installation involved a variable rhythm depending on the number of actuations which were ongoing at any point in time. This specifically depended on the number of people at any given time and the concentration of people below the surface. Physical activity rhythms were directly connected with the degree of actuation and the intensity with which an individual is connected with seeking his/her perfect reflection or is engaged in social game-play by means of actuating three dimensional patterns in space.

9.5 Conclusion and Discussion

The Chapter presents an intensive set of guidelines for the design of real-time interactive design environments (specifically in the form of physical interventions of variable scale) for enhancing urban health and wellbeing. Such environments go beyond the conception of clinically assistive technologies but rather bind them with socially interactive design systems of a more experimental nature. In doing so, such environments propose an enjoyment and immersive experience driven route to promote the active usage and positively impact user acceptance of otherwise insipid technologies. These guidelines have been built upon the authors' own experiences pertaining to evaluating observed user engagement and interviews with users who experienced the elaborated multi-scalar socio-technical interactive installations. The guidelines pertaining to Scale, Materiality, Range of movement, Spatial relations, Rhythm and Predictability of responses have been carefully chosen after understanding interaction design as a socio-technical instrument embedded within a spatial context. Interfacing technical aspects of mechanics, sensing, actuation and control systems with mental and physical attributes such as bodily awareness and interaction based sensory feedback, social dynamics and spatial relation, thus form the basis of the proposed guidelines. An active inclusion of social and psychological aspects of the relationship between the user and the interactive object/space rather than focusing specifically on functional/utilitarian aspects is thus proposed for the health and wellbeing sector.

A self-critique on the presented case studies relates to the nature of the experiments, which, are exclusively focused on enhancing overall physiological and psychological wellbeing, with hardly any interaction with users displaying a specific therapeutic need. Future experiments thus need to be conducted with this focus, in order to explore in practice how stricter medical guidelines can be embedded in the interaction dialogue while retaining a satisfactory degree of social interaction when this is needed. Furthermore, as the guidelines have been constructed with an intention to open the field of interaction design to other adjacent disciplines, a more interdisciplinary team structure will be pursued in future experiments, in order to actively incorporate input from collaborators with appropriate expertise in fields such as physiotherapy and rehabilitation robotics.

Future research direction for the authors shall also involve a steady refinement of the proposed guidelines while being actively engaged in developing such multi-scalar real-time interactive systems. However, the quantification of observed interactions in terms of interaction time, degree of engagement and attention span etc. would certainly be among the next steps to enrich the observed and interviewed experiences of users. This shall include capturing physiological data such as electrodermal activity, heart rate, skin temperature etc. and interfacing this with other heterogeneous data sets such as spatial location mapping, and mapping group dynamics. The measurement of affective responses through mapping facial expressions, eye movement and gesture tracking, will also assist in further decoding and quantifying social interaction. A future step would therefore be the enrichment of each category in the proposed guidelines with suggested means of evaluation of performance and unobtrusive measurement of the overall degree of bodily activity, the muscular actuation, the generated affects and the social interaction.

This shall enable a more structured identification of hidden relationships between space, people and technology, which instinctively activate the users at a mental and physical front to participate in and be motivated by such interactive experiences. An equal focus on individual behavior change and group level emergent engagements within such interactive environments shall thus become vital studies for the future of health and wellbeing initiatives.

Acknowledgements We would specially like to thank the research and design team members involved in the RoboZoo, Textrinium and FLUID projects: Dr. Jia Rey Chang, Javid Jooshesh, Guang Yang, Jan Paclt, Chris Pydo, Kasper Siderius, Radoslaw Flis, Bob Heester, Esther Slagter, Marien Teeuw, Veronika, Laszlo, Ricardo Galli, Chrysostomos Tsaprailis, Leslie Che, Jiarui Sun, Yağ ız Söylev, Tanya Somova, Nick van Dorp, Hua Fan, Y. Lyu, Danny Cheng, R. Chheda. Additionally, we would like to thank the European Union Culture Grant for providing us with the opportunity and for funding such interactive environments, as well as the Swedish School of Textiles from the University of Boras, and especially Dr. Delia Dumitrescu, Dr. Hanna Landin and Marjan Kooroshnia, for the provision of guidance and facilities for the construction of the interactive textiles.

References

Been-Lirn Duh, H., et al. (2010). Senior-friendly technologies: Interaction design for senior users. In *CHI extended abstracts* (pp. 4513–4516). New York: ACM.

Bilda, Z., Candy, L., & Edmonds, E. (2007). An embodied cognition framework for interactive experience. *CoDesign, 3*(2), 123–137.

Brewer, B. R., et al. (2007). Poststroke upper extremity rehabilitation: A review of robotic systems and clinical results. *Topics in Stroke Rehabilitation, 14*(6), 22–44.

Bullivant, L. (2007). Alice in Technoland. *Architectural Design, 75*(4), 6–13.
Delbrück, T., et al. (2007). A tactile luminous floor for an interactive autonomous space. *Robotics and Autonomous Systems, 55*(6), 433–443.
Fasoli, S. E., et al. (2003). Effects of robotic therapy on motor impairment and recovery in chronic stroke. *Archives of Physical Medicine and Rehabilitation, 84*(4), 477–482.
Fernaeus, Y., & Sundström, P. (2012). The material move how materials matter in interaction design research. In *Proceedings of the designing interactive systems conference* (pp. 486–495). Newcastle Upon Tyne.
Fiore, S. M., et al. (2013). Toward understanding social cues and signals in human–robot interaction: Effects of robot gaze and proxemic behavior. *Frontiers in Psychology, 4*, 859.
Gupta, A., et al. (2008). Design, control and performance of RiceWrist: A force feedback wrist exoskeleton for rehabilitation and training. *The International Journal of Robotics Research, 27*(2), 233–251.
Harris, Y., & Bongers, B. (2002). Approaches to creating interactivated spaces, from intimate to inhabited interfaces. *Organized Sound, 7*(3), 239–246.
Heerink, M., et al. (2010). Assessing acceptance of assistive social agent technology by older adults: The Almere model. *International Journal of Social Robotics, 2*(4), 361–375.
Heijden, H. (2004). User acceptance of hedonic information systems. *MIS Quarterly, 28*(4), 695–704.
Hirsch, T. et al. (2000). The ELDer project: Social, emotional, and environmental factors in the design of eldercare technologies. In *CUU '00 Proceedings on the 2000 conference on Universal Usability* (pp. 72–79). Arlington, Virginia, USA.
Hornecker, E., & Buur, J. (2006). Getting a grip on tangible interaction: A framework on physical space and social interaction. In *Proceedings of the SIGCHI conference on human factors in computing systems* (pp. 437–446). New York: ACM.
Javed, H. et al. (2015). Thomas and friends: Implications for the design of social robots and their role as social story telling agents for children with autism. In *2015 IEEE international conference on robotics and biomimetics (ROBIO)* (pp. 1145–1150). Zhuhai, China.
Kidd, C. D. et al. (2006). A sociable robot to encourage social interaction among the elderly. In *Proceedings of the 2006 IEEE international conference on robotics and automation* , (pp. 3972–3976). Orlando: IEEE.
Krebs, H. I., et al. (2007). Robot-aided neurorehabilitation: A robot for wrist rehabilitation. *IEEE Transactions on Neural Systems and Rehabilitation Engineering, 15*(3), 327–335.
Lahiri, U., et al. (2011). Design of a gaze-sensitive virtual social interactive system for children with autism. *IEEE Transactions on Neural Systems and Rehabilitation Engineering, 19*(4), 443–452.
Law, E. et al. (2017). A wizard-of-Oz study of curiosity in human-robot interaction. In *26th IEEE international symposium on robot and human interactive communication (RO-MAN)* (pp. 607–614). Lisbon, Portugal.
Lee, K. M., et al. (2006). Are physically embodied social agents better than disembodied social agents?: The effects of physical embodiment, tactile interaction, and people's loneliness in human–robot interaction. *International Journal of Human-Computer Studies, 64*(10), 962–973.
Leite, I., et al. (2013). Social robots for long-term interaction: A survey. *International Journal of Social Robotics, 5*(2), 291–308.
Luo, X. et al. (2005). An augmented reality training environment for post-stroke finger extension rehabilitation. In *Proceedings of the 2005 IEEE 9th international conference on rehabilitation robotics* (pp. 329–332). Chicago: IEEE.
Matarić, M. J., et al. (2007). Socially assistive robotics for post-stroke rehabilitation. *Journal of Neuroengineering and Rehabilitation, 4*, 5.
Oosterhuis, K. (2002). *Programmable architecture.* L'Arca Edizione.
Patton, J., et al. (2008). KineAssist: Design and development of a robotic overground gait and balance therapy device. *Topics in Stroke Rehabilitation, 15*(2), 131–139.

Pennycott, A., et al. (2012). Towards more effective robotic gait training for stroke rehabilitation: A review. *Journal of Neuroengineering and Rehabilitation, 9*(1), 65.

Polygerinos, P. et al. (2015). Soft robotic glove for hand rehabilitation and task specific training. In *2015 IEEE international conference on robotics and automation* (pp. 2913–2919).

Steele, R., et al. (2009). Elderly persons' perception and acceptance of using wireless sensor networks to assist healthcare. *International Journal of Medical Informatics, 78*(12), 788–801.

Sun, H., & Zhang, P. (2006). Causal relationships between perceived enjoyment and perceived ease of use: An alternative approach. *Journal of the Association for Information Systems, 7*(9), 618–645.

Taysheng, J. (2005). Advanced ubiquitous media for interactive space. *Computer Aided Architectural Design Futures, 6*, 341–350.

Turolla, A., et al. (2013). Haptic-based neurorehabilitation in poststroke patients: A feasibility prospective multicentre trial for robotics hand rehabilitation. *Computational and Mathematical Methods in Medicine, 2013*, 895492.

Wada, K., & Shibata, T. (2007). Living with seal robots-its sociopsychological and physiological influences on the elderly at a care house. *IEEE Transactions on Robotics, 23*(5), 972–980.

Yakub, F., et al. (2014). Recent trends for practical rehabilitation robotics, current challenges and the future. *International Journal of Rehabilitation Research, 37*(1), 9–21.

Part IV
Urban Living Labs

Chapter 10
Design Labs for Data-Driven Multivalence

Mathias Funk

Abstract Designing products, spaces, and services for the Everyday has become the focus of designerly research and practice over the last decade. As designers create complex systems that are space-aware, grow and dynamically morph, their tools and methods have to undergo a similar parallel transformation and extension–often towards and borrowing from technical disciplines. Current designers work with complexity and let data shape all facets and modalities of designed artifacts. This article investigates new challenges for design operating at macro, meso, and micro scales. A translational perspective is proposed together with new types of labs and design research infrastructure that address challenges and emerging needs of the design community.

Keywords Design labs · Multi-valence · Research through design · Research products · Industrial design · Systems design

10.1 Introduction

Different related areas of design, industrial design, product design and interaction design, have over the past years transitioned towards becoming more aware, concerned, and appreciative of environments. Spaces ranging from personal living to work, leisure and communal spaces are not anymore considered broader contexts that simply determine usage; instead, they have become part of the core business of design. The current situation in the broader field is that designers need to go beyond the past strengths in the design of products, systems, and services in the direct human context, where sensing of body and space connects to actuation and interaction with the human senses. The world for which we design became increasingly complex and multi-faceted, with different styles of interactivity and user (experience) needs. Technology has been integrated deeply in the world and, at the same

M. Funk (✉)
Department of Industrial Design, Eindhoven University of Technology,
Eindhoven, The Netherlands
e-mail: M.Funk@tue.nl

N. Biloria (ed.), *Data-driven Multivalence in the Built Environment*, S.M.A.R.T. Environments, https://doi.org/10.1007/978-3-030-12180-8_10

time, the world has been integrated with technology, i.e., algorithms have increasingly access to sense, know, and influence our Everyday. On the one hand, end-users comprehend more and aim to leverage computation in previously untouched fields and domains. On the other hand, autonomous and hidden computational processes work with personal, behavioral, and contextual data at an accelerating pace. We observe a growth of intricate relationships between information systems and associative material formations at variable scales.

As a response, designers became more confident in implementing designs in new application areas, based on emerging technologies. This paved the way for the move from conceptual design to a new form of applied, interventionist engineering of the relationships between humans, the context, and the world at large (Fischer et al. 2016). Consequently, what we design and research is not anymore confined to a singular space and shape: there is variety and diversity in the deployment contexts. Digital ubiquity in the contemporary environment is absorbed, modulated, processed, and actively used for enhancing the performance of all processes from the extra-ordinary to the mundane.

10.1.1 Multi-valence

The future Everyday is a distributed, decentralized design space that requires new design competencies: systemic understanding of design challenges, iterative translation into distributed prototypes, design explorations beyond a single product, and experiential working with data streams and analytics. This is crucial to embrace for design, as many challenges are too complex to leave to over-reductionist engineering views only. The state of design in this scope is characterized as a positive state of unfinishedness, as multi-valence. For years, products are released as *beta*, as data-driven design hybrids that functionally operate with lower fidelity while collecting data in-situ (Funk 2011) that is fed back to design and engineering to continue the design process, to specify follow-up products, or to even change the operational business model. At the same time, such hybrid products are vessels of temporary states determined by real-time data streams evolving from the creative fusion of social data, ubiquitous computing, parametric/relational design systems and material computing. The more products become physical and integrated in environments, the more interfaces to the Everyday are established – with unprecedented implications: "IoT sensors enable new sharing economy services that are personalized, hyperlocal, and can be delivered at short notice, for example food sharing among neighbors to prevent waste. Yet, there are many design challenges and ethical concerns that the HCI community needs to address to make these proactive services intelligible and accountable" (Fischer et al. 2016). This crucially contributes to multi-valence: products and systems change their shape, function, and purpose with the data they are fed and that they exchange with others products and systems. Their relations change according to collected, processed, and linked data, a multi-valence that shapes the perceived qualities of what is provided and meaningful for end-users.

Madeleine Akrich writes that "new technologies may not only lead to new arrangements of people and things. They may, in addition, generate and "naturalize" new forms and orders of causality and, indeed, new forms of knowledge about the world" (Akrich 1992). How can we contribute to the reality of contemporary living and working spaces with multi-domain research and design strategies? We need to define or rather re-define the scope of design and of what "environment" and "space" can mean for a design. At the same time, we need to embrace computational design strategies (e.g., stigmergy, biomimicry, algorithmic design, and generative design systems), we need to start designing eco-systems of products, systems, that build upon multi-agent systems, complex behavior, and emergence) and investigate their implications for the development of sustainable and resilient design of responsive spaces and products.

10.1.2 Designing with Data

To design systems for and in a real-life context, contextual parameters need to be available for design explorations and to design prototypes against. Such parameters are increasingly difficult to cover entirely, they are dynamic in nature and represent non-linear phenomena and mappings. Design now happens in a multi-dimensional space that cannot be left anymore to intuition and prior experiences and expertise; the variety in what a product might have to deal with in terms of sensed and communicated data and what it might influence in terms of actuation and, again, communicated data is beyond the scope of past design spaces. Data as design material is a crucial consideration, if not direct ingredient for most contemporary designs. The fact that machine sensing can now extend beyond the proximity of a single product or space, allows for interoperability in **understanding the context of use** and to build formal, structured knowledge as a product of gathering insights that can be compared and archived. Such data often enables the design as it drives a specific phase of the design process, but it might not take an integrated part in the final design. Other designs use data structurally, as **derivatives or models trained** before they are deployed. Data in these designs serves as an extensive body of examples against which the design or part of the design can be automatically trained. Such data and learning represent a different approach towards designing mappings: training by example in contrast to designed or programmed mappings. This approach has become en vogue with the recent availability of fast, efficient machine-learning techniques. However, the availability of data in the right quantity and quality is a severe bottleneck to applying machine-learning structurally in design. Finally, there is a class of **designs that leverage data** provided while they are used: this data can come from sensors in the context, e.g., temperature, weather, indoor-climate, and presence, or it comes from linked data streams that connect the product to a remote source of data, e.g., stock market or social media data. These designs range from data representation, i.e., visualisation, physicalisations, sonification, etc., (Funk 2016) with the aim to **communicate to end-users** and things in the context, to control systems that process data in a particular way to **control actuation in the context**. The crucial point is that data is the subject of design and without the availability of fresh, relevant data the product becomes considerably less useful or pleasant in its experience.

If the availability of data of a specific quality and quantity is decisive and determining for the success of a design process, designers need to focus on data acquisition and curation as well as ways to leverage the data in later stages of the design process successfully.

10.1.3 Designing with Complexity

Mirroring a more complex technological world, designers strive to understand and design with complexity in new ways. As discussed before, complexity has become a phenomenon of any current design context, not only because of designing for broader scopes and end-users repurposing products, but also due to the need to respond to the multiplicity of signals in contemporary environments. Hence the question: how to capture contextual complexity for design? We need answers beyond "go out, probe, bring back the data, design". We need to think in the direction of simulating data that matches the context to some degree and of involving scripted or data-driven (AI) agents to simulate the behavior. Synthetic data with well-defined levels of entropy can go a long way to develop data-driven generative meta-design systems (Khan and Angeles 2007).

In this article, we take the position that approaches scaling contextual spaces and involving complexity and data need labs and studio spaces to properly function, yet: labs are hard! How can a lab-based design approach look that maps fluently to different scales from materials and computation, products, and environments, towards buildings and cities? Contemporary industrial design is concerned with the products and systems directly within reach of individuals living in future smart spaces. While we observe an ongoing transformation from single product designs to more spatially, environmentally, and systemically aware products, traditional means to design, prototype and evaluate limit this progression. We investigate in this article how a new lab infrastructure for designing and researching smart environments could look like, and we propose a threefold classification of scales for designing systemic products and services. In the following, we will first introduce concrete challenges for design of current and near-future products and systems including related work on various forms of interaction, designing with data and systems design. After this, we define a set of criteria for framing new design research labs. We close with a discussion and general conclusions.

10.2 Challenges for Design

As described above, big challenges in design are how to design for systems, how to design at scale (for different scales) and how to design for the long-term mundane, the present and future Everyday. In other words, what does it mean to design spaces (1) that turn interactive, responsive, and dynamic, (2) that consist of a multitude of components, devices, products, and services whose composition changes dynamically, and (3) that must accommodate different, increasing needs over time up to the point when they must change or be eradicated (Rodden et al. 2004).

10.2.1 Designing Space-Aware Systems

Space-aware systems operate with and within specific (target) environments. Yet, what kinds of environments are we looking for? Environments have traditionally been rather stable, which is changing now. From a traditionally, general spatial meaning, we translate "interactive environment" commonly to a "place furnished with a specific set of interactive artifacts and systems" (Janlert and Stolterman 2017). Such a system are not anymore a "limited set of rather tightly organized artifacts […] in a fixed work setting with a fixed repertoire of recurring tasks" (Janlert and Stolterman 2017). Instead, the exposure is characterized by variety, both in devices and purposes. And this variety is not organized but dispersed in a "rather confusing and overwhelming dynamic multitude" (Janlert and Stolterman 2017). Although much effort was spent on designing spaces, from personal living and work places to public venues, this designed stability and order is breaking up, flattening out and becoming more fluid. While spaces traditionally have been characterized by different design units coming together, rather than being designed fully from scratch, our current reality offers new qualities of such bricolage and showing signs of an accelerating transition.

Interaction is part of this transition and will increasingly play a role in how "livable" our environments will be and can be perceived. Personal spaces nowadays house often a growing collection of devices, objects, and things that embody some form of smartness, intelligence, or cognitive abilities. Only in the future we will be able to turn this "collection" into a "system", through carefully designing new types of products that anticipate to realize collective behavior and perhaps emerging qualities. Such systems are not just interactive, but proactive and autonomous to serve us in a multitude of facets of the Everyday. In other words, "small digital devices that have become part of everyday life contain much complexity, much functionality to control, but there is very little surface available from controls and displays" (Janlert and Stolterman 2017).

As part of this transition, we need to tackle the problem of *cluttering*, which essentially refers to devices occupying visual, auditory, interaction and attention space and asking for focus and engagement. "With an increasing number of interactive devices, the situation is likely to get more cluttered, hampering or incapacitating user interactions." (Janlert and Stolterman 2017) When we look deeper, we can distinguish perceptual and behavioral cluttering: the former means that there is too much going on in a disorderly fashion, which threatens to confuse and mislead the user–occlusion, chaos and distraction ensue (Janlert and Stolterman 2017). Peripheral interaction might be a positive way to frame this phenomenon (Bakker et al. 2015), yet the problem remains. The latter, behavioral cluttering, refers to interference during interactions, in which several devices are involved, unintendedly. Proxemic or gestural interactions are and likely will be prone to this: the machines recognize gestures and commands where none were given. The example of a lively conversation comes to mind when suddenly a device picks up a command word and starts interjecting questions, confirmations, and notifications. The associations between what is meant and sent, and where and by whom is it received and interpreted are getting *multi-valent*, to close the loop from the beginning. While such multi-valence is a side effect of transforming and imbuing our space with complexity, it presents a problem to the general notion of ubiquitous computing (Weiser 1991; Rogers 2006).

10.2.2 Designing Systems

How to design an artifact for a specific space or situation traditionally relied on assumptions, a common sense, of what could be expected and could be required by the artifact to function well. If these needs were met, the artifact would do its job, if not, then performance would degrade, which is a well-accepted reality for end-users and stakeholders. For many places and situations, this is no longer viable. There are concepts that reject the notion of utility or least blur the line between utility and serendipity (Newman et al. 2002; Overgoor and Funk 2018). The stability of context and players in this context disintegrated, when the space became digital, dynamic, interactive, and autonomous. Two problems: first, the scope and context of interaction became less well-defined, with blurry boundaries, and second, different devices join and form ad-hoc systems in a context without order and regulation regarding interaction modalities, attention needs, and interactivity pollution (Janlert and Stolterman 2010, 2017).

Users might think that they are interacting with an environment, yet the meaning is in flux: in the past it was about a stable, spatially embedded system of interactive artifacts, now it means an ad-hoc collection of artifacts "making up" a growing system in a specific space *right now*. How long this system and its composition might last is not guaranteed nor is its functional scope and interactionality (Funk 2018).

10.3 New Design Labs

As we have seen before, three dimensions that challenge current and future design research and practice are space, time, and complexity. The next question is how we can support designers and design researchers in achieving break-throughs giving this complex terrain. Especially in making-focused approaches, materials, methods, and tools are key. The environment that combines, curates and consolidates these is often left out: the lab or studio where the action is (Lucero et al. 2012). Yet, such a place needs to achieve a lot (Lundsgaard and Chalmers 2013).

In the past, interaction labs have been designed about specific context like the home, e.g., to explore product concepts (Intille 2002) or to explore interaction in the area of ubiquitous computing (Kidd et al. 1999). The latter can serve as an example for what we attempt in this article, although with a different structure and technological maturity. Nevertheless, as design research matures as a discipline, labs need to fulfill different needs and meet more demands than before. In the following, we compile a structured list of requirements for new design labs, starting with the underlying purpose: creating and testing something in a controlled space with the assumption that it would fit an external purpose equally well. While labs have been seen traditionally as scientifically controlled spaces for experimentation, design research labs are dominated by often-messy engineering (exploring, making, hacking, tinkering) than by scientific experiments and their sterile, analytical needs.

10.3.1 Supporting Multi-faceted Approaches

With the advent of field studies, probes, and ethnographic approaches utilizing designed research products (Koskinen et al. 2008), labs have served mainly as technical staging grounds until an artifact is ready for deployment. The questions of validity and context-fit have not been solved through such approaches. Instead, they have been side-stepped and shifted from the product–market spectrum towards lab–deployment. The scope of a lab is still rather rigid and when the lab stops and the artifacts transitions beyond, reality bites. Alongside new labs, we need to think about how concept evaluation frameworks (Chai-Woo et al. 2010) need to be adjusted to (1) support both quantitative and qualitative data and meaningful linking between them, (2) strive for simplicity in how making and experimental procedures lead to high quality data, (3) provide a small, effective set of fine-tuning parameters, and (4) are open for and perhaps lead to extension.

10.3.1.1 Modularity and Data

(Conceptual) design is characterized by the rapid generation of variants and evaluating them in context. With variants of a modular system, we need to shift between the whole and its components, and consider that all relations among design components are qualitative. To assess the validity then involves understanding the change and evolution of components within the designed system, either through design action or through computational techniques such as complex adaptive behavior or learning. For this purpose, we also need to document sensed, reported, and linked data. New design labs will allow us to store and collect streaming data at will, and allow for simulation and deferred computation using such data. The more complex a concept becomes, we can observe increasingly resulting from external complexity, which in turn leads to increasing internal complexity. This generally means a greater need for some sort of verification, i.e., the test whether the designed system accomplishes what it was designed for. New design research labs will to perform such checks at will and seamlessly across scales.

10.3.1.2 Perspectives

When designing data-intensive systems, e.g., systems that harness the power of ubiquitous computing, streaming data, and human machine interaction, we often observe non-linear design processes spanning not only different phases, but also different levels of abstraction when working with data. If we want to maintain a highly experiential design process and enhance human awareness and actively engage stakeholders in iterations, from explorative and synthesizing to analytical, academic activities, participatory design and collaborative practices are a part of contemporary design research and thus their support criterion for a lab (Binder et al. 2015). Although we take a more technological perspective in this article, the requirements for new design research labs are not limited to the technological stance.

Perspectives in design research nowadays often refers to diverse views that different end-users have of a system, moderated by the environment and other participants in a longitudinal interaction process. Especially, we designing for applications that are meant to enhance social interaction and collaboration in a shared space, perspectives emerge and need not only to be considered, but also actively pursued in design, through logging, recording, simulation and generation. New design research labs should readily support this way of working.

10.3.2 Space Scales

Systems and system components are dependent on proximity, to communicate but also to define their boundaries. Apart from that, the physical scale of an environment can help in exploring, designing, and validating multi-valent systems and interfaces. For the sake of simplicity, we can distinguish three scales relating to smart environments: micro scale–the room, the close context; meso scale–the building, the protected community space; and macro scale–the city, the open. Each scale is characterized by different aspects of interaction, and relations between actors in the space.

10.3.2.1 Micro

Traditionally, interaction design is confined to a user-product relationship and if one takes the environment around this relationship into account, we think of rooms with functional and experiential qualities. As mentioned above, such definitions have changed and have been extended towards connected spaces with ubiquitous artifacts embodying different capabilities, from sensing to actuating. What we also associate with the micro scale are qualities like protection, privacy, intimacy, personalization, and predictability. When mapping this to a lab environment, the controlled, clean lab spaces of the past fit. Still, we can envision situations even within the micro scale that traditional labs could not address, e.g., multi-person domestic disputes and messy technological debugging, to give two diametral examples. The micro scale is home to various interaction styles and techniques, such as proxemic interaction (Marquardt et al. 2011, 2012; Greenberg et al. 2014), peripheral interaction (Bakker et al. 2015), faceless interaction (Janlert and Stolterman 2015), multimodal interaction and mixed-reality interactivity.

Here, we need labs that are not only built with flexibility in most spatial and technological aspects – from walls to furniture to media and communications, down to the technological stack of sensing, processing, and actuation. We need flexibility in how components and data streams within the environment can be connected, interlinked, and enriched. Presumably ubiquitous data is often limited to specific application scenarios cannot be fluently, seamlessly linked in creative ways. This results from platforming and engineering the technological underpinnings of the space, which are preplanned and a layer below where design activities happen. Given the needs of designing connected spaces, such limitations feel oddly out of place.

10.3.2.2 Meso

If we leave the micro scale of rooms and closed spaces, the building, the community, and the campus open up and form the meso scale. This design scale is more architectural (Wiltse and Stolterman 2010; McCullough 2004) and it is at the same time characterized by more fluctuation and share of space and resources. Yet, designing connected system at this scale is different than at micro scale: issues of identification, authorization and privacy start to play bigger roles, we need to deal with communication in both noise and signal, and the environment needs to deal with devices and things that are more transitional. This is the scale where buildings learn (Brand 1995), where links between people join places (Jones et al. 2004), and new interactions emerge (Alavi et al. 2016): environmental interfaces and interaction styles such as proxemic and peripheral interaction that are commonly situated at micro scale give way to more usage of personal, mobile devices and navigational interfaces. This is a space where digital nomadic patterns start to emerge.

At this scale, we need a lab that provides powerful means to design with positioning, orientation, and movement. Likewise, resources that might be easily accessible and abundant at micro scale, such as energy, networking, and display space, might need different consideration at meso scale. Finally, the lab should provide ways to interface with the building more directly. Since the lab is usually in a different place than the final deployment place, such interfaces need to reproduced and simulated to allow for fidelity in the design.

10.3.2.3 Macro

The macro scale is beyond the building context and opens up to the city and society. While the meso scale introduces an architectural perspective to the design of artifacts, the macro scale embeds designed artifacts in a traditionally largely architecturally planned context (Houben et al. 2017) interfacing with societal issues and high degrees of fluctuation, openness and traditionally few interfaces available for direct, meaningful interaction. Designing at macro scale has been practiced for decades and this scale is in constant progress with consideration of social (Hillier and Hanson 1984), digital (Mitchell 1996) and interactive dimensions (Schnädelbach 2003). What if we want to span the city, for instance, when designing an artifact with medical purposes that needs to transfer data from a patient to doctors in a hospital and back? Designing for the out and open has legal implications, unknown adverse actors and technological challenges. In the future, we need to consider any communication over the Internet as macro scale–as this consideration reiterates the importance of data security, privacy, and the awareness that data travels across an unsafe medium. Even just assuming this, might prevent future product flaws at macro scale.

10.3.2.4 Translation

The three scales–micro, meso, and macro–should not be seen and treated in isolation. It is crucial to be aware of how to design across the boundaries of a scale and to take concepts from scale to scale without losing essential elements and meaning. Consequently, new design labs need to facilitate translation of designed concepts across scales. Ideally, proximity translated to different qualities of relations between objects and interactive artifacts, without breaking connections and communication threads that would need to be re-established again.

An artifact might enter temporal relations with other artifacts depending on scale and use. It might reveal and give access to different kinds of data and information, and even limit itself to sensing collecting only certain types of data depending on where it is. While distributed interfaces (Bongers et al. 2014; Bongers 2015) are well-understood, transitional use of different displays and changing associations between artifacts is yet to researched exhaustively. New design research labs can cater for a better understanding of how artifacts and displays play together at different scales, e.g., how an artifact can make itself heard, seen, or experienced leveraging displays that are in current temporary proximity.

From a user perspective, technological needs regarding entire buildings or multi-room installation have been researched (Poole et al. 2008a, b). Yet again, a transitional perspective is lacking, for which new labs could provide important impulses. What does it mean to instruct or control technology within a room and how do these instructions translate to a larger context of an entire floor or building. What is the multi-performative nature (Fasoulaki 2005) of a meso or macro scale environment, where agency and modularity emerge? How can we take our preferences our of a close context and have systems at macro scale react and adhere to them? This is a problem recognized in designing for important transitions in life, such as how to age in place (Mynatt et al. 2000). However, transitions can and will happen faster and more rapidly in the future as places adapt and we adapt to such new flexibility. Concepts like pace layering and shearing layers might help here (Brand 1995).

10.3.3 Technology and Infrastructure Stacks

Finally, new design labs need to advance our understanding and making with new technologies. Even traditionally, labs provide technological, computational infrastructure deeply integrated with experiential methods. The way designers learn about contemporary technologies was and still is highly mediated by labs and the choices made those who run the labs. Increasingly, technology dominates news and hype cycles, which has consequences on how designers might learn about and embrace them. New design labs need to give access to evolving or emerging technologies (Mennicken et al. 2015), yet need to moderate: without the mediating role of labs and careful consideration of what works how and why – and the interplay with existing technologies and infrastructure, designers run the risk of following short-lived techno trends that ultimately slow down their progress and might even lock them into unintended technology stacks. Consequently, labs maintain an authority in guiding exploration and facilitating making which enabling data-driven exploration of design in various multi-stable environments.

More concretely, design labs that match the vision outlined in different spatial scales need to foremost support local spatial navigation ("where am I?") and exploration ("what can I do here?"), connectivity ("who else is there?") and communication ("how can I talk to __?"), and facilities for cognition ("how can I make sense of what is around me?"), learning ("how I can improve?") and sharing ("what can I contribute?"). Such making infrastructure needs to be delivered and taught in a way that support rapid iterations and bursts of exploration especially at early stages of a design process. At the same time, it needs to be stable, reliable, and robust to withstand transitions in scale and deployments that last days and weeks. Finally, technological infrastructure needs to support incompleteness: when a modular design is evolving through iterations, it will often only deliver the desired experience when it reaches completeness. New design labs need to sidestep this issue and provide for functional, behavioral, and experiential scaffolding that allows to design with and within incompleteness.

10.3.4 Summary

As a corollary of the above, new design research labs need to transcend specific technology, experimental operations, space, and data. They need to operate at four levels continuously and occasionally provocatively:

At the **data level**, labs will facilitate the sensing and tracking of data internal and external to the designed product or system. The data flows within the lab are recorded, visualized and potentially fed back into the design. Data becomes a design material that is just as malleable as other materials that are intuitively available to designers.

At the **spatial level**, labs will mediate the interaction between the designer on the one side, and the system, user, and the environment at different scales on the other side. Designers will be able to transition fluently between scales to investigate and manipulate their design – both through their senses and through abstract means (data and simulation).

At the **process level**, labs will support rapid iterations and various processes, but also allow for branching and versioning of designs with their data and meta-data repositories.

At the **technological level**, labs will support the creation of high-fidelity prototypes that are always-ready to be deployed, or even remain constantly deployed while the design process continues. The labs will help achieve experiential qualities that match the complexities of context and scale.

Finally, design research labs will have a **transformative** quality. If we see the above levels as dimensions of labs practice, transformations of lab practice mean the free movement within this four-dimensional space. With such design research labs, designers will be free to make their own choices in how to instantiate a design research space with specific qualities that match the desired design, design process, target contexts and complexity.

10.4 Discussion

The above describes considerably less than a blueprint for design research labs. Detailed sketching was not the intention as it would prescribe a monoculture of infrastructure starving the creative environment of variety and entropy that it inherently requires. We need diverse implementations of the above that differ in details and particulars. The remaining challenges are not unlike other efforts to build and maintain long-term installations: the amount of resources and support needed, the spatial limitations and cross-cutting concerns of managing the building around the lab, the technical expertise required to plan, implement, and operate the lab, and also the requirements to collect data, to protect it and leverage it as limited by international legal frameworks.

Research labs and infrastructure frame and bind resources in particular ways: their instantiation represents choices made at an earlier time that project a possible future. Such projections of research needs and operationalizations are often far from obvious. Forecasting given constraints of evolving research lines, research funding, political landscape and other external influences is difficult and represents risks in planning lab infrastructure on the long run. What we can do is stay flexible, anticipate changes early and communicate well with stakeholders.

The new labs outlined above consider and allow for many possible implementations and (technical) operationalizations of current and rather near-future needs. Nevertheless, it is entirely possible that new technologies emerge that have widespread consequences on how design research will operate. Yet, we see the evolving of design research and its lab infrastructure as a necessary precursor of that–or another–future reality.

How to start? In most cases, it is unrealistic to assume the availability of huge budgets and purpose-built space for labs. Yet, we can find ways to design such a lab, for instance, by starting small to explore and demonstrate the needs. An example of a research product that fits such an approach description is the IoT sandbox (Frens et al. 2018), a scaled context (1:20) that allows for design research action in-situ without the need for large-scale facilities and the necessary investments. The key aspect of the IoT sandbox is to easy the process of designing with materials and technology without simplifying too much. Designing products that are highly contextualized, embedded and linked to a particular environment needs to be fed the inherent complexity of this environment to prevent oversimplification in the process that designers are prone to.

10.5 Conclusion

In this article, we have revised the literature on how design, interaction and architecture and proposed a tentative framework for specifying, designing and evaluating meaningful lab spaces in the future, for the future. We aimed at a better understanding of what it means to design at scale at adequate levels of complexity and for long-term application. This area of design that has considerable overlaps with architecture, but also computer science and other engineering disciplines. Yet, it is currently not well supported through infrastructure and making spaces. We not only show that such design spaces are thinkable, but also provide a set of considerations detailing how existing infrastructure and emerging technologies can be fused to facilitate new environments that help design for systems at different scales. All these measures need to be embedded in a social and political structure that grounds, scopes, and protects the space. We hope to see more diverse enablers of new types of design and design research appearing and flourishing in the future.

References

Akrich, M. (1992). The de-scription of technical objects. In *Shaping technologybuilding society* (pp. 205–224). https://doi.org/10.1111/j.1365-2621.1989.tb07952.x.

Alavi, H. S., Lalanne, D., Nembrini, J., Churchill, E., Kirk, D., & Moncur, W. (2016). Future of Human-Building Interaction. In *Proceedings of the 2016 CHI conference extended abstracts on human factors in computing systems – CHI EA '16* (pp. 3408–3414). New York, NY, USA: ACM Press. https://doi.org/10.1145/2851581.2856502.

Bakker, S., van den Hoven, E., & Eggen, B. (2015). Peripheral interaction: characteristics and considerations. *Personal and Ubiquitous Computing, 19*, 239–254. https://doi.org/10.1007/s00779-014-0775-2.

Binder, T., Brandt, E., Ehn, P., & Halse, J. (2015). Democratic design experiments: Between parliament and laboratory. *CoDesign, 11*, 152–165. https://doi.org/10.1080/15710882.2015.1081248. Taylor & Francis.

Bongers, B. (2015). Interactive infrastructures: Towards a language for distributed interfaces. In *Proceedings of the ninth international conference on tangible, embedded, and embodied interaction* (pp. 481–484). https://doi.org/10.1145/2677199.2683585.

Bongers, B., Eggen, B., & Oosterhuis, K. (2014). Interactive infrastructures—Distributed interfaces for the built environment. *Next Generation Building, 1*, 101–112.

Brand, S. (1995). *How Buildings Learn: What happens after they're built*. London: *Penguin Books*. https://doi.org/10.2307/990971.

Chai-Woo, L., Suh, Y., Kim, I. K., Park, J.-H., & Yun, M. H. (2010). A systematic framework for evaluating design concepts of a new product. *Human Factors and Ergonomics in Manufacturing & Service Industries, 20*, 424–442. https://doi.org/10.1002/hfm.20193.

Fasoulaki, E. (2005). *Integrated design: A generative multi-performative design approach*. Cambridge, MA: Massachusetts Institute of Technology.

Fischer, J. E., Colley, J. A., Luger, E., Golembewski, M., Costanza, E., Ramchurn, S. D., Viller, S., Oakley, I., & Froehlich, J. E. (2016). New horizons for the IoT in everyday life: Proactive, shared, sustainable. In *Proceedings of the 2016 ACM international joint conference on pervasive and Ubiquitous computing: Adjunct* (pp. 657–660). UbiComp '16. New York, NY, USA: ACM. https://doi.org/10.1145/2968219.2968347.

Frens, J., Funk, M., van Hout, B., & Le Blanc, J. (2018). Designing the IoT sandbox. In *Proceedings of the 2018 designing interactive systems conference* (pp. 341–354. DIS '18). New York, NY, USA: ACM. https://doi.org/10.1145/3196709.3196815.

Funk, M. (2011). *Model-driven design of self-observing products*. Eindhoven: Eindhoven University of Technology. doi:978-90-386-2427-3.

Funk, M. (2016). *Design and data: Strategies for designing information products in team settings*. In *Collaboration in creative design: Methods and tools*. Cham: Springer. https://doi.org/10.1007/978-3-319-29155-0_17.

Funk, M. (2018). Designing the fog: Towards an intranet of things. In F. Müller, D. Schnelle-Walka, S. Günther, & M. Funk (Eds.), *2018 CHI workshop on interacting with smart objects* (Vol. 2082, pp. 31–38). Montreal: CEUR Workshop Proceedings.

Greenberg, S., Boring, S., Vermeulen, J., & Dostal, J. (2014). Dark patterns in proxemic interactions: A critical perspective. In *2014 conference on Designing Interactive Systems (DIS'14)* (pp. 523–532). https://doi.org/10.1145/2598510.2598541.

Hillier, B., & Hanson, J. (1984). *The social logic of space* (Vol. 53). *Cambridge University Press*. https://doi.org/10.1017/CBO9781107415324.004.

Houben, M., Denef, B., Mattelaer, M., Claes, S., & Moere, A. V. (2017). The meaningful integration of interactive media in architecture. In *Proceedings of the 2017 ACM Conference companion publication on designing interactive systems* (pp. 187–191). New York, NY, USA, ACM Press. https://doi.org/10.1145/3064857.3079143.

Intille, S. S. (2002). *Designing a home of the future. IEEE Pervasive Computing* 1. Piscataway, NJ, USA: IEEE Educational Activities Department, pp. 76–82. https://doi.org/10.1109/MPRV.2002.1012340.

Janlert, L.-E., & Stolterman, E. (2010). Complex interaction. *ACM Transactions on Computer-Human Interaction, 17*, 1–32. https://doi.org/10.1145/1746259.1746262.

Janlert, L. E., & Stolterman, E. (2015). Faceless interaction – A conceptual examination of the notion of interface: past, present, and future. *Human-Computer Interaction, 30*, 507–539. https://doi.org/10.1080/07370024.2014.944313.

Janlert, L.-E., & Stolterman, E. (2017). *Things that keep us busy: The elements of interaction*. Johanneshov: MIT Press.

Jones, Q., Grandhi, S. A., Terveen, L., & Whittaker, S. (2004). People-to-people-to-geographical-places: The P3 framework for location-based community systems. *Computer Supported Cooperative Work: CSCW: An International Journal* 13. Kluwer Academic Publishers, pp. 249–282. https://doi.org/10.1007/s10606-004-2803-7.

Khan, W. A., & Angeles, J. (2007). The role of entropy in design theory and methodology. In *Proceedings of the Canadian Engineering Education Association*.

Kidd, C. D., Orr, R., Abowd, G. D., Atkeson, C. G., Essa, I. A., MacIntyre, B., Mynatt, E. D., Starner, T., & Newstetter, W. (1999). The aware home: A living laboratory for ubiquitous computing research. In *Proceedings of the second international workshop on cooperative buildings, integrating information, organization, and architecture* (pp. 191–198). CoBuild '99. London, UK: Springer.

Koskinen, I., Binder, T., & Redström, J. (2008). LAB, FIELD, GALLERY, AND BEYOND. *Artifact* 2. Routledge, pp. 46–57. https://doi.org/10.1080/17493460802303333.

Lucero, A., Vaajakallio, K., & Dalsgaard, P. (2012). The dialogue-labs method: process, space and materials as structuring elements to spark dialogue in co-design events. *CoDesign, 8*(1), –23. https://doi.org/10.1080/15710882.2011.609888. Taylor & Francis.

Lundsgaard, C., & Chalmers, S. A. (2013). *NEW WAYS OF NETWORKING: A hands on workshop exploring the workspace: Lab and its equipment* (pp. 463–465).

Marquardt, N., Diaz-Marino, R., Boring, S., & Greenberg, S. (2011). The proximity toolkit: Prototyping proxemic Interactions in Ubiquitous computing ecologies. In *Proceedings of the 24th annual symposium on User Interface Software and Technology (UIST'11)* (pp. 315–325). https://doi.org/10.1145/1979742.1979691.

Marquardt, N., Ballendat, T., Boring, S., Greenberg, S., & Hinckley, K. (2012). Gradual engagement : Facilitating information exchange between digital devices as a function of proximity. In *ITS '12 Proceedings of the 2012 ACM international conference on interactive tabletops and surfaces* (pp. 31–40). https://doi.org/10.1145/2396636.2396642.

McCullough, M. (2004). *Digital ground: Architecture, pervasive computing, and environmental knowing*. Cambridge, MA: MIT Press.

Mennicken, S., Hwang, A., Yang, R., Hoey, J., Mihailidis, A., & Huang, E. M. (2015). Smart for life. In *Proceedings of the 33rd Annual ACM conference extended abstracts on human factors in computing systems – CHI EA '15* (pp. 2377–2380). New York, NY, USA: ACM Press. https://doi.org/10.1145/2702613.2702631.

Mitchell, W. J. (1996). *Excerpts from city of bits: Space, place, and the infobahn*. Cambridge, MA: MIT Press.

Mynatt, E. D., Essa, I., & Rogers, W. (2000). Increasing the opportunities for aging in place. In *Proceedings on the 2000 conference on universal usability – CUU '00* (pp. 65–71). New York, NY, USA: ACM Press. https://doi.org/10.1145/355460.355475.

Newman, M. W., Sedivy, J. Z., Neuwirth, C. M., Keith Edwards, W., Hong, J. I., Izadi, S., Marcelo, K., & Smith, T. F. (2002). Designing for serendipity: Supporting end-user configuration of ubiquitous computing environments. In *Proceedings of the 4th Conference on designing interactive systems: Processes, practices, methods, and techniques* (pp. 147–156). DIS '02. New York, NY, USA: ACM. https://doi.org/10.1145/778712.778736.

Overgoor, C., & Funk, M. (2018). IdleBot: Exploring the design of serendipitous artifacts. In *DIS 2018 companion – Proceedings of the 2018 ACM conference on designing interactive systems*. Hong Kong: ACM.

Poole, E. S., Chetty, M., Grinter, R. E., & Edwards, W. K. (2008a). More than meets the eye: Transforming the user experience of home network management. In *Proceedings of the 7th ACM conference on designing interactive systems* (pp. 455–464). DIS '08. New York, NY, USA: ACM. https://doi.org/10.1145/1394445.1394494.

Poole, E. S., Le Dantec, C. A., Eagan, J. R., & Keith Edwards, W. (2008b). Reflecting on the invisible: Understanding end-user perceptions of Ubiquitous computing. In *Proceedings of the 10th international conference on Ubiquitous computing* (pp. 192–201). UbiComp '08. New York, NY, USA: ACM. https://doi.org/10.1145/1409635.1409662.

Rodden, T., Crabtree, A., Hemmings, T., Koleva, B., Humble, J., AAkesson, K.-P., & Hansson, P. (2004). Between the dazzle of a new building and its eventual corpse: Assembling the ubiquitous home. In *Proceedings of the 5th conference on designing interactive systems: Processes, practices, methods, and techniques* (pp. 71–80). DIS '04. New York, NY, USA: ACM. https://doi.org/10.1145/1013115.1013127.

Rogers, Y. (2006). Moving on from Weiser's vision of calm computing: Engaging Ubicomp experiences. In *Proceedings of the 8th international conference on Ubiquitous computing*, pp. 404–421. UbiComp'06. Berlin/Heidelberg: Springer. https://doi.org/10.1007/11853565_24.

Schnädelbach, H. (2003). Adaptive Architecture. *Interactions* 23. ACM, pp. 62–65. https://doi.org/10.1145/2875452.

Weiser, M. (1991). The computer for the twenty-first century. *Scientific American, 265*, 94–104. https://doi.org/10.1145/329124.329126.

Wiltse, H., & Stolterman, E. (2010). Architectures of interaction. In *Proceedings of the 6th Nordic conference on human-computer interaction extending boundaries – NordiCHI' 10* (p. 821). New York, NY, USA: ACM Press. https://doi.org/10.1145/1868914.1869038.

Chapter 11
The Role of Living Labs in Developing Smart Cities in Indonesia

Suhono Harso Supangkat, Arry Akhmad Arman, Yuti Ariani Fatimah, Ryan Adhitya Nugraha, and Hendra Sandhi Firmansyah

Abstract This chapter studies the role of living labs in smart city development in four Indonesian cities: Depok, Semarang, Bekasi and South Tangerang. Since 2012, Indonesian cities have started to incorporate the smart city approach for solving urban problems. One of the main similarities between these cities in implementing the smart city approach is the adoption of information and communication technology to improve public services by making citizens' applications easier and better traceable. This research showed that despite political and technical support from the national government to develop smart cities, its implementation was obstructed by silos between different institutions and the persistence of non-digital documents, which make them difficult to analyze and share. Through action research in these cities, it was shown that the smart city is best approached as a 'living lab', i.e. a continuous-collaboration space between various stakeholders to sense city conditions (needs, problems, future limits) based on real-time data and to react to these conditions accordingly. The analysis showed that one of the success factors for such living labs is to find a balance between social forms of support, for example political, financial or cultural, and technical forms of support, for example infrastructure and technology.

Keywords Action research · Collaborative space · Dynamic · Living lab

11.1 Introduction

Globally, cities are becoming more and more attractive to live in compared to the countryside. In 2008, people who lived in cities exceeded the number of people who lived in the countryside (UN 2008). In Indonesia, this occurred in 2015, when people who lived in cities reached 53.35% (bps.go.id). Regionally, Asia has one of the highest rates of urbanization in the world (GSMA 2017). The growth of city

S. H. Supangkat · A. A. Arman · Y. A. Fatimah (✉) · R. A. Nugraha · H. S. Firmansyah
Institute of Technology Bandung, Bandung, Indonesia
e-mail: suhono@lpik.itb.ac.id; arman@stei.itb.ac.id; yuti.ariani@sappk.itb.ac.id

N. Biloria (ed.), *Data-driven Multivalence in the Built Environment*, S.M.A.R.T. Environments, https://doi.org/10.1007/978-3-030-12180-8_11

populations brings pressure to the cities due to their limited capacity. As noted by Nam and Pardo (2011), despite only occupying less than 2% of the earth's landmass, urban people consume over three quarters of global natural resources and are mostly responsible for producing green-house gases. This leads to problems such as traffic congestion, pollution and social inequality (Kim and Han 2012). Additionally, GSMA (2017) notes that South East Asia and the Western Pacific have the highest air pollution related death rate and have huge transport and energy problems.

The smart city concept is one of the approaches that policy makers are adopting to solve urban problems by using information and communication technologies (ICT) in order to make better use of urban resources (Neirotti et al. 2014). Despite ICT adoption being generally accepted, smart-city practices vary from using an integrated ICT system that can produce real-time information to optimize operations (cf. IBM 2009; GSMA 2017) to the smart city as an urban innovation platform in management and policy (Nam and Pardo 2011). In this chapter, we define the smart city as 'a city that has good capability to manage all its resources effectively and efficiently to solve all city problems using innovative, integrated, and sustainable solutions by delivering good city services to improve the quality of life' (Supangkat et al. 2018). This definition allows us to work with both ICT and urban innovation in management and policy.

Since 2012, Indonesian cities have started to adopt the smart city approach to solve urban problems such as traffic jams, lack of security, waste disposal, clean water scarcity and poverty. The adoption came in different forms, such as by implementing an e-government system, developing apps to improve public services, building a command center, using CCTV in public areas, etc. Despite the potential of such initiatives to solve urban problems, our experience in working with several Indonesian cities has shown that their implementation is still limited to inventorying urban problems without further mechanism for tackling these problems beyond displays of technology and gimmicky apps. Our previous research (Supangkat et al. 2018) on the Smart City Index showed that among criteria such as economic development, environmental problems, social issues, health, mobility, safety and security, digital government, infrastructure readiness, innovation ecosystem and competitive ecosystem, urban development and management have the lowest score, followed by integration readiness. This implies that technical solutions may not be sufficient due to a lack of data integration and coordination between government bodies.

In this chapter, we aim to gain an understanding of smart-city practices in 4 Indonesian cities through action research. This method was selected due to the character of smart-city implementation, which happens in a continuously changing situation, and our relationship with city stakeholders as researcher-consultants. The latter places us in a unique situation, where the city stakeholders had an interest in the activities we carried out in the city. Through action research, we were not passive spectators who observe and analyze from a distance, but rather active actors who got response and feedback from the city stakeholders.

This chapter is divided into 4 sections, including the foregoing introduction. Section 11.2 explains the conceptual framework and methodology, using action research as approach for collecting data. Section 11.3 presents the general conditions of the cities of Depok, Semarang, Bekasi and South Tangerang; their experiences with smart city development; and how the living lab approach has been incorporated in their activities. We end this chapter with a conclusion section.

11.2 Conceptual Framework

11.2.1 Literature Review on Living Lab

The term 'living lab' emerged in the scientific literature in 2006 through the European movement that promoted innovation systems based on 'living labs' (Schuurman et al. 2016). Since its emergence, the definition of the living lab and its approach have varied from the living lab as an innovation lab to a real-life monitoring system of a social setting or a participatory approach to involving users in a development process and an organization facilitation network for the European movement itself (Dutilleul et al. 2010). Moreover, Pallot, cited by Van der Walt et al. (2009), described the living lab as a traditional research or innovation platform that brings together all stakeholders, such as end users, researchers, industrialism policy makers and others, to conduct an experiment. ENNOL (European Commission) defines the living lab as a system and environment for building a future economy with real-life user-centric innovation to create techniques for new products, services and social infrastructures (Van der Walt et al. 2009).

In general, living labs are a new way of handling problems that emerge in a community. Based on community-driven information, livings lab are fueled by knowledge sharing, collaboration and experiment in an open, real environment (Van der Walt et al. 2009). Additionally, Van der Walt et al. (2009) built a living-lab framework with the objective of creating a prosperous community based on system thinking. This objective is translated into the following operational objectives: (1) to create a learning platform; (2) to allow experimentation; (3) to support collaboration and virtualization; and (4) to use action research. These definitions and conceptualizations show that the key point of living labs is human-centric involvement in developing new ICT-based services and products. This is done by including different stakeholders in a co-creative way. This conceptualization aligns with Larios et al. (2016), who showed how the living lab concept introduced by Prof. Bill Mitchel in 2003 supports innovation and citizen-centered solutions. They suggest that for cities and smart cities, the citizens are the most valuable assets and therefore the design of solutions in living labs should be human-centered and driven by innovation.

In the context of urban life, smart cities and living labs have become a popular phenomenon all over the world, referring to various local experimental projects with a participatory approach that are characterized by being user-centered and based on an open innovation ecosystem (Steen and Van Bueren 2017). These characteristics allow city stakeholders to solve their problems, as shown by some projects presented by Larios et al. (2016). The living lab in Singapore initiated by Nanyang Technical University (NTU) has a strong focus on reducing carbon footprint, energy usage and water wastage. In Europe, London Living Labs have initiated a dynamic series of test-bed sites for the urban environment, including a school, a park and a city neighborhood supported by a wireless sensor network to develop Internet-of-Things (IOT) solutions that measure air quality, water quality, noise pollution, light pollution, and citizen engagement. In North America, the Metro Lab Network initiated by Carnegie Melon University built a network connecting 34 cities, 44 universities and several industries to develop innovative smart-city solutions to address data management challenges. The same also happened in Canada and Latin America, where living labs and smart cities have created smart solutions for a number of cities. For example, Guadalajara Living Lab focuses on innovation derived from the use of sensors, data management, and open data as assets to support adequate data analysis for decision makers (Larios et al. 2016).

According to Larios et al. (2016), each project in a living lab has 5 principles: scalability, interoperability, modularity, resiliency and security. These characteristics are similar to the characteristics of the living labs proposed by Vale et al. (2018), who identify living labs as having a co-creation philosophy, an open innovation environment, stakeholder management, a realistic environment, and interoperability to create better cities. Meanwhile, Steen and Van Bueren (2017) state that each urban living lab should have the following components, such as a **goal** (innovation, knowledge development for replication and increasing urban sustainability) as a target to reach, **activities** (development of innovation, co-creation and iteration between activities) as initiatives to reach the goal, **participants** (users, private actors, public actors, knowledge institutions, decision-makers) for user-centric development, and a **context** (real-world implementation). Based on the characteristics mentioned above, it can be said that the idea behind the living lab concept is to stimulate the development and demonstration of initiatives/activities/applications/services as solutions for smart cities considering regional characteristics or needs.

Based on the literature above, the living lab concept is very useful in developing cities for the following reasons:

1. A living lab is a highly evolving theory and practice, which relates to almost any managerial problem and can help organizations find out where to focus on when tackling problems (Van der Walt et al. 2009).
2. A living lab enables users to take active part in research and innovation (Van der Walt et al. 2009; Vale et al. 2018).
3. A living lab aims to produce additional value for realistic environments, so the product has greater chance to satisfy real needs (Vale et al. 2018).

11.2.2 Methodology

Based on our experience in supervising Indonesian cities, problems and challenges that arise in the implementation of a smart-city approach are as follows:

- Partial and incidental implementation
- Incompatibility between smart-city concept and city conditions
- Implementation scope too broad
- Too focused on technology development while neglecting governance and improvement of the mindset of human resources
- Lack of implementation evaluation

Due to these and other issues, we propose to see the city as a kind of living lab, as shown in Fig. 11.1.

Smart City Living Lab is an approach of smart-city implementation in a small (or very small) area of a city so that the impact of the implementation can be directly felt by the community and is measurable. What is important for living labs is the existence of indicators of the initial conditions and measuring the impacts of interventions on these indicators. The initiatives and programs of a living lab are continuously evaluated and adjusted to reach the aims.

This approach allowed us to questioned the local government and other city stakeholders as a way to understand their initial condition and after some time provided feedback based on the real situation of the cities. We balanced the process of

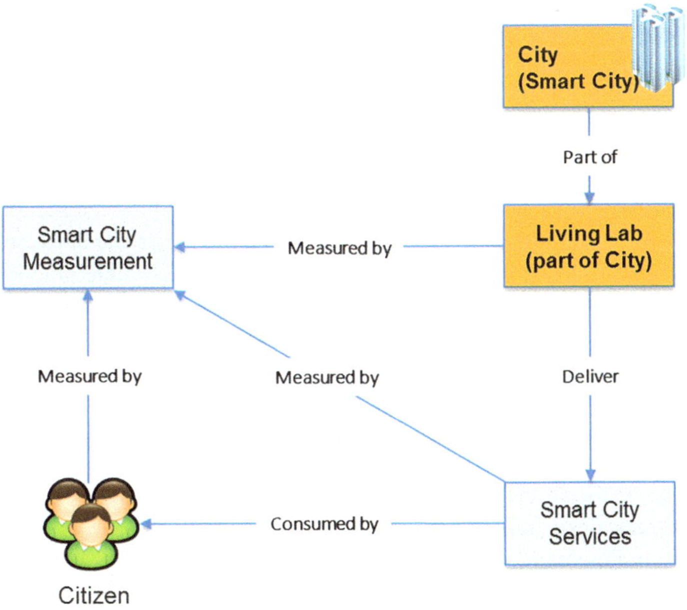

Fig. 11.1 Living lab approach in GSCF. (Source: Authors)

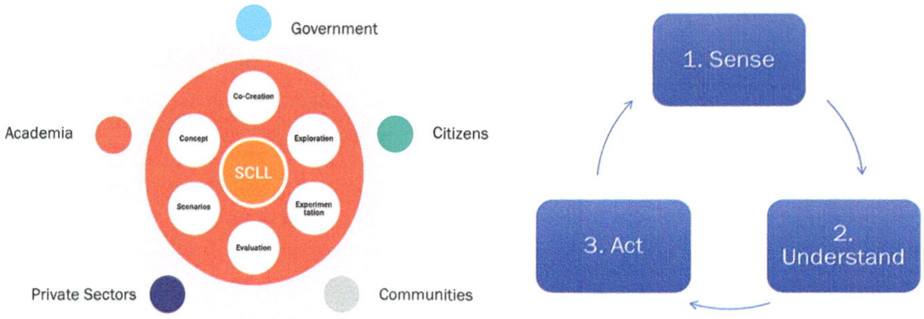

Fig. 11.2 Living lab approach in GSCF (2). (Source: Authors)

research design and collecting data and adjusted our approach based on feedback from the city stakeholders. (Fig. 11.2)

In collecting information on urban conditions, evaluating and providing recommendations to improve the quality of urban services, a living lab uses the following principles (Supangkat et al. 2015):

1. Sensing – A process to capture data on urban conditions. This process is done through collection of statistical data, direct survey as well as data generated by Internet-of-Things devices, social media, platforms, etc.
2. Understanding – A process of analyzing urban conditions based on existing data. This process is done by analyzing the gap between ideal models (such as the Garuda Smart City Model) and current urban conditions.
3. Acting – A process to take action based on the gap analysis. Actions taken may include: development and/or adjustment of services, policy and regulation development, socialization and training, introduction of role models, or enforcement. This can be done by humans, for example through policies, or by machines, for example through automation.

We selected action research (AR) to investigate and analyze living-lab development in 4 Indonesian cities. Stinger (2014) defines AR as either a research initiated to solve problems or a reflective process between the subject who does the research and the object of research. It works in changing situations, where practices within organizations or institutions, or between these organizations, are continuously evaluated and adjusted to reach the aims. In our research, we incorporated the idea of AR through our role as consultants of the cities involved. This role allowed the local government and other stakeholders questioned to give feedback to our analysis and to change the way we understood things and the type of recommendations we were giving to the city stakeholders. We balanced the process of research design, collecting data and adjusting the approach based on the feedback of the city stakeholders.

We conducted AR in Depok in 2015, in Semarang in 2017, in Bekasi in 2016, and in South Tangerang in 2017. Each research was done over 4–6 months. Our interactions with the city stakeholders were done in the form of focus group discussions (attended by 20–30 people), in-depth interviews with local government representatives, workshops with researchers and city stakeholders, and a questionnaire with a total of 400 respondents in each city (in 2017). Apart from primary data we also collected secondary data, such as policy/planning documents, news from the media and regulations.

11.3 Living Lab Implementation in Indonesian Cities

11.3.1 Depok City, West Java, Indonesia

11.3.1.1 General Conditions and Problem Identification

Each regional organization (OPD) in the Depok City government, as a public department, has the duty to build and develop information and documentation systems properly and efficiently so that they can be accessed easily. However, these efforts are still done independently and stand-alone, so the following issues arise:

- Data are spread in the information systems of each OPD but are not accessible in other OPDs;
- Data management through electronic systems is done separately in each OPD on various platforms;
- Data duplication often occurs over all OPDs, with overlapping or uncoordinated resources;
- Synergy is difficult to achieve between OPD digital information in the absence of standard terminology as a reference and because of information system platform differences;
- Validation of electronic data cannot be done to ensure data accuracy;
- Security against damage to the digital data is not assured;
- Lack of confidence in the information level;
- Summaries of important information are difficult to get from various OPDs in real time.

11.3.1.2 Proposed Solution

The information systems of each of the government departments are on different platforms and use different data formats. Therefore, to establish synergy of these information systems, it is necessary to integrate them and enable data sharing among government departments through interoperability management and interconnectivity of information systems that support decision-making in every government department. The Communication and Informatics Department as the leading sector of e-government development in Depok City has started implementing application integration in 2014.

In the context of information systems, system integration is a series of processes executed to connect several computerized systems and software applications, both physically and functionally. The integrated system will incorporate all of the sub-system components in one system and ensure that the functions of the sub-systems are part of the main system. System integration is an interesting challenge in software development because its development must continue to refer to the consistency of the whole system, so that the existing sub-systems can still be operated and function properly during the process of integration and once the sub-systems have been integrated. The challenge is how to design the mechanism to integrate these systems with minimum effort and even, if necessary, without refactoring or re-developing systems that already exist.

The information system integration process in Depok City has the two following components:

- **Service integration**
- Integration of the service system with the objective to improve services to the customer. In Depok City, integration of services will be done on the existing system in all government departments by providing convenience to entry users in registering the identity of the applicant, patient, or participant. In addition, service integration is also done for data verification in certain government departments.
- **Reporting integration**
- In contrast to service integration, reporting integration is aimed at collecting information (reports) from some of the government departments in Depok.

11.3.1.3 Evaluation

After the system has been implemented, the government departments of Depok City that are involved in the implementation phase can share data and information easily, real-time and efficiently. For the system to be utilized to the maximum it is necessary to do the following:

(a) **Supporting human resources training**
The data system integration process needs to be supported by human resources who master the platform and the environment used in the integrated data system. For this purpose training is needed related to the technology used, i.e. ESB, SOA, Webservice, among others.

(b) **Increased network capabilities and reliability**
The digital network is an important element in data system integration. The support network should always be able to serve the needs of the integrated data system in Depok City. With a well-functioning network, the data exchange information system and the information system in the form of a dashboard can work well.

(c) **More government department integration**
At this moment there are still government departments that are not yet connected to the information system to improve the service and performance of Depok City. Government departments that are not yet connected need to be integrated.

Based on the citizen survey, we got the following result:

- 54.10% of respondents were familiar with smart city programs in Depok
- 57.81% of respondents think smart city applications provided by the local government were effective in solving city problems
- According to its citizens, the smartness level of Depok city is 66.77%

11.3.2 Semarang City, Central Java, Indonesia

11.3.2.1 General Conditions and Problem Identification

Semarang City is a developing city with a continuously increasing infrastructure to serve its population of 1,765,396 people. Infrastructure is important for the quality of life in a city. The infrastructure improvement activities of Semarang City require good management in terms of implementation and supervision. For implementation and monitoring these activities, technology is a solution that is continuously developed by Semarang to provide transparency to the public. Technology provides tools that simplify the management and processing of data quickly and accurately. Providing transparency to the public is expected to contribute to good government and good governance.

The Public Works Department as one of the official departments of Semarang City is committed to supporting the application of the smart city concept in Semarang City, especially regarding infrastructure. The Public Works Department has a strategic function in managing the public works field, which includes basic infrastructure such as roads and bridges. This task is essential as it greatly influences the rate of Semarang City's development. An integrated information system and excellent resources are needed to meet expectations. Therefore, it is necessary to build a smart Public Works system, i.e. integration of the latest information and communication technology with government governance and qualified human resources.

The first thing to do is to group entities based on their main function and not on the actors in the organizational structure. The identified functions potentially have the same name as the work unit within the Public Works Department. The business processes of the Public Works Department are divided into 3 (three) entities, i.e. the core entity, the support entity, and the operational entity. The core entity represents a group of functions that deal directly with the main function. The support entity is a group of functions that supports the implementation of the main function. The operational entity is a functional group that aims to ensure that internal processes can run well to support the main tasks of the Public Works Department in performing its duties and functions. This entity includes functions such as financial management, budget management, data and information management, asset management, human resources management, procurement, correspondence, public relations, evaluation and report preparation.

In general, the existing condition of the information system in the Public Works Department of Semarang City is as follows:

Area	General condition overview
Support for transactional business processes	Information system support for transactional business processes that is still not optimal
	A lot of data and information are still collected manually in the form of paper and digital files kept by staff members separately
	The system is not integrated yet
	Transactional data are not yet flowing from one agency to the others
Support for analytical business processes and decision-making	Information system support for analytical business processes and management decision-making is still very limited
Network infrastructure	The network infrastructure is not well-structured and is not able to cover all personnel in the work units
	The existing network infrastructure in the Public Works Department City is provided by the Communications and Informatics Department but the number of connection points and bandwidth provided are not sufficient
IT governance	All rules and policies related to the utilization of ICT are compiled by the Communications and Informatics Department so that the Public Works Department's position is as a user of the services provided by the Communications and Informatics Department
	In the case of the development of a specific information system with official duties and functions, the Public Works Department should have the authority to develop the system while coordinating with the Communications and Informatics Communications and Informatics so as to avoid redundancy of initiatives of other departments

11.3.2.2 Proposed Solution

The architecture of the Public Works Department system should be structured by considering the development of ICT to enable users to access various IT services using various devices or delivery channels. Considering the complexity of the various applications that will be owned by the Public Works Department in the future, the selection of an application platform that facilitates deployment, maintenance and integration is an absolute requirement. Related to this, the entire application software development for the Public Works Department is implemented on a web-based main platform for the presentation layer (Figs. 11.3, 11.4 and Table 11.1).

The information system architecture is designed to meet the requirements of information system architectures for businesses and at the same time is a solution

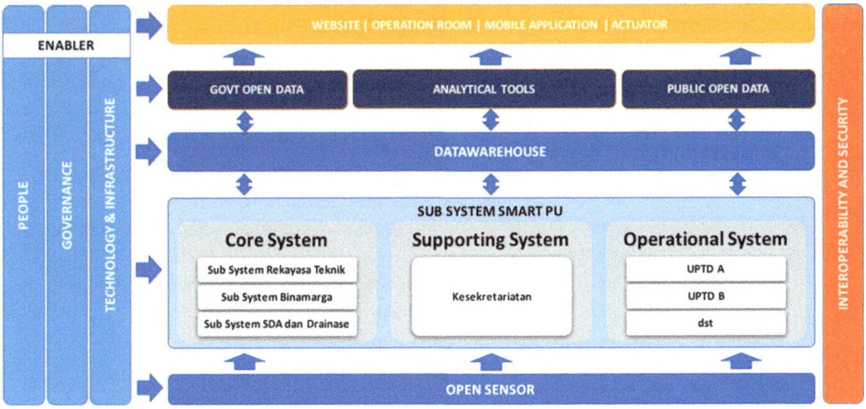

Fig. 11.3 Integration architecture

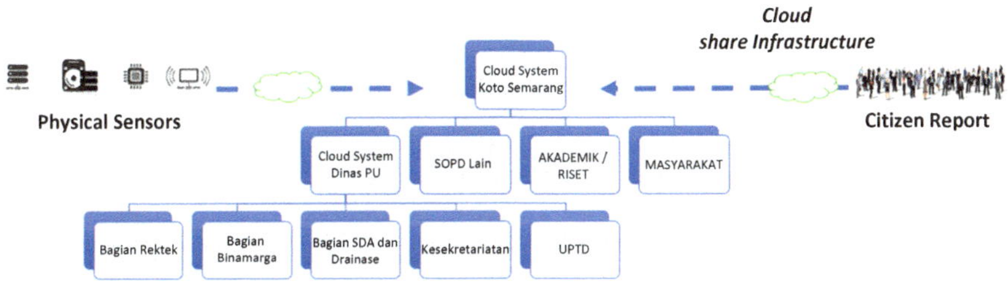

Fig. 11.4 Big Data and cloud architecture for Public Works Department, Semarang

for existing technical problems. Below is an image from the Smart PU Dashboard, Semarang (Figs. 11.5 and 11.6).

11.3.2.3 Evaluation

For the system to be utilized to the maximum the following actions are necessary:

(a) **Supporting human resources training**
The data system integration process needs to be supported by human resources who master the platform and the environment used in the integrated data system. Also human resources are needed to improve data digitalization in the Public Works Department of Semarang City.

(b) **Increased network capabilities and reliability**
The digital network is an important element in the integration of the Public Works Department of Semarang City. The support network should always be able to serve the needs of the integrated data system. With a well-functioning network, the data exchange information system and the information system in the form of a dashboard can work well.

Table 11.1 Integration architecture

No.	Component	Description
1	Open sensors	Utilizing various sensors as a means of sensing both by internet-of-things devices and humans.
		Data can be obtained actively and passively from the community:
		Actively, derived from community reporting by providing a hotline service via phone/text messaging or complaints from the community > requires operator support to receive complaints and enter them into the system.
		Passively, extraction from news media or social media > requires operator support to run the process of collecting the data.
		Some of the tools that can be used are:
		Cameras / CCTV to be placed in multiple points in the city.
		GPS trackers on multiple devices.
		Certain sensors such as environmental condition sensors and disaster early warning systems.
2	Subsystem Smart PU	Window for each field to find and enter information and support the process of understanding (comprehension of the condition)
3	Data warehouse and analytical tools	Analysis begins with processing a large amount of complex data (Big Data) from different sources that serve as the basis for making quick and accurate decisions in solving problems in the region. The basic approach is data collection, data modeling, and data processing to provide information for decision-making.
4	Open data	Data and information stored in the data warehouse can be utilized by other organizations in the field as well as by the public with predefined access and information security settings (information security management system – ISMS).

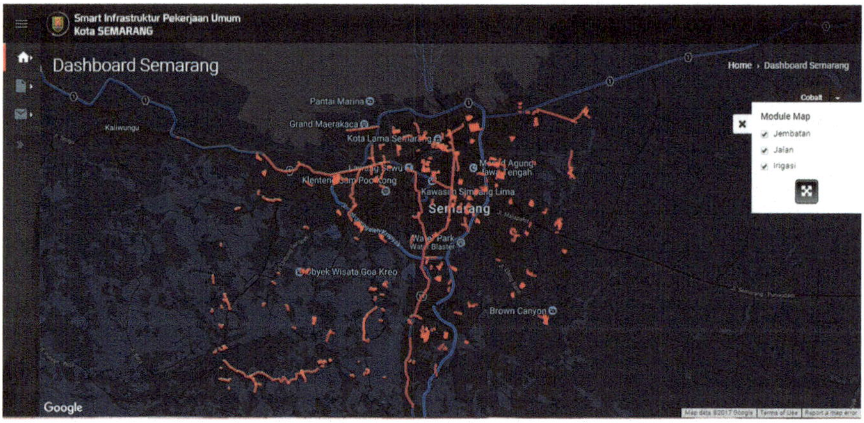

Fig. 11.5 Smart PU dashboard (1)

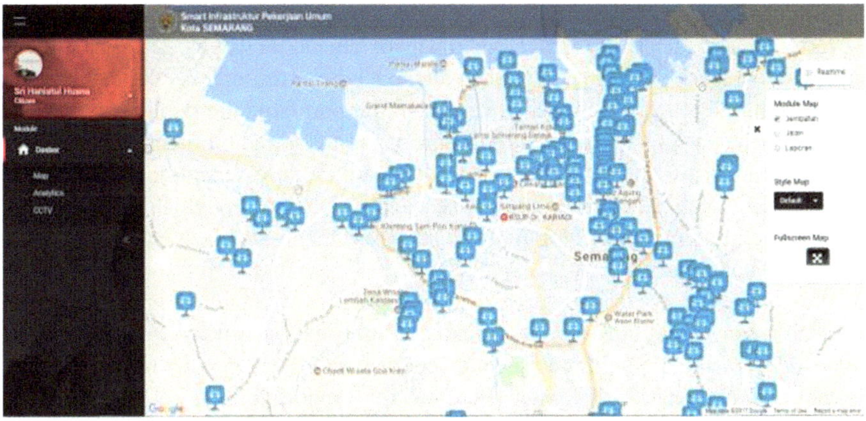

Fig. 11.6 Smart PU dashboard (2)

Based on the citizen survey:

- 55.18% of respondents were familiar with smart city programs in Semarang.
- 60.15% of respondents think smart city applications provided by the local government were effective in solving city problems.
- According to its citizens, the smartness level of Semarang City is 67.33%

11.3.3 Bekasi City, West Java, Indonesia

11.3.3.1 General Conditions and Problem Identification

Bekasi City is one of the major cities in Indonesia that began to realize the smart city concept to combat a variety of urban problems. A smart city is able to manage its resources effectively and efficiently with the support of information technology to achieve a comfortable and sustainable urban life. However, the problems in every city are different, influenced by geography, population, community education, economy, and so on. Geographically, the city of Bekasi is located in West Java and has a strategic location because it is directly adjacent to Indonesia's capital city Jakarta. It is usually referred to as a satellite city of Jakarta and thus Bekasi is crossed by numerous vehicles going to or out of Jakarta. Usually there is congestion in the Cikampek area due to the dense traffic in and out of Jakarta via Bekasi. In addition to being connected with the city of Jakarta, Bekasi is also connected with the city of Bogor through the Bekasi River. River water coming from Bogor with a very high discharge can cause flooding in Bekasi. Various other problems are also felt by Bekasi, such as waste disposal problems, social problems such as beggars, homeless people, etc.

Solving these problems requires the cooperation of various parties, both from the government and the private sector, and the involvement of citizens. The government cannot solve these problems on its own due to a lack of resources. Public participation is required to support better governance. Support from the public can be realized in various ways, such as citizens reporting incidents and problems that occur in the community, proposing innovations and creative improvements of the city, not committing violations of law, paying taxes, and so forth. Although public participation can be implemented, communities and governments still face challenges from on-the-ground reality.

One of the efforts to realize Bekasi Smart City was establishing an operation control center to monitor city resources and information in real time in order to make decisions in a quick, precise, and accurate way. The operation control center is called Patriot Operation Center (POC) and is supported by various smart infrastructures, such as wall display, a PC and other hardware equipment. It is expected that with the Patriot Operation Center, Bekasi City can improve the comfort and quality of life for its citizens with the support of information technology.

To be able to monitor public participation issues we are doing an ongoing survey. The survey successfully identified the challenges faced by the government and communities, who collaborate to resolve various problems:

- The complexity of the process involved in reporting by the community
- Late response to reports from the community
- Measurable Key Performance Indicators for report handling by OPD
- Planning not based on report mapping.

11.3.3.2 Proposed Solution

The purpose of implementation of Patriot Operation Center in Bekasi City government is:

1. Implement a situation space that can:
   (a) Provide an overview of the current state of Bekasi City with information obtained in real-time from the field, thereby enhancing the understanding of decision-making officials in solving a problem or determining a policy.
   (b) Give warnings when there are things that require special attention, thereby enhancing the government's ability to respond to unforeseen phenomena in the city.
   (c) Provide information that is a common reference for the government of Bekasi City.
2. Improving the ability of the Bekasi City government to adopt information technology to carry out government activities more accurately, effectively, and efficiently (Fig. 11.7).

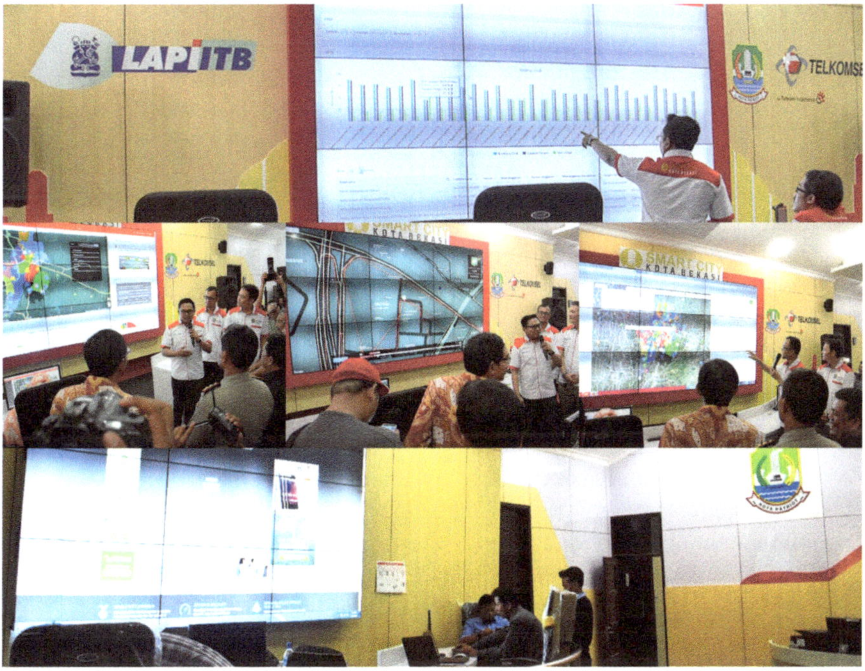

Fig. 11.7 Patriot Operation Center, Bekasi

Currently there are two applications for conveying reports and aspirations by the public that have been integrated with POC, i.e. POT (Integrated Online Reporting) and SOROT (Smart Online Reporting and Observation Tool). POT is a special application provided by the Bekasi City government to its citizens, while SOROT is a reporting application developed from the results of research at the Institute of Technology Bandung (ITB). Citizens can freely choose to report and make their aspirations known through POT or SOROT. Every report conveyed by the public to the government through POT or SOROT via POC is directly followed up by a local or village official. To provide a report or feedback, the public can use the web or download an app from Google Play.

In the development of Bekasi Smart City, apart from software development activities, implementation of hardware is also involved. Hardware is useful for sensing, working by providing real-time online information from the field. The type and number of installed smart devices is the result of a discussion between a telecommunication provider, as the Corporate Social Responsibility (CSR) program provider, and Bekasi City, as the CSR program recipient. Based on the results of the discussion, an agreement was reached that the Bekasi City government needed the following equipment:

1. FFWS (Smart Tech4Water)
2. VTS and OBD (GPS Tracker)
3. MPos Tax

11.3.3.3 Evaluation

For the system to be utilized to the maximum the following actions are necessary:

(a) **Supporting human resources training**
The data system integration process needs to be supported by human resources who master the platform and the environment used in the integrated data system. For this purpose training is needed related to the technology used, i.e. ESB, SOA, Webservice, among others.

(b) **Increased network capabilities and reliability**
The digital network is an important element of integration of the Bekasi City agencies. The support network should always be able to serve the needs of the integrated data system. With a well-functioning digital network, the data exchange information system and the information system in the form of a dashboard can work well.

(c) **More government department integration**
At this time some government departments have not been integrated in the information system yet. To improve the service and performance of Bekasi City, more departments need to be integrated with POC.

Based on the citizen survey:

- 46.52% of respondents were familiar with smart city programs in Bekasi.
- 50.13% of respondents think smart city applications provided by the local government were effective in solving city problems.
- According to its citizens, the smartness level of Bekasi City is 59.93%.

11.3.4 South Tangerang, Banten, Indonesia

11.3.4.1 General Conditions and Problem Identification

For the people of Indonesia, the concept of public participation (co-creation) is part of their culture, known under the name of *gotong royong*. Co-creation is a concept whereby various stakeholders work together and get involved to solve various problems that exist. In co-creation all stakeholders have their respective roles, therefore the more stakeholders involved, the better the outcome that can be expected. Stakeholders involved in smart-city co-creation include the government, academia, the community and businesses.

Globally, one of the smart-city solutions that have been widely applied by cities to overcome urban problems is to involve public participation ('smart citizens'). Communities are involved in working with governments by providing input for planning and policy. Given the importance of public participation in the improvement of urban services, an application system is needed to facilitate collaboration and communication between the public and the government for the realization of public participation. This system helps knowing problems, understand problems, and solve problems in the community. It is hoped that with this collaborative platform, the community can participate by being able to easily convey their aspirations and reports to the city government, so the government can understand the problems and aspirations of the people quickly and accurately, and all parties have the same sense of responsibility toward fixing urban issues.

11.3.4.2 Proposed Solution

The concept of this participation and collaboration system in South Tangerang City is called SIARAN (Reporting and Assignment Application System). The development of SIARAN aims to:

- Improve the ability of the South Tangerang City government to handle public complaints in real time;
- Improve the ability to monitor the performance of parties in handling public complaints;
- Facilitate citizens of South Tangerang City to convey reports to the South Tangerang City government;
- Facilitate urban analysis and planning through problem analysis mapping.

11.3.4.3 Evaluation

For the system to be utilized to the maximum the following actions are necessary:

(a) **Supporting human resources training**
Training for operators who will undertake reporting as well as to those who will follow up on reporting coming from the community.

(b) **More analysis for standard operation procedures in each government agency**
There is a need for further coordination related to the suitability of the system and business processes, or Standard Operation Procedures (SOPs), in every government agency in South Tangerang due to differences between SOPs and business processes between each government agency.

Based on the citizen survey:

- 52.90% of respondents were familiar with smart city programs in South Tangerang
- 56.08% of respondents think smart city applications provided by the local government were effective in solving city problems
- According to the citizens, the smartness level of South Tangerang city is 67.26%.

11.4 Concluding Remarks

From the four cases above, the main concern in the implementation of the smart city concept, especially related to living labs, is how data owned by the city can be used optimally by integrating different applications and various OPDs. Apart from the importance of community participation in giving feedback, technical issues still occurred in one of the cities caused by a lack of back-up servers, while all surveyed cities need to increase their network capability and reliability.

Apart from these technical issues, all cities need human resources training to teach personnel how to master the platform and the environment used in the data integrated system. Coordination between local government departments and the presence of formal regulations that encourage data integration are other critical issues in the four cities. Additionally, our research showed that despite political, technical and financial support from the national government to develop smart cities, only around half of the citizen (51.93%) were familiar with the local government smart city programs. As for the use of apps in solving city problems, an average of 56.03% respondents think it is useful. According to the respondents, the smartness level is 64.64%.

Based on these results, we conclude that the four cities have different readiness levels both from a technical and a social point of view. The citizen surveys showed that despite the local government activities to adopt the smart city concept, only half of the respondents knew the program and felt the use of Smart City apps was useful. The low level of citizen awareness towards the smart city concept calls for a participatory approach where the smart city is developed using a citizen-cantered approach. This result is in line with Nam and Pardo (2011), who proposed that a smart city is not a situation but rather a process.

In this paper, we proposed the role of living labs can play in smart city development as a process. Through the living lab approach, the evaluations and recommendations that we delivered to the four local governments should be addressed and used as a learning process for future projects. Furthermore, the living lab approach includes citizens as main actors in modulating the city trajectory. By including various representatives from the local government, citizens, academia and businesses in a collaborative space called a living lab, the city can be developed based on its local potential and real-time situation.

References

Dutilleul, B., Birrer, F. A., & Mensink, W. (2010). Unpacking European living labs: Analysing innovation's social dimensions. *Central European Journal of Public Policy, 4*(1).

GSMA. (2017). *Maximising the smart cities opportunity: Recommendations for Asia-Pacific policymakers*. https://www.gsma.com/iot/maximising-smart-cities-opportunity-recommendations-asia-pacific-policymakers/

IBM. (2009). *A vision of smarter cities: How cities can lead the way into a prosperous and sustainable future*.

Kim, H. M., & Han, S. S. (2012). City profile: Seoul. *Cites, 29*(2), 142–154.

Larios, V. M., Gomez, L., Mora, O. B., Maciel, R., & Rosales, N. V. (2016). *Living labs for smart cities: A use case in Guadalajara city to foster innovation and develop citizen centered solutions*. 2016 IEEE Smart Cities Conferene (ISC2).

Nam, T., & Pardo, T. A. (2011). *Smart City as urban innovation: Focusing on management, policy, and context*. *ICEGOV2011*, September 26–28, 2011, Tallinn, Estonia.

Neirotti, P., De Marco, A., Cagliano, A. C., Mangano, G., & Scorrano, F. (2014). Current trends in Smart City initiatives: Some stylised facts. *Cities, 38*, 25–36.

Schuurman, D., Marez, L. D., & Ballon, P. (2016). *Living labs: A systematic review*. Ghent University. https://biblio.ugent.be/publication/7026155/file/7026171

Steen, K., & Van Bueren, E. (2017). *Urban living lab: A living lab way of working*. Amsterdam Institute for Advanced Metropolitan Solutions.

Stinger, E. T. (2014). *Action research* (4th ed.). Thousand Oaks: SAGE.

Supangkat, S. H, Arman, A. A., Nugarah, I. G. B., et al. (2015). *Pengenalan dan Pengembangan Smart City*. Bandung, e-Indonesia Initiatives.

Supangkat, S. H., Arman, A. A., Nugraha, R. A., & Fatimah, Y. A. (2018). The implementation of Garuda Smart City framework for Smart City readiness mapping in Indonesia. アジア太平洋討究, *32*, 169–176.

United Nations. (2008). *World population prospects: The 2008 revision*. Population Division of the Department of Economic and Social Affairs of the United Nations Secretariat. Department of Economic and Social Affairs, Population Division.

Vale, T., Carvalho, E., Souza, M., Raimundo, P., Faria, I., Spinola, R., & Elberzhager. (2018). *A mapping study on Living Lab: Characteristics, smart cities initiatives, challenge and software architecture aspect*. Third International Conference on Fog and Mobile Edge Computing.

Van der Walt, J. S., Buitendag, A. A. K., Zaiman, J. J., & Van Vuren, J. C. J. 2009. *Community living lab as a collaborative innovation environment*. Informing science and information technology.

Part V
Disruptive Technologies

Chapter 12
Algae Building: Is This the New Smart Sustainable Technology?

Sara J. Wilkinson, Peter J. Ralph, and Nimish Biloria

Abstract Building energy use contributes around 40% of total greenhouse gas (GHG) emissions (UNEP F, Fiduciary responsibility: Legal and practical aspects of integrating environmental, social and governance issues into institutional investment. NEP FI, Geneva, 2009, September) and reducing building-related GHG emissions could mitigate global warming significantly. With a three degree increase in global temperature by 2100 predicted by the United Nations Intergovernmental Panel on Climate Change we need to explore ways to mitigate these impacts. An option for the built environment is to build and retrofit using innovative technologies to adopt onsite energy generation and reduce energy use (UN 2015). Increasing energy efficiency and using renewable energy are ways to reduce GHG emissions.

Technological innovations change over time, and innovations that start as expensive and inefficient can become economic and highly productive, solar energy is an example. In the mid 1800s the photovoltaic (PV) effect was discovered but it took a century to invent a suitable storage device, after which rapid innovation in efficiency and costs followed. Could the same happen for bio-energy? Global biomass energy production reached 88 GW in 2014 (Rosillo-Calle F, de Groot P, Hemslock SL, Woods J: The biomass assessment handbook, 2nd edn. Routledge. ISBN 978-1-138-01965-2, 2016); and bio-energy is no longer a transition energy source. In 2013, a residential building in Hamburg Germany adopted algae, as a renewable energy source. Several questions arise; how does algae produce energy for buildings? How much energy is produced? How does it compare to other renewable

S. J. Wilkinson (✉)
Faculty of Design Architecture and Building, School of Building, University of Technology Sydney, Sydney, Australia
e-mail: Sara.Wilkinson@uts.edu.au

P. J. Ralph
Faculty of Science, C3, University of Technology Sydney, Sydney, Australia
e-mail: Peter.Ralph@uts.edu.au

N. Biloria
Faculty of Design Architecture and Building, School of Architecture, University of Technology Sydney, Sydney, Australia
e-mail: Nimish.Biloria@uts.edu.au

N. Biloria (ed.), *Data-driven Multivalence in the Built Environment*, S.M.A.R.T. Environments, https://doi.org/10.1007/978-3-030-12180-8_12

energy sources? Furthermore, which building types are suited to adoption of algae as an energy source? This chapter explores the feasibility of algae building technology explaining the technology and how it works; the strengths and weaknesses. Then the chapter sets out the drivers and barriers to adopting Algae Building Technology, and; to assesses opportunities across a range of building types.

Keywords Algae building technology · Solar thermal energy · Biomass · Climate change · Technical issues · Design issues · Architecture

12.1 Introduction

The environmental impact of human's manifest in various ways, for example, greenhouse gas emissions (GHG) contribute to the greenhouse effect where temperatures increase and the Earth warms. Buildings, and energy used therein, contributes around 40% of total GHG emissions (UNEP 2009). Reducing building-related GHG emissions could mitigate global warming significantly. The United Nations Intergovernmental Panel on Climate Change predicts a three degree increase in global temperature by 2100. As we explore ways to mitigate these impacts, one option for the built environment sector could be build and retrofit using innovative technologies to reduce energy use and provide onsite energy generation (UN 2015). Increasing energy efficiency is one way to reduce GHG emissions; another option is to use renewable energy, which are expected to dominate energy production in the twenty-first century (Goldenberg in Rosillo et al. 2016).

In 1839, Becquerel discovered the photovoltaic (PV) effect, however energy generated using PV technology was inefficient and prohibitively expensive until a century later in 1941, when Ohl invented the solar cell. In the 75 years that followed, developments in battery storage, smart electricity grid management, greatly reduced production costs, and transitioned PV to become a viable alternative to fossil fuels. In the 1950s, PV cost AUD$2723.32 per watt in 2016 money. Slowly, then swiftly, the cost of solar cells had fallen to less than AS$1.14 per watt by 2016 (The Guardian Sustainable Business 2016). This is evidence of the sudden, disruptive and largely unpredictable technology shifts that occur to make technologies viable and attractive (Davila et al. 2012), this occurred with solar; and could happen for other 'new' renewable energy technologies. Global biomass energy production reached 88 GW in 2014 (Rosillo et al. 2016); and as such bio-energy is no longer a transition energy source. In 2013, a residential building in Hamburg Germany adopted algae, as a renewable energy source for the residents. Several questions arise; how does algae produce energy for buildings? And how much energy is produced? How does it compare to other renewables such as wind and solar? Furthermore, which building types are suited to adoption of algae as an energy source?

The built environment is extremely varied in scale as well as size and in form and function. For example, housing can be low rise and low density, detached with one or two floors to high rise and high density, with 80 plus storeys housing thousands of people. Similarly, commercial buildings vary from low rise load bearing construction to high rise framed construction. Industrial buildings are characterised by external walls with few openings, single story and wide span construction, whereas retail buildings range from small individual high street shops to large out of town shopping centres with car parks, restaurants, cinemas and gyms. Regardless of size and construction, all buildings consume energy. A lot of energy. Not only do we need to reduced operational energy consumption, but we also need to consider construction forms and whether, and which, buildings could accommodate biotechnology systems.

Given population growth and the UN predictions on temperature increase, it follows that actions that mitigate GHG emissions now, matter more than those 20 years from now, as we are liberating GHG that lock in warmer temperatures. This chapter explores the feasibility of Algae Building Technology by explaining the technology and how it works; the strengths and weaknesses. Then the chapter sets out the drivers and barriers to adopting Algae Building Technology, and; to assesses opportunities across a range of building types.

12.2 Biofuels

Globally renewables represented 22% of total energy production in 2013 (Rosillo et al. 2016) although distribution of adoption is very unequal, with the European Union having a 72% share of renewable energy. Australia is currently lagging behind in adoption of energy innovation with just 13.5% renewables in 2014 (Clean Energy Council 2014). Of the various renewable energy technologies, hydro contributes the most (6.2%) to total Australian energy, followed by wind (4.2%), solar (2.1%) and bioenergy (1%) (Clean Energy Council 2014).

Bioenergy in Australia has had a tumultuous history with support waxing and waning between Governments and consumers. Bioenergy encompasses biogas (methane) from landfill, covered anaerobic ponds, and in vessel waste treatment; and liquid fuels (predominantly biodiesel and ethanol) from a range of sources. Ho et al. (2014) provides a good overview of the sustainability issues of a number of these biofuels. Methane and ethanol are other forms of biogas and liquid fuel. Traditionally, the raw biomass materials for liquid fuels have been produced on arable land in Australia or use precious freshwater that would otherwise be used for crop or animal production (Brennan and Owende 2010), and thus a conflict exists. However, there are signs of change.

The Clean Energy Council's Bioenergy Roadmap (Clean Energy Council 2008) proposed that by 2020 the contribution from Australian biomass for electricity generation could be 10,624 GWh/y; six times the 2013 generation. The estimated long-term potential for electricity from biomass in 2050 could be 72,629 GWh/y, approximately 40 times the 2013 level (Clean Energy Council 2008). Furthermore, CSIRO noted the potential for second-generation biofuels to replace between 10% and 140% of current petrol only usage over time (Bio fuels in Australia, RIRDC

2007). This chapter explores the potential for algae biomass to provide a renewable source of energy for buildings. To date, one building has adopted Algae Building Technology (ABT) and the next section of the chapter examines ABT and how it works in detail.

12.3 Algae Explained to Non-specialists

Algae are either single-celled microbes (microalgae) or multi-celled organisms (macroalgae or seaweeds) that photosynthesise. Algae grow from the tropics to the poles, in freshwater, saltwater and in the soil. For the most part, we are only describing microalgae in this chapter. Algae need light, nutrients and CO_2 to grow and produce new biomass. The biochemical diversity of cellular products produced by algae is immense and therefore the products that can be "grown" in these cells can also be used across a wide range of industries. Algal biomass can be used in biofuels, human food supplements, functional foods, feedstock for livestock, fishmeal for aquaculture, bioplastics, industrial enzymes, pharmaceuticals, nutraceuticals, the list of applications is virtually endless (Wilkinson et al. 2016).

To convert algae from cells growing in water to a final product requires some process engineering. First, the cultured cells are filtered, flocculated or centrifuged (de-watering) once the cells are more concentrated, usually they need to be ruptured to access compounds such as omega-3 oils or proteins. The product must be chemically separated from the cell debris and purified to the level required for the specific product. To convert the oils (lipids) into a biofuel requires additional chemical processing, such as hydrothermal liquefaction (high temperature and high-pressure conversion of oil to hydrocarbon).

12.4 Existing Algae Building Technology

The BIQ House, designed by Arup was constructed in Hamburg in 2013. Hamburg has a cool temperature of a Northern European climate. The BIQ comprises 15 apartments located over four floors plus a penthouse level, with apartment sizes ranging from 50 m^2 to 120 m^2. Gross floor area is approximately 1600 m^2 (Arup 2013). Energy is provided by 200 m^2 of integrated photo-bioreactors (PBRs) in 120 panels on two façades, which generate algal biomass and solar thermal heat as renewable energy resources in a low-energy residential building (Sarda and Vicente 2016) (see Fig. 12.1). The algae façade panel system provides a thermally controlled microclimate around the building, as well as noise abatement and dynamic shading (Arup 2013; Elnokaly and Keeling 2016). The construction costs of the BIQ House were approximately five million euros (Buildup 2015) which was higher than conventional residential apartment costs at the time.

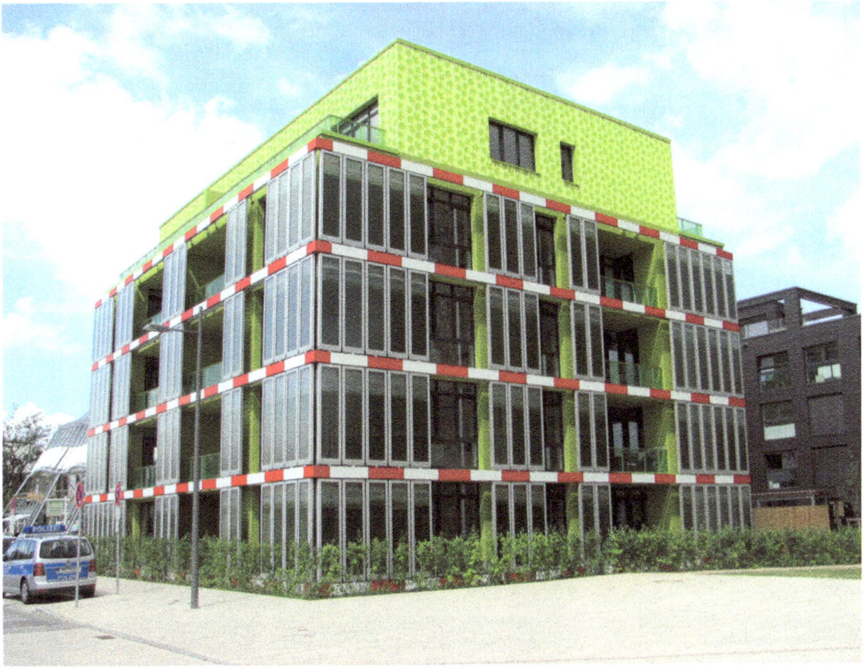

Fig. 12.1 BIQ House, Hamburg. (Source: NordNordWest, Lizenz: Creative Commons by-sa-3.0 de [CC BY-SA 3.0 de (https://creativecommons.org/licenses/by-sa/3.0/de/deed.en)])

Microalgae are cultivated in flat panel glass bioreactors, shown in Fig. 12.2 (Photo Bio Reactors (PBRs). Sunlight and constant turbulence of the fluid with injection of air, causes the microalgae to grow sequestering carbon, producing heat and a food source such as phosphorous. The heat produced by the panels a has 38% efficiency compared to 60–65% in a conventional solar thermal source and the biomass has a 10% of efficiency compared to 12–15% with a conventional PV (Buildup 2015).

The algae biomass and heat generated are transported via pipework to an energy management centre where the biomass is harvested and heat is recovered by a heat exchanger. The bioreactor façade removes up to six tonnes/y of carbon dioxide (CO_2) using flue gas delivered in the gas burner to produce biomass in the PBRs. Excess heat from the PBRs pre-heats domestic hot water, which warms interiors, or is stored in an underground aquifer. The algae biomass, resulting from growth (30KWh/m^2/y), is harvested through an algae separator and collected (Buildup 2015). Up to 80% of the biomass is converted into methane, at an offsite outdoor biogas plant, after which it is returned to the building to generate electricity and heat for the residents.

Factors that need to be considered in PBR design include temperature, lighting, rates of dilution, water quality and pH level, CO_2 sequestration and removal of oxygen (Kunjapur and Eldigre 2010). The effects of algae culture density and the geometry of the PBR panel on daylight penetration was examined by Decker et al.

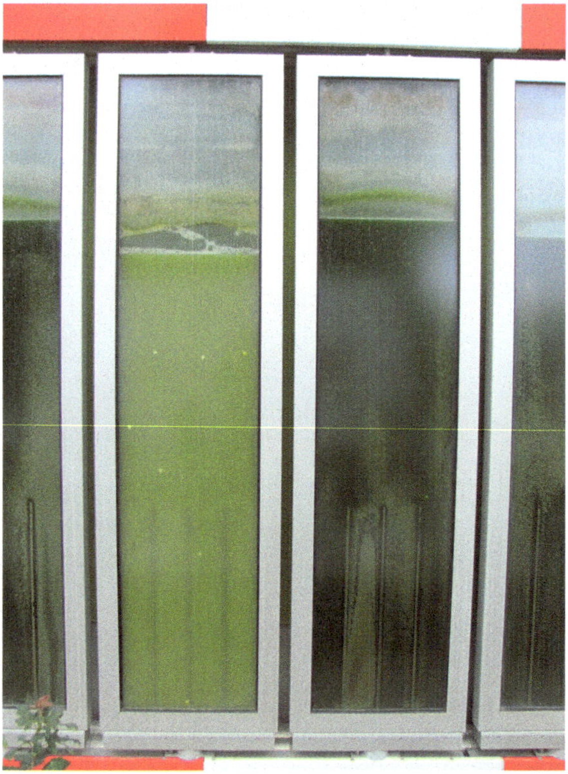

Fig. 12.2 PBR Panel BIQ Hamburg. (Source: Colt Arup SCC)

(2016) who concluded remote control of the PBRs would reduce the chance of algae dying and PBR failure occurring. Another consideration is the interaction between the façade and the PBR, Pruvost et al. (2014) concluded that optimum design enhances microalgae production rates, energy savings and thermal regulation of the building. The quality of the PBR glazing can affect production rates (Vasumathi et al. 2012). Where flat PBR panels are used across window or door openings on a façade there is an issue of levels of daylight penetration and illuminance to be considered with some studies finding enhanced luminance (Kim 2013) and other studies focused on tubular bioreactor design finding that daylight penetration is reduced (Elnokaly and Keeling 2016). The design of the PBR panel affect production rates and the geometry will affect the existence of dead culture zones, where the algae dies off (Iqbal et al. 1993). Iqbal et al. (1993) concluded V shaped flat sided PBRs could produce high mixing rates and minimise dead zones. In summary the microalgae growth issues can be categorised as biological, chemical, physical, operational and health and safety.

Health and safety also relates to the design and construction of the façade and panel. Issues are live and dead loadings; where live loads include wind and, in some regions, seismic activity or snow. The building will have to meet minimum requirements in respect of fire safety too. Dead loads are the weight of the panel and the method of fixing to the façade. For the PBR, the design must ensure that leakage does not occur and the sealants do not react with the microalgae. The panel should accommodate any building settlement and movement without failure of the seals or connections to the façade (Kim 2013). The materials used in construction should be sufficiently durable to have an expected lifecycle comparable to conventional façade designs. Finally the design should protect the PBR from accidental or impact damage as leakage of the microalgae could be hazardous to human health and/or cause odours and contamination (Kim 2013).

12.5 Energy Production Levels and Sustainable Design Services

The associated heat production of about 40 °C (150KWh/m^2/y) is reintroduced to the building system via a heat exchanger in the heating network or, stored in below ground geothermal boreholes. The boreholes store the heat from 16 °C to 35 °C depending on the season. When a higher temperature is required for heating and/or hot water, a heat pump moves the water back into the system. A unit is operated to provide the CO_2 (flue gas) required by the microalgae in the bioreactor façade and, to cover the supply of hot water at 70 °C or heating into the energy network (Buildup 2015; Arup 2016).

Microalgae absorb sunlight and the bioreactor panels provide dynamic shading, with the amounts of sunlight absorbed and shading, dependent on the algae density (Elnokaly and Keeling 2016). When there is more sunlight, the algae grow faster providing more shading for the building (Arup 2016). According to Arup (2016), the flat PBRs on the Hamburg building are highly efficient for algal growth and require minimal maintenance. The PBRs have four glass layers: a pair of double-glazing units creating a cavity, filled with argon gas to minimise heat loss.

The water temperature in the PBRs is controlled by the speed of the fluid flowing through the panel, with lower flow rates allowing a greater time for the sunlight to warm the water as it passes through, and by the amount of heat extracted via heat exchangers in the central plant. The maximum temperature within the BIQ PBRs is around 40 °C, as higher temperatures could harm that species of microalgae. The relatively low maximum PBR temperature limits the practical use of the extracted heat to mainly a pre-heating function for building systems, which is then boosted by an additional energy source. Temperature constraints pose challenges to applying the BIQ system in Australia as the maximum growing temperature for algae used may limit use to the cooler regions of Australia as air temperatures can exceed 40 °C in much of the country. However, it is possible to use other algae species, which tolerate higher temperatures.

The specific algae species used in panels will need to be selected for the particular extremes of the Australian climate. Australians could operate the PBRs on buildings all year round; however, it may be necessary to have two species, a summer and winter specialist. Cold temperature species would be similar to those used in the BIQ; however, summer temperatures would dictate a different species that tolerates temperatures in excess of 40 °C. Cho et al. (2016) examined the thermal tolerance of a range of freshwater algae species. They showed that *Dictyosphaerium* spp. was able to tolerate a wide range of thermal conditions from 15 °C to 35 °C; whereas other species grew better in low temperatures such as *Pediastrium* spp. Thermally tolerant species include *Chlorella* spp., *Scenedesmus* spp. and *Desmodesmus* spp. Endemic Australian species would need to be bio-prospected, cultured and then screened to identify the elite strains that match the thermal conditions, as well as provide high energy yielding biomass for combustion.

The total energy conversion efficiency of the entire building system is 27% relative to the fully available solar radiation that is incident upon an unobstructed building roof (Arup 2016). By way of comparison, contemporary PV systems yield an efficiency of 12–15% and solar thermal systems 60–65%, when placed optimally to capture the total available solar radiation. Total energy conversion of the BIQ algae system is lower than that of conventional solar hot water panels. However, the BIQ building's bio-responsive façade necessarily aims to provide energy directly to several building services systems, as well as providing additional energy benefits through summertime shading, and by providing a biomass stock for additional energy production. The BIQ is designed to Passiv Haus standards which means it is thermally very efficient and has lower energy demands to bring temperatures to comfortable levels, residents claim energy bills are around 1000 euros per year. Energy costs in Germany are high, in the first half of 2016, the average electricity price for households was 29.69-euro cents per kWh (Statistica 2018), which equates to 48 cents per kWh, whereas electricy cost 33.1118c per kWh in NSW (Canstar 2018).

12.6 Experimental Applications of Algae Technology Within the Built Environment

Apart from the aforementioned BIQ Hamburg building, other attempts to incorporate algae building technology within building components, structural photobioreactor elements and self-sustaining localised energy production systems show a globally positive trend in investigating the benefits and limitations of such technologies. Another category of spatial experimentation with algae technology concerns the production of spatial experiences by using algae technologies as an inherent part of hybrid (art and science) physical installations, which present unique narratives for mental wellbeing. Some such installations also acquire a participatory nature and thus provide an opportunity to educate and sustain ecosystems of algaetecture. This section specifically explores the diversity of such applied research projects within the contemporary built environment. Three cases using three different algae cultivation techniques connected with achieving respective outputs shall be elaborated upon: An Algae Farm deployed over a freeway, An Urban Canopy Structure and an Exposition using small-scale algae production techniques while encouraging participatory cultivation.

The Urban Alage farm prototype (Fig. 12.3a, b, c, d), developed by a French-Dutch based 'Cloud Collective' in 2014 showcases an interesting example of deploying Algae Building Technology on public infrastructure. The prototype was developed expressly to exploit the fundamental property of Algae to consume sunlight and CO_2 to produce oxygen. These two environmental conditions are amply satisfied over intensively used transport corridors which are extensive open spaces with high CO_2 emission levels. The project focused on producing biomass by positioning a PBR glass tube-based Algae farm prototype on a highway overpass in Geneva, Switzerland (for the Genève: Villes et Champs garden festival).

The farm consists of a closed system of transparent glass PBRs attached to a specially designed steel structure which also hosts essential equipment such as pumps, filters and solar panels. This setup and the orientation of the overpass enables the installation to capture CO_2 from the intensively used and polluted highway below, while being exposed to ample sunlight on the sides of the overpass where it is mounted. The primary purpose of the installation is the filtration of air as well as the production of combustible biomass and raw material for the cosmetics industry (https://inhabitat.com/overpass-algae-garden-turns-co2-emissions-into-combustible-biomass-in-switzerland/). The supporting steel structure doubles as an educational medium, providing process related information to cyclists and pedestrians using the overpass. The project, more than operating as a scientific tool, professing the filtration of air and its benefits, stands testimony for a plausible future where

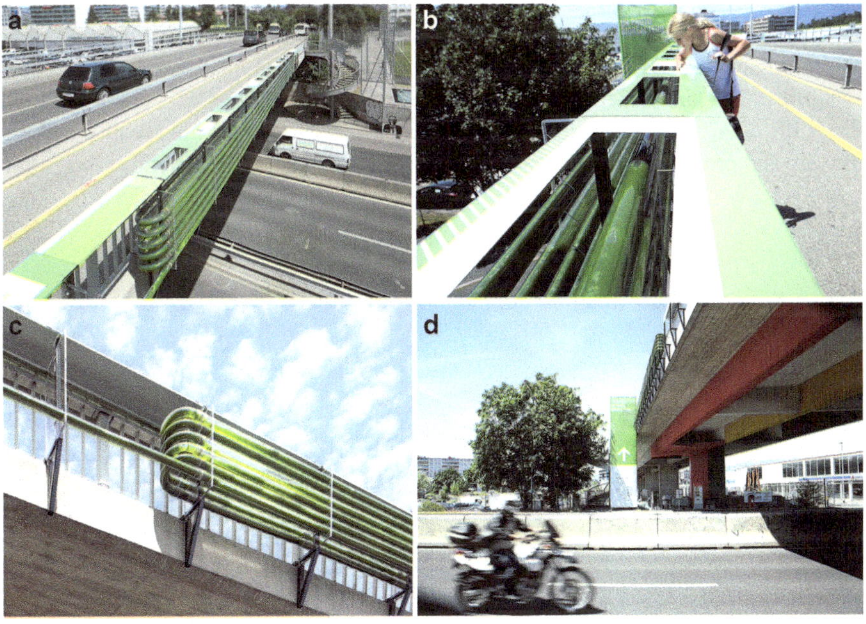

Fig. 12.3 (**a**, **b**, **c**, **d**) The Urban Algae Farm prototype designed by The Cloud Collective and photographed by Olivier Arandel. The prototype was deployed on top of freeway in Geneva, Switzerland

large-scale infrastructure can be used in a multi-performative manner rather than serving a utilitarian function. Production of energy, aiding education and research opportunities, purification of our environment, re-interpretation of infrastructure use within dense urban environments and, acquiring a new perspective on the conservation of green areas using retrofitting of the built environment as a credible channel, are all bundled into the case of this prototype.

After this Macro-scale public infrastructure deployment scale, the next case examines the Messo-scale wherein the development of an urban algae canopy and an urban algae façade are conceived as retrofitting systems at a building scale. These two systems were designed and exhibited at the Milan Design Week in 2014. Here, it is speculated that micro-algae photosynthesis can be used to produce the same amount of oxygen as four hectares of woodland (https://newatlas.com/urban-algae-canopy-milan-expo/37480/). The two projects exploit the accelerated and efficient rate of photosynthesis performed by microalgae as compared to other prominent modes of vegetation to its advantage and use the available abundant surface area potential in the built environment to clean the air we breathe. The two prototypes are conceived under an "Algaetecture" research umbrella by the Architect, Cesare Griffa and the ecoLogicStudio. Cesare Griffa (https://cesaregriffa.com/) recognized the potential of cultivating microalgae on billions of square metres of architectural surfaces such as roofs and facades, which can be transformed into clever photosynthetic surfaces within dense urban environments. Architectural cladding systems which double up as innovative energy and food production systems within our cities is a vision which is tested by these two projects.

The Urban Algae Façade (Fig. 12.4a,b) builds upon an earlier prototype of a Micro-Algae vertical farm in the form of an architectural cladding system called Waterlilly 2.0 developed by Cesare Griffa (https://cesaregriffa.com/waterlilly/waterlilly-2-0/). The proposed micro-algae façade can help in absorbing carbon dioxide and producing oxygen, while acting as a second skin of buildings, boosting

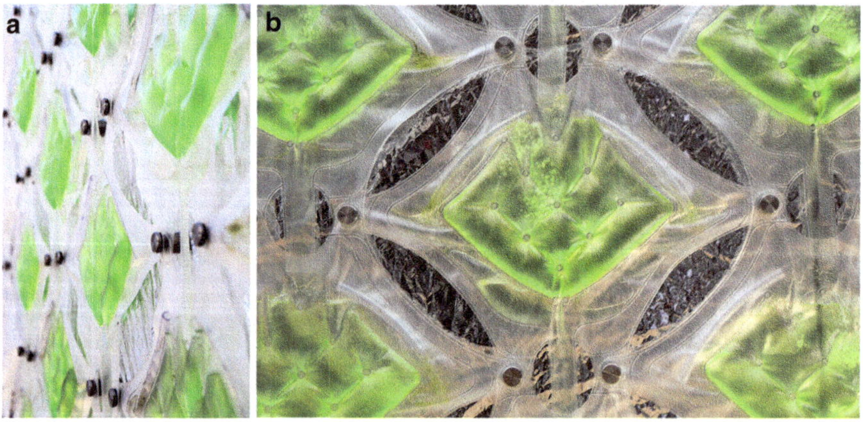

Fig. 12.4 (**a**, **b**) The WaterLily 2.0, as a microalgae cultivation system on architectural surfaces by Cesare Griffa architetto

passive cooling and increasing shading of the facade. The Urban Algae Canopy (Fig. 12.5a, b), developed by ecoLogicStudio (Claudia Pasquero and Marco Poletto) in collaboration with specialist ETFE manufacturing contractor Taiyo Europe, was developed as a 1:1 scale prototype for the Milan Design week 2014. It is often referred to as the world's first bio-digital canopy since it integrates micro-algal cultures and real-time digital cultivation protocols into one comprehensive system (http://www.ecologicstudio.com/v2/project.php?idcat=7&idsubcat=59&idproj=129). The microalgae, in this case, are cultivated within a 3 layered ETFE cladding system which is enabled due to a special CNC welding technology. This technology not only enables the accurate control of the morphology of the ETFE cushion but also enables the controlled regulation of the flow of water, CO2 and energy based on specific contextual conditions such as weather conditions and the movement of visitors. For instance, the visitors can influence the growth of the algae even on a sunny day in real-time, and thus control the amount of shading despite the high photosynthesis level based exponential growth of the algae. This is done by connecting the presence of people with the act of triggering electro-valves to alter the speed of algal flow through the canopy component (ETFE cushion) thus producing variations of algal density in their vicinity. A symbiotic relationship between people, space, technology and context are thus achieved, which ultimately controls the colour, shading and transparency levels of the entire canopy.

The last case in this section, looks at a micro scale project, in the form of a participatory public installation called H.O.R.T.U.S (Hydro Organisms Responsive to Urban Stimuli), set up at the Architectural Association, London, the UK by ecoLogicStudio (http://www.ecologicstudio.com/v2/project.php?idcat=7&idsubcat=71&idproj=115). The installation (Fig. 12.6a, b) consists of photosynthetic colonies of cyanobacteria, which visitors are encouraged to feed with carbon dioxide in order to generate oxygen and growing biomass. This installation was conceived as an urban garden prototype which promotes ideas of urban renewable energy and was accompanied with sensing technologies and a virtual interface which simulates a digital

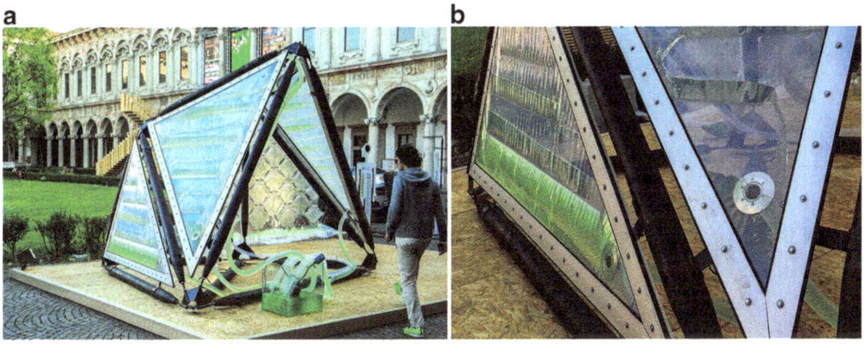

Fig. 12.5 (**a**, **b**) The Urban Canopy prototype developed by ecoLogicStudio at the Future Food District project curated by Carlo Ratti Associatti, Milan Design week. (Image courtesy Carlo Ratti Associatti)

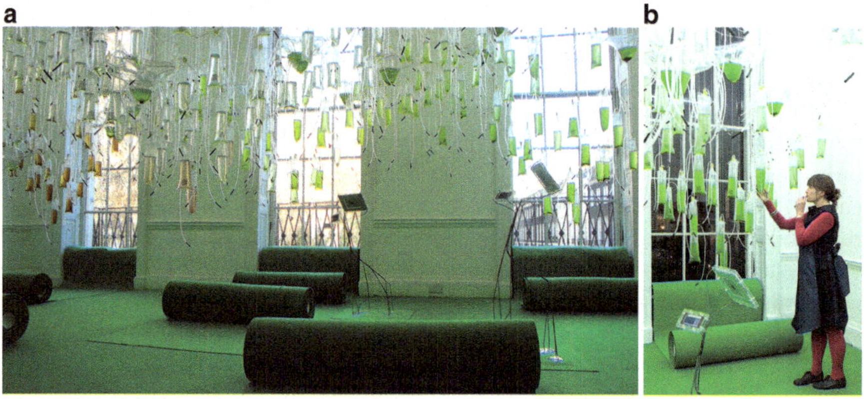

Fig. 12.6 (**a**, **b**) The H.O.R.T.U.S. Installation by ecoLogicStudio. The installation encourages users to interact with it on a daily basis and in-turn produces Oxygen to nourish other electro-luminescent bacteria within the exhibition space

image of the garden (https://www.youtube.com/watch?v=Rgnix2RDCqQ). The sensing system takes the form of ambient light sensors which are connected to containers with Bio-luminescent bacteria. According to ecoLogicStudio, flows of Energy [light radiation], Matter [biomass, CO2] and Information [images, tweets, stats] are triggered during the 4 week long growing period, inducing multiple mechanisms of self-regulation and evolving novel forms of self-organisation. Participation within the entire exhibition was a crucial means of engaging people on a daily basis by physically blowing air inside the photobioreactor containers, thus contributing CO_2 as well as adjusting their nutrient contents, resulting in the production of oxygen, which feeds other bioluminescent bacteria in the space. Besides this, the data harvested by the installation (in the form of observations posted by visitors, lighting levels, human interaction in real-time) feeds the emergent growth of its virtual garden interface, which is accessible via smartphones. An interesting interdependence of physical and digital infrastructures combined with a central agenda of raising awareness about microalgae cultivation and its benefits via participatory modes of engagements thus drives the project.

12.7 Drivers and Barriers to Adoption of ABT

Algae Building Technology is completely new to practitioners and therefore there is an imperative to understand the drivers and barriers to adoption from their perspective (Wilkinson et al. 2016). Having this understanding will enable us to promote and target the technology more effectively amongst these stakeholders. One major issue is the lack of examples to benchmark performance and cost against. Although some stakeholders will be attracted to this, to be perceived as leaders and innovators, others will be more risk averse.

The drivers and barriers to adoption are categorised under the headings political, economic, social, technological, legal and environmental and based on a City of Sydney feasibility study canvassing built environment stakeholders in 2016 (Wilkinson et al. 2016). Twenty-three interviews were conducted with built environment professionals from architecture, civil engineering, construction, certification, project management, structural engineering, chemical engineering, façade engineering, services engineering, mechanical engineering, property development, sustainability, valuation, quantity surveying, planning and building surveying. These stakeholders have varying degrees of influence over client decisions at different stages of the building lifecycle, and therefore they will have different perspectives framing their views. Semi-structured interviews enabled the researchers to explore this innovative technology and stakeholder views of the potential drivers and barriers to adoption.

12.7.1 Political and Regulatory Issues

Within Australia, the political influence of the coal and gas industries makes it hard for new renewable energy sources to emerge (Wilkinson et al. 2016). In terms of planning regulations, the market could help develop renewable on-site energy technology, including biomass, by making it a requirement of certain types of development. Another planning aspect is loss of net lettable area within buildings as a result of the façade area and plant room requirements and incentives may be needed (Wilkinson et al. 2016). Currently, this technology would require an alternate solution approach to building code compliance, which is expensive and time consuming.

In terms of maintenance, commissioning, and operation, directives and guidelines in respect of Health and Safety are needed to ensure the safety of building operators, occupants, and passers-by. Furthermore, there may be a requirement for certification of installations by Health and Safety officers. Guidelines for planners, building certifiers and other bodies such as Sydney Water, Department of Health NSW guidelines are needed to ensure officers give appropriate advice as none exist currently (Wilkinson et al. 2016).

A retrofit issue would occur where an original structure is built to the boundary line, because the retrofitted façade would overhang boundary line. It is possible to negotiate permission to overhang the boundary for a fixed period, however, it adds time and cost to projects. Some developers and owners would avoid additional unnecessary legal arrangements if the technology did not add substantially to capital or rental values (Wilkinson et al. 2016).

12.7.2 Economic Issues

The economic issues raised were extensive and related to design, construction and operation. Current plant and panel cost is very expensive compared to other renewables. An unknown is the scale or size of installation needed to make algae building economically viable. Larger installations may make algae technology more economically viable, for example at precinct level. The relative costs of the centralised and shared system elements influence scalability. The majority of participants felt cost is the main barrier to algae system adoption. The façade cost on the BIQ building was US \$2200–2300 m^2, approximately ten times more expensive than conventional facades (Wilkinson et al. 2016).

However, this technology will help position NSW in a low-carbon economy. Another barrier here is that the value of positioning NSW in a low-carbon economy is delivered to the State generally, but is born entirely by the property developer or owner. Structural disconnects between investment and return, or split incentives, abound in the world of renewables and energy conservation. This needs to be resolved to promote up take of this technology.

Additional costs are incurred in the design, construction, operation and maintenance. There is only one complete building to inform industry on probable costs for this technology. Only after several ABT buildings are completed will there be sufficient cost data to draw reliable conclusions. Without reliable data, cost management risks are significantly higher, a factor that is an additional barrier to adoption. There are long-term cost savings through on-site energy production and increasing energy costs over time. The economic loss of NLA from the additional thickness of the façade and the plant room also makes the technology less attractive as land costs are high. The economic payback period is unknown, but certainly needs to be within the building services typical lifecycle of 25 years to be competitive.

A critical economic factor from an investor's perspective is the return on investment, and for smaller scale installations, the return will most likely be poor due to high installation costs and high operation and maintenance costs. There is very little energy cost savings, relatively speaking, to generate income that recoups the investment (Wilkinson et al. 2016). Also, relative to other renewable energy sources, the return is even worse, since PV continues to improve its economic return and the energy is in a more useful form, because it is electricity. The only way to get a financial return with algae in the foreseeable future is to sell the algae into a high-value market, which is complicated and beyond the business model and capability of most medium/high rise buildings. If adopted on a wider scale over time, economies of scale will result in driving down unit costs of algae product production.

12.7.3 Social Issues

Surprisingly, the social factors comprised the fewest number of concerns. The most frequently raised concern was the negative perception of algae as 'slime', which was also associated with odours (Wilkinson et al. 2016). There were concerns raised also about the potential health impacts caused by leakage of algae or damage to PBRs and this risk needs to be managed.

On a positive note, it was a widely held view that this technology would engage people's minds about biomass and renewable energy – although large scale production may be better in peri-urban locations where it is important to educate and to remind the wider community about the importance of these technologies (Wilkinson et al. 2016).

12.7.4 Technological Issues

Technological issues arise over algae production rates. The amount and intensity of sunlight in NSW could lead to higher rates of biomass production which was a positive; however, the lifespan and durability of the technology is unknown. For example, the glazing panels and pipes with valves require cleaning and periodic replacement (Wilkinson et al. 2016). Maintenance training and education in the trades and professions is needed with regards to ABT. Maintenance may be onerous and few have experience with such technology and therefore costs might be high.

An important structural issue is the weight of the algae façade requiring support for dead and live loads. Building adaptation occurs often, after occupation and drivers can be technological, economic, social, environmental, locational or regulatory (Wilkinson et al. 2016, Wilkinson and Langston 2014). This can be unpredictable in many instances. Alterations to facades are less common due to costs (Wilkinson and Remoy 2015).

The absence of a 'blueprint' means algae panel information and design guidelines are needed for all stages of the development process. Green washing is the practice of making unsubstantiated or misleading claims about the environmental benefits of a product, service or technology. There is a danger that algae technology, because of its' novelty, is perceived as 'green wash' by industry who do not appreciate the potential of the technology. Reliability of the installations was raised and algae technology would need to approach the reliability of static systems, performing consistently to succeed. Many participants summed up the technological issues as 'complex'. This is because the technology is new and unknown; and no one has direct experience yet of the technology, on which to draw.

12.7.5 Environmental Issues

Environmental drivers and barriers focus on carbon abatement, innovation, bio-building technology, environmental rating tools, competing renewables and potential contamination (Bell and Codd 1994). Adoption of this technology would lead to lower operational GHG emissions; however, concerns were raised about the total carbon footprint. If implemented on a larger scale, the potential to mitigate the Urban Heat Island effect exists (Subhadra 2011) and; for reduced loading on existing energy infrastructure. There is the possibility of selling biomass to chemical, polymer companies. Potential food production exists however, food health and safety regulations may inhibit this option. Possible revenue from biomass sales may offset energy costs. Another driver might be innovation points in the Green Star building-rating tool. With new technologies the risks are that the innovation fails to perform as anticipated.

Other renewables; solar, PV and wind produce more energy than algae. Australian algae production rates may be higher than Hamburg as there is more sunlight, over longer periods. Building shutdown due to lack of sunlight would not be an issue in NSW, however overheating may be a problem (Wilkinson et al. 2016). The costs of new technologies compared to established technologies are always relatively more expensive. Concerns about contamination and leaks exist as some algae species contain hepatotoxins and neurotoxins, which are deleterious to human health (Bell and Codd 1994). Furthermore, damage or leakage could cause odours.

The benefits arising from the technology and the barriers identified in the literature and by the research participants, are summarised in Table 12.1.

12.8 Different Building Types & Suitability for ABT

Another aspect considered was which building types might suit ABT? The BIQ is a medium density residential building. Would economies of scale and greater production be achieved by either using high density property or considering other property types? Commercial, retail, industrial and other buildings were evaluated.

With regards to economies of scale, adopting this technology on medium to high-rise residential buildings would make more sense financially. There are opportunities to consider precinct scale energy and water systems, such as Sydney's Central Park development in Ultimo. Algae can provide some of the heating energy and hot water demand, and using algae to bioremediate greywater is another possibility. Furthermore, high and medium density residential property is often accompanied with retail property, such as cafes and restaurants which might be able to use algae products. The challenge in this sector is that Strata law in Australia complicates ownership of centralised building energy systems; however, as more models are developed, familiarity with this approach deepens.

Table 12.1 Perceived Drivers and Barriers to ABT

Issue	Driver	Not clear	Barrier
Political and regulatory	Incentivising technology Building certification	Retrofit issues	Power of vested interests Health and safety
Economic		Value of the end product Scalability Capital value	The cost of production Costs
Social	Innovation Aesthetically different Engage peoples minds		'Slime' Contamination risks Lacks aesthetic appeal
Technological	Heat transfer and shading	Building adaptation Algal production rates Cleaning (exterior and interior surfaces) Green wash Reliability	Climate Lifespan and durability Maintenance Competition with other renewables Structural issues and façade design Blueprints and guidelines needed Performance clauses in green leases needed Intentional and accidental damage Education of stakeholders Complexity
Environmental	Carbon abatement, Innovation, Bio building technology, Environmental rating tools		Competing renewables Potential contamination

Commercial buildings are an option, especially those at the top end of the market and rated under sustainable building tools such as Green Star to denote the levels of sustainability achieved. Some office buildings also embody dead facades, with no fenestration or doors, in addition unused roof areas. These can become excellent locations for deploying ABT. The uncertainty around the costs of maintenance and operation of ABTs within such set-ups is the only hurdle foreseen in such scenarios.

Major retail centre owners, especially those in urban centres, increasingly have ambitious sustainability commitments that may make them more interested in adopting innovative technology, particularly visible technology that reduces environmental footprint. Furthermore, retail centres have a fair component of tenants selling food and beverages, that could make direct use of algae as a locally grown food for consumption on the premises – with almost zero carbon food miles. Retail centres would also have a high demand for the heat produced in the ABT. The challenges in the retail sector are, that maintenance and operation staff do not currently have the knowledge and skills needed to operate ABT.

Industrial warehousing might be a good option for ABT, as there are large areas of facades without openings or glazing and large roof areas. In these respects, the facades of industrial buildings share characteristics with 'big box' retail buildings. They could afford cost effective installation of ABT, furthermore some industrial properties accommodate industries who could use the algae, for example, micro-breweries. Furthermore, there is potential to adopt circular economy paradigm whereby industrial waste becomes the raw material for another adjacent industry, The challenge in this sector is the structural capacity to retrofit or fit the technology may increase build costs. Another issue is that industrial locations often have heavy vehicles moving around and the potential for accidental damage is higher, and installations would need to be protected. Most industrial buildings would not need the heat produced by the ABT, which is another issue for industrial buildings. Aircraft hangers might offer a potential site for installation of ABT, with the heat produced being used in other airport buildings such as terminal, retail and office buildings.

Finally, there are public sector buildings, which might present an opportunity to showcase new technologies. Local government authorities are keen to lead by example, and have a variety of buildings such as libraries, sports buildings, town halls and offices. Depending on the use, there are varying demands on heating, which could be partially, or possibly, fully met, by ABT. At a smaller scale, public buildings in parks, such as cafes and toilets might offer potential to showcase the technology at a more modest scale. However, a concern is that some buildings might be vulnerable to impact damage or vandalism if not adequately protected.

There is considerable potential, in a range of land uses and buildings to adopt the technology at various scales. With a new and unfamiliar technology, such as ABT, there is a period of educating other stakeholders from building owners, investors, occupiers and the public about the benefits of the technology, before it can transition into the mainstream. If ABT is adopted across a range of building types, as indicated above, and at different scales to meet a variety of energy and other needs, this period is likely to be shorter than otherwise.

Clearly some barriers affect all typologies, and these are associated with the innovative qualities of the technology and lack of stakeholder familiarity. Thus, planning and regulatory aspects (for example, building certification) require development of clear guidance notes for stakeholders before ABT can be accepted as a viable option.

Further barriers exist with regards to the scale of development, with costs and payback periods and maintenance costs diminishing with increasing scale. Economies of scale are more likely with medium and high-density housing developments and large-scale retail and commercial properties. Although the legal issues associated with OH&S issues and maintenance will be more complex for owners. These upfront costs need to be traded against the economic savings within the operational phase.

The social acceptance factor for ABT could go either way, with some seeing the technology as exciting and innovative, whereas others would be risk-averse and see the technology as 'slime' on a façade with potential odour and contamination issues. Positive marketing and promotion of the technology is essential to promote the positive and demonstrate how issues around potential contamination and odours are managed.

Physically, retrofit will be more complex than integrating the technology into new buildings. Where retrofit is considered there are issue around load bearing capacity of the original facades and elevations. Orientation affects viability, as the ABT needs to have maximum access to sunlight for photosynthesis to occur.

Environmentally, there are clear gains in terms of reduced energy consumption and generation of onsite biomass and solar thermal energy. The scale of the installation may affect economic viability; and it is speculated that the sharing paradigm might offer a solution, whereby a number of houses or buildings in a street adopt the technology and share the costs of plant. This may make the technology more viable economically, although it is much more complex legally.

12.9 Conclusions and Where to Next?

This chapter has set out the case for adoption of ABT in new build and retrofit of properties to mitigate the impacts of climate change. The scene was set by discussing the evolution and transition of solar energy from non-viable technically and economically in the 1950s to becoming efficient and affordable in the second decade of the twenty-first century. Furthermore, advances in bioenergy have led others to state that the twenty-first century will see the domination of biofuels and the demise of fossil fuels. ABT as an innovative technology that could be a means of delivering the GHG emissions reductions needed to mitigate a 3 degree increase in global temperature predicted by the UN before 2100 (UN 2015).

Given the novelty of the technology, ABT was explained in the context of one building which currently uses ABT for heating and hot water energy; the BIQ Hamburg. Some experimental applications of ABT in the built environment such as urban algae farms above highways, an urban canopy structure and an exposition encouraging participatory cultivation of algae were also discussed. The literature review, identified the political, economic, social, technological, legal and environmental issues associated with the adoption of ABT in the built environment. This understanding was further analysed through interviews with 23 professional stakeholders in Sydney during 2016 and summarised in Table 12.1. There are various drivers and barriers which need to be acknowledged and managed, if the stakeholders are to feel comfortable adopting and recommending this innovative technology.

There are clear barriers to address identified in this research, with some issues being either, a barrier or a driver, depending on the circumstances. All of the issues identified require further research and experimentation so that empirical data can support design decisions. Further, opportunities to adopt algae also became apparent, for example, biomass remediation of black and greywater is possible, and; in taking buildings partially, or totally, off grid it is possible to extend the life of existing water and power infrastructure in our towns and cities. With population growth and increasing urbanisation, retrofitting current building stock with ABT could mitigate the predicted 3-degree temperature increase which we would be subjected to.

Action needs to be taken in respect of generating some empirical data on performance in different locations, so that design can be informed. Concurrently there is a need to develop design guidance, maintenance manuals, education for tradespeople and professional practitioners, as well as vocational education in colleges and university programmes. Regulations and legislation need to be introduced and/or amended and guidance in respect of OH&S is required. With up to date resources and guidance notes, decisions can be made with confidence and awareness of risks, as well as benefits. There is no doubt of the damage that use of fossil fuel energy systems has brought about, it is time to explore and adopt new paradigms; and the possibly of widespread use of ABT is one of them.

References

Arup. (2013). *World's first microalgae façade goes 'live'*. Retrieved on 4th February, 2016, from http://www.arup.com/News/2013_04_April/25_April_World_first_microalgae_facade_goes_live.aspx

Arup. (2016). *World's first microalgae façade goes 'live'*. Retrieved February 4, 2016, from http://www.arup.com/News/2013_04_April/25_April_World_first_microalgae_facade_goes_live.aspx

Bell, S. G., & Codd, G. A. (1994). Cyanobacterial toxins and human health. *Reviews in Medical Microbiology, 5*(4), 256–264.

Brennan, L., & Owende, P. (2010). Biofuels from microalgae—A review of technologies for production, processing, and extractions of biofuels and co-products. *Renewable and sustainable energy reviews, 14*(2), 557–577.

Buildup. (2015). *The BIQ House: First algae-powered building in the world*. Retrieved September 21, 2016, from http://www.buildup.eu/en/practices/cases/biq-house-first-algae-powered-building-world

Canstar. (2018). *Average electricity costs per kWh*. Retrieved September 25, from https://www.canstarblue.com.au/electricity/electricity-costs-kwh/

Cho, D.-H., Choi, J.-W., Kang, Z., Kim, B.-H., Oh, H.-M., Kim, H.-S., & Ramanan, R. (2016). Microalgal diversity fosters stable biomass productivity in open ponds treating wastewater. *Scientific Reports, 7*, 1979.

Clean Energy Council. (2008). *Australian Bioenergy Roadmap: Setting the direction for biomass in stationary energy to 2020 and beyond.* Clean Energy Council, September 2008. ISBN: 978-0-9805646-0-0 (print), 978-0-9805646-1-7 (online PDF)

Council, C. E. (2014). *Guide to installing Solar PV for business and industry.* Clean Energy Australia report.

Davila, T., Epstein, M., & Shelton, R. (2012, November 9). *Making innovation work: How to manage it, measure it, and profit from it.* Upper Saddle River: FT Press.

Decker, M., Hahn, G., & Harris, L. M. (2016). Bio-enabled façade systems-managing complexity of life through emergent technologies. In *Proceedings of the 34the CAADe conference on complexity and simplicity.* Oulu: Finland: University of Oulu.

Elnokaly, A., & Keeling, I. (2016). An empirical study investigating the impact of micro-algal technologies and their application within intelligent building fabrics, in social and behavioral sciences. In *Proceedings of the urban planning and architecture design for sustainable development conference.* Lecce, Italy.

Ho, D. P., Ngo, H. H., & Guo, W. (2014). A mini review on renewable sources for biofuel. *Bioresource technology, 169,* 742–749.

Iqbal, M., Grey, D., Sarkissian, F. S., & Fowler, M. W. (1993). A flat-sided photobioreactor for continuous culturing microalgae. *Aquacultural Engineering, 12*(1993), 183–190. https://doi.org/10.1016/0144-8609(93)90010-9.

Kim, K. H. (2013). A feasibility study of an algae façade system. In: *Proceedings of international conference on sustainable building Asia (SB13).* Seoul, South Korea, 8–10 July 2013.

Kunjapur, A. M., & Eldigre, R. B. (2010). Photobioreactor design for commercial biofuel production from microalgae. *Industrial and Engineering Chemistry Research, 49*(2010), 3516–3526. https://doi.org/10.1021/ie901459u.

Moser, C. A., & Kalton, G. (2017). *Survey methods in social investigation.* London: Routledge.

Patton, M. Q. (2002). *Qualitative research and evaluation methods.* Thousand Oaks: Sage Publications.

Pruvost, J., Gouic, B. L., & Legrand, J. (2014). Symbiotic integration of photobioreactors. In *A factory building façade for mutual benefit between buildings and microalgae needs, 21st international congress of chemical and process engineering CHISA 2014 Prague 17th conference on process integration, modelling and optimisation for energy saving and pollution reduction PRES 2014,* Praha, Czech Republik. https://doi.org/10.13140/2.1.2076.1920.

Robson, C., & McCartan, K. (2016). *Real world research.* John Wiley & Sons.

Rosillo-Calle, F., & Woods, J. (2012). *The biomass assessment handbook.* London: Routledge.

Rosillo-Calle, F., de Groot, P., Hemslock, S. L., & Woods. J. (2016). *The biomass assessment handbook* (2nd ed.). Routledge. ISBN 978-1-138-01965-2.

Sarda, R. C., & Vicente, C. A. (2016). Case studies on the architectural integration of photobioreactors in building facades. In F. P. Torgal, C. Buratti, S. Kalaiselvam, C. G. Granqvist, & V. Ivanov (Eds.), *Nano and biotech-based materials for energy building efficiency* (pp. 457–484). Cham: Springer.

Statistica. (2018). *Electricity prices for households in Germany from 2010 to 2017, semi-annually (in euro cents per kilowatt-hour).* Retrieved September 25, 2018, https://www.statista.com/statistics/418078/electricity-prices-for-households-in-germany/

Subhadra, B. (2011, January 15). Algal biorefinery-based industry: An approach to address fuel and food insecurity for a carbon smart world. *Journal of the Science of Food and Agriculture, 91*(1), 2–13.

The Guardian Sustainable Business. (2016, February 2). *Solar power what is holding back growth in clean energy?* http://www.theguardian.com/sustainable-business/2016/jan/31/solar-power-what-is-holding-back-growth-clean-energy?CMP=new_1194&CMP

UN. (2015). The Paris Agreement. Retrieved on 13th June 2018 from; https://unfccc.int/sites/default/files/english_paris_agreement.pdf

UNEP F. (2009, September). *Fiduciary responsibility: Legal and practical aspects of integrating environmental, social and governance issues into institutional investment.* Geneva: NEP FI.

Vasumathi, K. K., Premalatha, M., & Subramanian, P. (2012). Parameters influencing the design of photobioreactor for the growth of microalgae. *Renewable and Sustainable Energy Reviews, 16*(2012), 5443–5450. https://doi.org/10.1016/j.rser.2012.06.013.

Wilkinson, S. J., & Langston, C. (2014, January 21). *Sustainable building adaptation: Innovations in decision-making*. Chichester: Wiley.

Wilkinson, S., & Remoy, H. (2015). *Sustainable conversion adaptation: An international comparison of best practices*. RICS COBRA conference UTS Sydney July 8–10 2015. ISBN 978–1–78321-071-8.

Wilkinson, S. J., Stoller, P., Ralph, P., & Hamdorf, B. (2016). *The feasibility of algae building technology in Sydney*. City of Sydney Environmental Performance Grant 2015. https://doi.org/10.13140/RG.2.1.4349.6560.

Yin, R. K., 2011. *Applications of case study research*. Los Angeles: Sage.

Chapter 13
The Qualitative Image: Urban Analytics, Hybridity and Digital Representation

Linda Matthews

Abstract High-precision analytical software, such as that used for medical imaging, can be also applied productively to the assessment of urban conditions such as pedestrian and vehicular flow. A prominent feature of this tool is its ability to offer a new and more abstract understanding of the material nature of the city. Drawing upon a range of scaled-up software procedures to illustrate capability, the chapter reveals how an analytical medical software tool can be adapted for use in alternative interdisciplinary contexts such as urban design. Using imagery captured from public domain webcams, it demonstrates how the upscaling and transferal of this digital tool from its original disciplinary role provides a new way of assessing the appropriateness of a proposed built intervention. It also reveals that the extension of this tool's fine-grain, image-based analysis capabilities into a broader, more complex urban scale allows the more ambiguous and often-disregarded properties of city life to form part of a comprehensive and wholistic data set. The chapter concludes with the proposal that the synthesis of quantitative and qualitative data facilitated by this analytical platform exceeds the capability of urban assessment tools currently used by the discipline.

Keywords Medical imaging · Protocol · Pixel · Cross-disciplinary · Qualitative · Patterns · Digital · Colour · Luminosity

13.1 Introduction

To engage with the contemporary city is now to engage with the relationship between its built surface and the visioning technology that presides over it. Urban space has been transformed by new modes of navigation and perception that are amplified by the camera's ability to traverse the urban landscape in an

L. Matthews (✉)
School of Architecture, Faculty of Design Architecture and Building,
University of Technology Sydney,
Sydney, Australia
e-mail: Linda.Matthews@uts.edu.au

N. Biloria (ed.), *Data-driven Multivalence in the Built Environment*, S.M.A.R.T. Environments, https://doi.org/10.1007/978-3-030-12180-8_13

unprecedented way. While the effect of the zoom lens extends the opportunity to correlate camera focal increments with the effects of a vast range of physical conditions, the streaming image-making process delivers this urban data to a global audience as an uninterrupted video stream, with a frame-rate capture indistinguishable from the perception of real time. As a consequence, both technology and the image assume a highly instrumental role in relation to the assessment and determination of conditions that arise from this new type of engagement with urban space.

With digital camera protocols mimicking many of the functions of the human visual system (HVS), optical cues based upon colour, brightness and shape become the principal determinants of image assembly and perceptual hierarchy. This means that the pixel not only radically shifts the rules by which representation is constructed and perceived, but these properties set new criteria according to which the city's operation and physical properties are able to be indexed and quantified. In this new digital frame, it is therefore the data array of the pixel grid that serves as a supplementary portal for the admission of new modes of urban information gathering and assessment.

Visual analytics play an important role in analysing the phenomena and processes that evolve in contemporary physical space and, by extension, the diverse decisions that are made based upon this data. Through an overview of current methods, tools and procedures, Andrienko et al. (2010) identify variations of movement data as the main focus of urban analytics, speculating that the answer to overcoming the representational shortcomings of these tools lies in cross-disciplinary cooperation (Andrienko and Andrienko 2013). Many recent software developments in visual analytics are concerned with overcoming problems associated with visualization complexity and clutter (Andrienko et al. 2010, Scheepens et al. 2011; Wongsuphasawat and Gotz 2012; Zeng et al. 2016), with the express purpose of rapid commercialization (Scheepens et al. 2016). However, as an alternative approach to these types of proprietary software tools, many independent freely available open-source platforms also offer highly efficient, targeted data analysis capabilities to produce an index of reality. Diagnostic or medical imaging software, currently the principal mode of scientific image-based analysis, demands a high degree of data precision to track and map the progression or remission of disease. Using image-based analysis, these independent, high-performance tools are specifically configured to analyse images in ways that resist the deliberate intervention of manufacturers' promotional strategies.

However, the transposition of this software from a medical to a design application calls for a new understanding of what types of disciplinary contribution the image might now be able to make. If the specific problem-set addressed by medical imaging is the representation and analysis of change over time, then the adaptation of similar criteria to the assessment of urban conditions, understood as color, luminosity/contrast and density, is simply an increase in the scale of analysis. Furthermore, the digital translation of these properties into digital data releases their potential to incorporate highly qualitative and affective data in the information-gathering processes of the contemporary city.

This chapter will discuss the interdisciplinary adaptation of software to the assessment of urban conditions. It will reveal how the precision of an open-source medical imaging toolset can be applied productively, not only to the assessment of pedestrian and vehicular flow, but to a new and more abstract understanding of the material nature of the city. Using a range of scaled-up interdisciplinary software procedures, it will reveal how this approach can set a new standard for the assessment of complex urban conditions that, through the synthesis of quantitative and qualitative data, exceeds the disciplinary capabilities of urban assessment tools currently available.

13.2 The Distributed City

The diverse urban data-gathering capabilities of the Internet webcam network currently remain largely unexplored. As John Macarthur (2000) observes, while Modern painting transposed the relation of pictorial depths into a relation of surfaces, then so too does the aerial vantage point transpose the variation of landscape contours into a relation of patterns and textures that awaits further release. Traces of ownership of public space are clearly demonstrated by the textural patterns of images produced from these new aerial viewpoints. As one example of many, Google Earth views of politically sensitive zones are heavily edited and pixelated below a certain elevation, producing a *specific* pattern recognizable by its association with a *specific* type of activity and located in a *specific* place. Conversely, less sensitive zones are neither pixelated nor traceable through any particular pattern type at corresponding elevations. (Fig. 13.1).

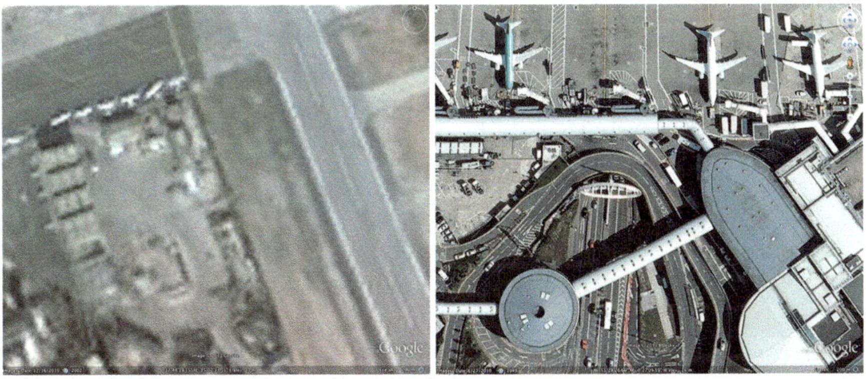

Fig. 13.1 Google Earth images of Haifa Airport Israel (left) and Heathrow airport United Kingdom (right) at identical altitudes, showing Google intervention in image definition of Haifa airport. (Image: Google Earth)

The types of patterns that emerge at certain elevations also bear an historical trace of the impact of different political regimes and cultural mores upon individual land ownership. The diversity of patterns that appears at corresponding aerial elevations in different locations thus sets up an indexical relationship between the vertical representation of space and the material nature and scale of its content. Figure 13.2 reveals a correspondence between the physical occupation of the landscape and the magnification index of the camera. In both cases, the left-hand image was taken from exactly the same altitude above the earth as the right-hand image, revealing an observable relationship between the image patterning and the camera's vertical viewpoint.

Similarly, the *guerilla* tactics of urban groups like the New York–based Institute of Applied Autonomy indicate how the webcam platform might contribute to the formation of new landscape usage patterns. As Laura Kurgan observes, thanks to the Internet platform interdisciplinary mechanisms of digital data manipulation are now broadly accessible across global digital space. 'Many military technologies have gone from classified to omnipresent, from expensive to free, and from centralized to distributed, downloadable on our desktops anywhere on earth with access to the Internet.' (Kurgan 2013, 24).

This group's *i-SEE* program is a web-based application (21st Century Digital Art) which maps the locations of CCTV cameras in urban environments with the express purpose of providing a hidden route for the user that avoids Internet camera surveillance. The software reveals that there is a strong correlation between areas with the highest incidence of cameras and the presence of politically, morally or economically sensitive property. (Fig. 13.3).

By avoiding detection and reversing the idea of personal visibility promoted by urban Internet camera networks, the individual *i-See* user therefore subverts the original intent of the system. The selection of a *path of least resistance* that uses unorthodox routes across the urban landscape thus potentially not only eventually aligns the inhabitation of these spaces with non-conforming citizens but links the image-making platform to the material evolution of the city. In this respect, it is both the data in the image in combination with the network system that simultaneously influence urban growth patterns and bear witness to their evolution.

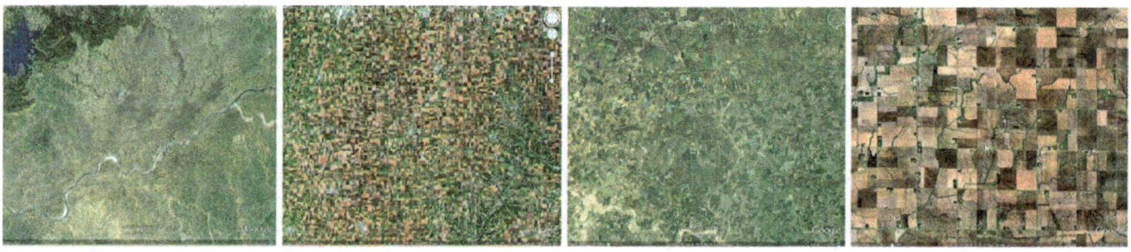

Fig. 13.2 Google Earth images of India (left) and Israel (right) showing relative variations in patterns at identical altitudes. (Image: Google Earth)

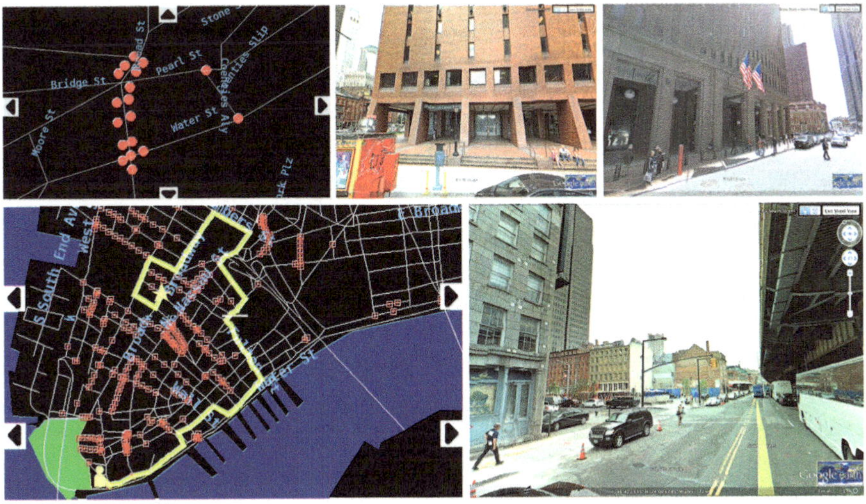

Fig. 13.3 Top left to right: i-See software map of lower Manhattan showing area of concentrated surveillance cameras; corresponding Google Street View of this area showing Morgan Chase Bank; Goldman Sachs. (Image: Google Earth)
Bottom left to right: i-See software map of lower Manhattan showing route avoiding surveillance cameras; Google Street View of this area showing currently degraded zone and sparse inhabitation. (Image: Google Earth)

13.2.1 The Open-Source Digital Imaging Platform and New Opportunities for Data Analysis

The replication by camera manufacturers of the cues of the human eye within camera technology re-presents similar optical conditions and vulnerabilities to which the HVS is subject. In both personal camera and public webcam terms, image-processing malfunctions associated with environmental conditions such as reflection, refraction and diffraction are all targeted for removal by camera manufacturers to ensure that the individual snapshot and the public capturing of urban space are smooth and flawless. An example of this are the camera's shape-sensitivity patterns, which are extrapolated algorithms of HVS saliency factors relating directly to coarse or low-resolution peripheral vision (Kruegle 2011). This mimicked scanning process is engineered specifically to use shape-scanning algorithms that can enhance pre-selected areas of an image (Foley et al. 2014). In a context of urban space, this inevitably produces a predetermined image of the city aligned with the politics of site ownership. It also excludes peripheral data relating to what are classified as *aberrations* from the city image that could potentially add enormous insight and value for data-gathering. The precise strategies hardware and software manufacturers employ for camera applications are therefore predictably difficult to access (Klette and Rosenfeld 2004). Not only are they concealed from the viewer, but they do not disclose the history of the processes to which image data has been subject.

However, the fundamental image properties of the HVS and the digital image, colour, luminosity and shape, can be released from the constraints of embedded proprietary hardware and software through the availability of open-source code, which is free to users as well as to developers. Many of these software programs enable the image to be captured directly from the Internet in *raw* file format before it is subject to reductive optimisation and culling processes and then re-cycled as an *authentic* and comprehensive basis for urban analysis. Also most open-source software has associated collaborative communities for development support and therefore the benefit of future enhancements that are not dependent on a single organisation (Chen 2005). Many open-source software programs have availed themselves of the open-source GNU/Linux code to either avoid or correct the numerous image enhancement decisions embedded within commercial software. *GIMP* (GNU Image Manipulation Program), is a freely distributed program that is expandable and extendable, allowing the user to undertake image manipulation at all levels of complexity, including photo retouching, image composition and image authoring. Other programs like *Color Blender* (Color Blender) and *Pipette* (Charcoal Design) operate exclusively to override any default hardware colour choices, allowing the user to access the internal colour geometries of the image, and thus to have control of the predictive assemblies of multiple colour palettes (Fig. 13.4). The use of this type of code, in combination with the relentless generative capacity of the Internet camera, therefore means that the ability to produce a reductive, stable image of urban space is severely diminished.

However, it is the hidden choices embedded in the more inaccessible aspects of both the image processing pipeline and its final contextual location that pose the greatest obstacle to the opening up of the image-making process. Proprietary software manufacturers have been able to discourage intervention because the colour demosaicing or interpolation process involves the interaction between software and camera hardware, both of which are tied to the copyright of the product and also automated. 'In practice, it is extremely rare to have access to any history of the processes to which image data has been subject, so no systematic approach to enhancement is possible' (Poynton 2012, 383). However, another cross-platform

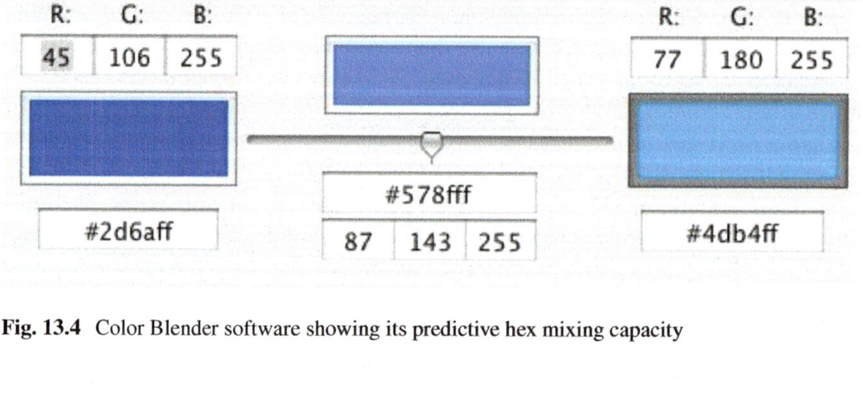

Fig. 13.4 Color Blender software showing its predictive hex mixing capacity

image-processing program, *Raw Therapee* (Raw Therapee), intervenes in this process at its origin, allowing *raw* or untampered files to be read by the computer. This program gives the user advanced control over the colour-demosaicing process, enabling use of a variety of different algorithms rather being subject to the camera's built-in code.

The assignation of highly specific and layered integer values to the basic image unit, the pixel, means that the primary compositional and structural elements of the image are color, contrast and brightness data. In the case of colour images, pixel values are represented by triples of scalar values such as red, blue, green or hue, saturation and intensity, and these values alone determine the relationships that each pixel can have with another. Circumventing the concealed manoeuvres of commercial image-processing pipelines, open-source imaging toolsets such as *PixelMath* (PixelMath Software), *ImageJ* (ImageJ: Image Processing and Analysis in Java) *and Fiji* (ImageJ) instead provide high-precision insights into this type of image geometry. *PixelMath* is able to perform a series of pixel-level arithmetic and logical operations between images. *ImageJ* is a Java-script software that allows custom acquisition, analysis and processing plug-ins to be developed using its internal editor and Java compiler. A public domain open-source software, *ImageJ* delivers Richard Stallman's four essential software freedoms to the user.[1] *Fiji* is a distribution of *ImageJ* focused on biological image analysis. *Fiji* is *open* not only in respect to its source code but its inter-connectivity to other platforms. The ambition of its developers is to integrate with other bioimage analysis software that outperforms it in particular tasks, seen in its integration with MATLAB and ITK (Schindelin et al. 2012). *Fiji* facilitates the transformation of novel algorithms into *ImageJ* plugins that can be shared with end users through an integrated update system.

13.2.2 The Numerical Indexing of Urban Space

The application of image analysis software to the city means that image content, in this case an urban scene, is represented by an array of pixels, all distributed in a specific numeric relationship to each other. By extension, it also means that complex urban conditions captured by Internet webcam technology are assigned specific numeric values and locations on the picture-plane grid that are recognisable according to a unique array pattern of pixel values. Conditions relating to urban pedestrian and vehicular flow and material surfaces, mediated according to intrinsic pixel values of colour and brightness, thus become a primary mechanism for urban data gathering and assessment, while the temporal nature of this platform's content capture allows the shape-based evolution of urban conditions to be similarly quantified.

[1] '(1) The freedom to run the program, for any purpose; (2) The freedom to study how the program works and change it to make it do what you wish; (3) The freedom to redistribute copies so you can help your neighbor; (4) The freedom to improve the program, and release your improvements to the public, so that the whole community benefits.' (Ferreira and Rasband 2011, 1).

Using open-source software *PixelMath* to identify individual pixel values, the following example draws upon unique numeric arrays to identify particular urban conditions which can be distinguished according to the precise contextual distribution of pixel values. This can be seen in Fig. 13.5 where a portion of blurred image content is translated into a numeric matrix which then serves as the means by which the distribution of numbers that compose this particular represented condition, in this case atmospheric diffraction, can be readily identified.

Diffraction artefacts are another example of aberrant and normally disregarded images that represent the city in all of its variable conditions. While an image such as this would normally be rejected and not considered as part of this city's formal, curated *iconic* image library, the webcam's automatic capture of this event nevertheless presents it as just another of the city's many shifting conditions. By establishing a means whereby the complex conditions of urban space can be documented in numeric form, a reproducible platform is thus established that indexes the properties of the city according to a new range of user-determined qualitative criteria that in proprietary circumstances would have been otherwise discarded.

Another example of the type of inclusion made available through the proliferation of the Internet are webcam glitches, or transmission errors which are often highly abstracted, affective representations of urban conditions (Fig. 13.6). The webcam's automatic inclusion of these images within the daily urban image portfolio further reveals the extraordinary potential diversity of translatable digital arrays into the city's material surfaces.

The incorporation of non-traditional representations of the city's many conditions as part of its visual documentation can also be understood within a broader disciplinary context. If the designer's role is to understand complex urban conditions through the mapping of urban space, then the inclusion of diversity, aberrant or otherwise, responds to this brief. Furthermore, at the forefront of urban representation and analysis, it is therefore the introduction of new mapping and data-gathering tools contesting the city as a singular, normative space that sets this process in motion.

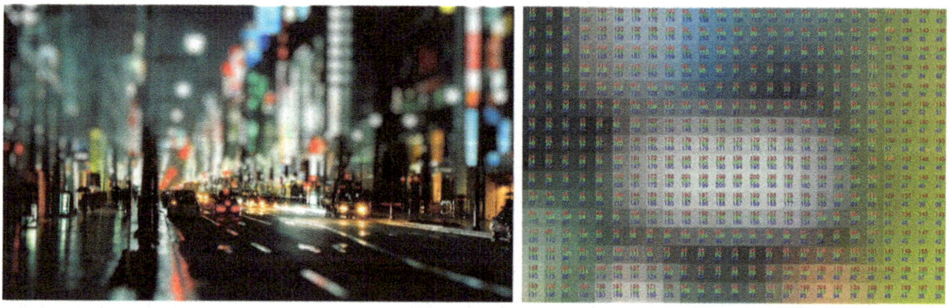

Fig. 13.5 Image of urban street scene, showing diffraction artefacts and areas of content selected for *PixelMath* analysis (left). Numeric distribution of RGB pixel values of a diffraction artefact from the same image produced using *PixelMath* software (right). (Image: Creative Commons)

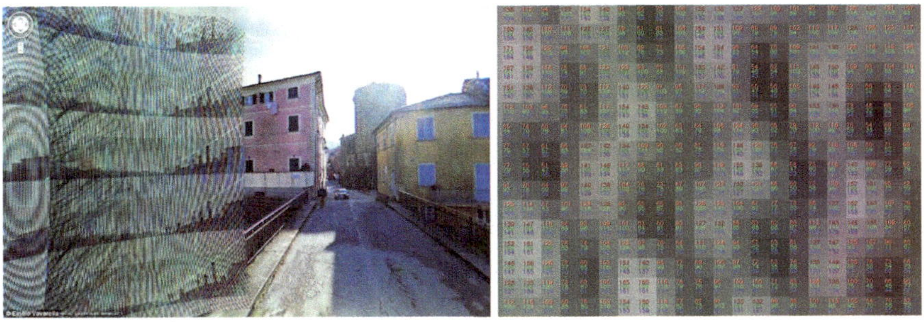

Fig. 13.6 Image of urban scene showing transmission or glitch error artefacts (left) and close-up of the artefact area in a *PixelMath* analysis showing numerical distribution of RGB pixel values (right). Left-hand image: Emilio Vavarelle. Google StreetView

13.3 The Temporal City

The distributed nature of the city means that the formation of either a continuous or comprehensive image from any single vantage point is not possible. Unlike the traditional static images of the city, the webcam's progressive revealing of contemporary urban space can be extracted as a projective analytical tool to reveal the evolutionary pattern of diverse and yet simultaneously occurring urban conditions. The two key determining factors in this procedure are time and place.

ImageJ addresses the first of these factors. The adaptation of this software as an urban analysis tool calls for a reassessment of what types of information the image might provide. The specific problem set addressed by medical imaging is the analysis and representation of change over time, which can easily be transposed to the assessment of transformative urban conditions. *ImageJ* has the capacity to organise streaming video footage into manageable image sets or *stacks*. Image stacks are multiple, spatially and temporally related images or slices displayed in a single window that can be easily manipulated, rotated and reassembled according to user specifications. The three-dimensional visualisation of an image stack thus extends its functionality well beyond the realm of two-dimensional analysis into more projective analytical functions in which the evolution of environmental and material properties associated with colour and luminosity can be traced.

The proliferation of Internet webcams in Tokyo addresses the second factor owing to the ability to capture multiple readings of the same place over controlled intervals of time. The density of this urban space also presents an ideal opportunity to observe and assess simultaneously occurring complex activity.

A stack of webcam images extracted from streaming webcam video footage of Shibuya Crossing, Tokyo clearly shows the evolution of programmatic activity over a relatively brief time-frame (approximately 13 s) across multiple image axes (Fig. 13.7). A development in different degrees of colour and luminosity can also be seen. The visual capture of the city across multiple, simultaneously evolving axes

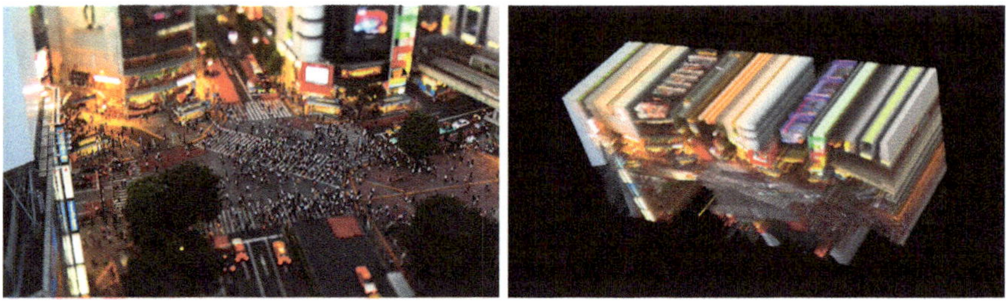

Fig. 13.7 Still from webcam footage (left) and rotated stack of webcam images (right) extracted from streaming webcam video footage of Shibuya Crossing, Tokyo, Japan. (Left-hand image: Forrest Brown/Shutterstock.com)

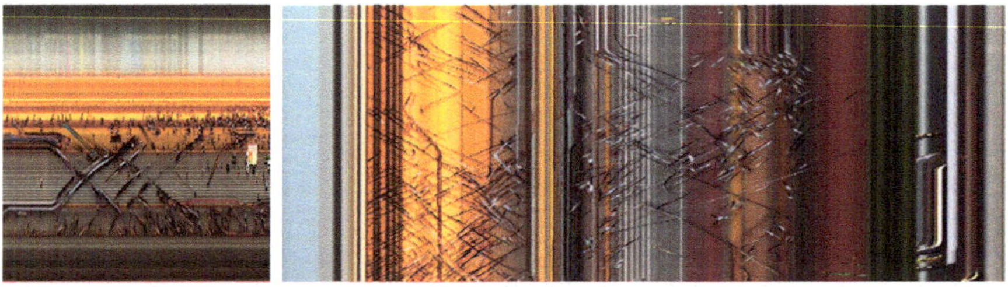

Fig. 13.8 Interior slice of image stack of Shibuya Crossing, Tokyo Japan on XZ (left) and ZY (right) axes. Original image: Forrest Brown/Shutterstock.com

thus allows a specific temporal point within the image stack, not only to be identified, but assessed according to its qualitative properties of colour and brightness.

ImageJ facilitates the type of visual journey that moves the viewer through a series of orthogonally intersecting *x,y* axes that progressively evolve along a third *z* axis to produce a complete reconfiguration of the formal content of the image stack (Fig. 13.8). These new image *slices* are the synthesis of axial cuts that collectively form a new urban spatial map that interrogates the more traditional representations of the city's activities and its material surfaces. Reminiscent of the analytical model proposed by Ferreira et al. (2013), in which access to a specific urban data set relating to taxi trips is facilitated by a visual query model that allows users to select data slices and explore them, here instead the slices record more qualitative data, foregrounding hitherto unseen variants of the city in terms of its colour and brightness properties. The capacity for the user to *step inside* the image stack releases the city's multiple viewpoints and its conditions in unprecedented ways that, on the one hand profoundly transform the understanding of the city as a complex condition, and on the other endow the designer with comprehensive analytical agency.

13.3.1 Urban Flow as Qualitative Brightness

A comprehensive solution for the visualisation of arbitrary origin–destination flows has long eluded researchers (Andrienko et al. 2010). Rejecting conventional visualisation methods such as flow maps because of their propensity to generate visual clutter, Zeng et al. (2016) nevertheless concede that the aggregate movements of objects between different locations could have huge spatial and temporal variations. In addition to this, these authors observe that existing visual analytic methods generally focus on global OD flows across regions and ignore OD flows constrained along specific locations/paths. Proposing their waypoints-constrained OD visual analytics model as a partial, temporary solution, they identify the need for a way of visualizing OD flow volumes along with the movement paths of the OD flows.

Acting as a supplementary urban visualisation tool, *ImageJ*'s capacity to transform activity into degrees of brightness presents a new analytical means by which the city can be understood. Using the *Z Project* function, the conflation of an image stack comprising thousands of single urban *snapshots* into a single image, means that traditional modes of representing the city's flow are relinquished in favour of the blurred trajectories of motion over time (Fig. 13.9). Precise temporal readings are available for either single or comparative analysis in one or several locations respectively.

Depending upon the location, the compressed images can demonstrate different types of activity. While Fig. 13.9 reveals distinct variations mostly relating to the volume of pedestrian traffic through the Shibuya Crossing location at different times of day, another Tokyo webcam seen in Fig. 13.10 mainly discloses information about the density of vehicular traffic. This is just one instance of how this type of software application can add informative and comparative insights into specific locations and demographics, particularly if data extractions were conducted at key intervals throughout the day.

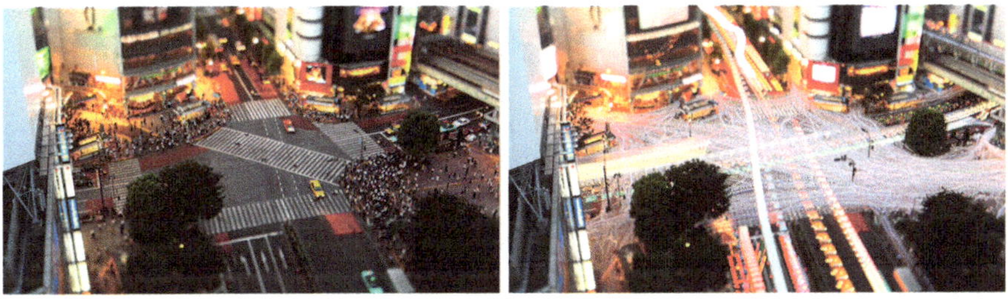

Fig. 13.9 Single still from webcam footage of Shibuya Crossing, Tokyo, Japan (left) and a conflated projection of same image stack along *z* axis according to maximum luminosity for a 13 s interval showing mainly pedestrian flow (right). (Left-hand image: Forrest Brown/Shutterstock.com)

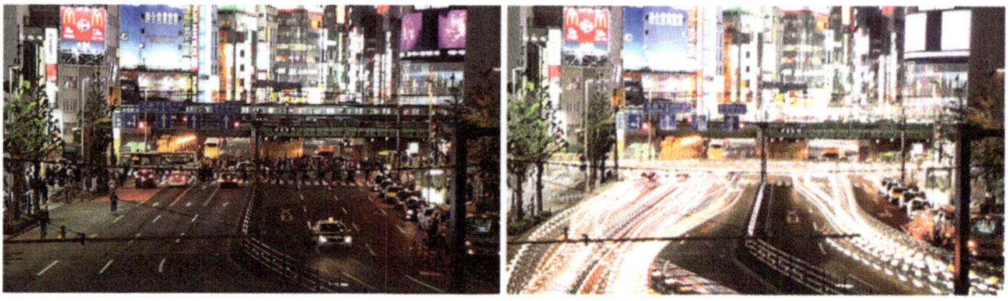

Fig. 13.10 Single still from webcam footage of Shinjuku district, Tokyo, Japan (left) and a conflated projection of same image stack along z axis according to maximum luminosity for a 13 s interval showing mainly vehicular traffic flow (right). (Left-hand image: Tokyo Motion/Shutterstock.com)

In design terms, this type of representation also offers the opportunity for a design intervention within this space to be contextualised according to the many urban properties made visible by viewing technology. In other words, the image stack serves as a mechanism for a new type of design decision that is, at once, qualitative and time-based. To position this within a global context, the *ImageJ* image stack establishes a new means and criteria by which both the properties of the city and any intervention within this space can be assessed. Because the stack is but one small part of an evolving continuum, it therefore produces a collective *montage* of the distributed global city, where new volumetric representations of qualitative urban space continually cross-pollinate and evolve. The ability of this software to foster new modes of observing the inhabitation of urban space thus raises the possibility of pre-testing a design intervention according to whether it is either complementary or antagonistic to existing site use. The deliberate and strategic activation of program-related brightness within a webcam-viewed urban context could therefore profoundly affect the experience of the city for a global audience.

13.3.2 Urban Flow as Quantitative Luminosity

However, the numeric basis of the conflated urban image also means that it can be subjected to comprehensive, traditional modes of analytical scrutiny. The visible trails of pedestrian meandering discussed previously, described within the image as colour and brightness levels, can also form the basis of a scaled-up PIV analysis, a block-based optic flow, used to cross-correlate between specific areas of diagnostic images. In this case, the pattern generated by particles is used to compute the velocity field based on what direction and to what extent a section of an image has moved between two successive instants.

In Fig. 13.11, the optic flow analysis of the two different extremities of the image stack of Shibuya Crossing reveals highly specific visual data about the direction of traffic flow in this space. Although the images are extracted from opposite ends of the image stack, the overall displacement of traffic between the images is not sig-

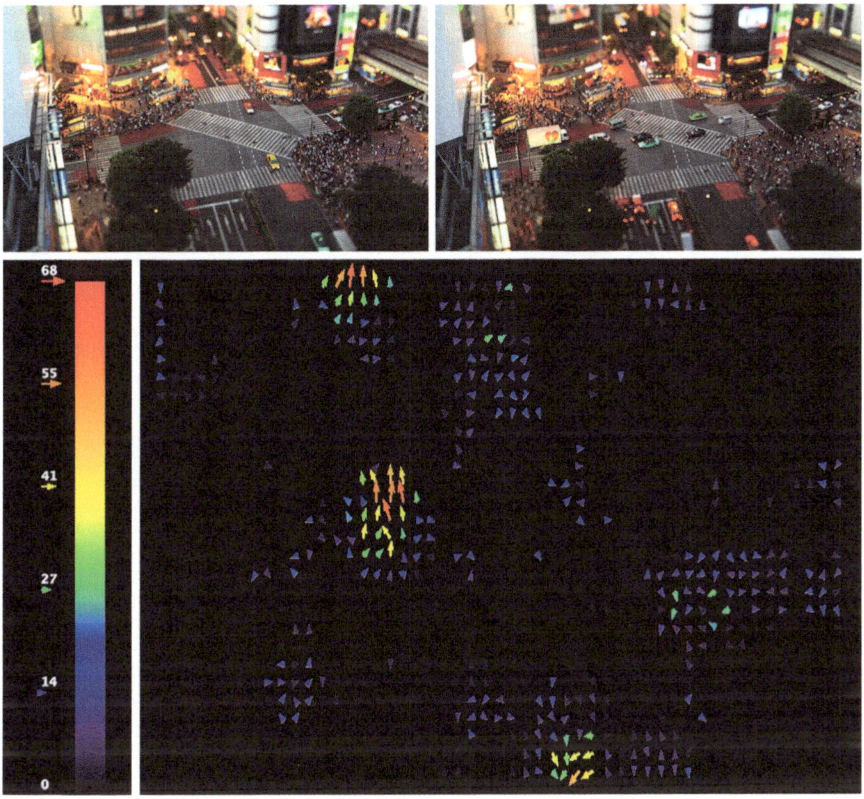

Fig. 13.11 Top: Single stills from webcam footage of Shibuya Crossing, Tokyo, Japan. (Image: Forrest Brown/Shutterstock.com. Bottom: PIV analysis of optic flow between the same two images)

nificant. The PIV analysis nevertheless provides a detailed analysis of this displacement according to both motion direction and intensity. Extended into a design context, the application of this analytical process could provide invaluable insights into urban planning through the provision of highly nuanced and assessable data over any predetermined time interval.

Levels of image colour and luminosity therefore underpin this type of image-based analysis. The capacity to describe spatial luminance as height for a three-dimensional surface plot allows these values to be visualised and tested against those of another. The benefit of this function is that it allows the status of the individual colour channels to be observed well as the relative luminosity levels of different spaces to be easily compared. This function is, in turn, supported by a binary converter and a particle assessment function, the Floyd Steinberg Dithering Algorithm (Fig. 13.12). Similar to a recent approach outlined by Scheepens et al. (2016), in which directions of traffic flows are visualized using a particle system on top of the density map, here the image data is converted to binary form and subsequently counted and measured according to the maxima of luminance. In this case

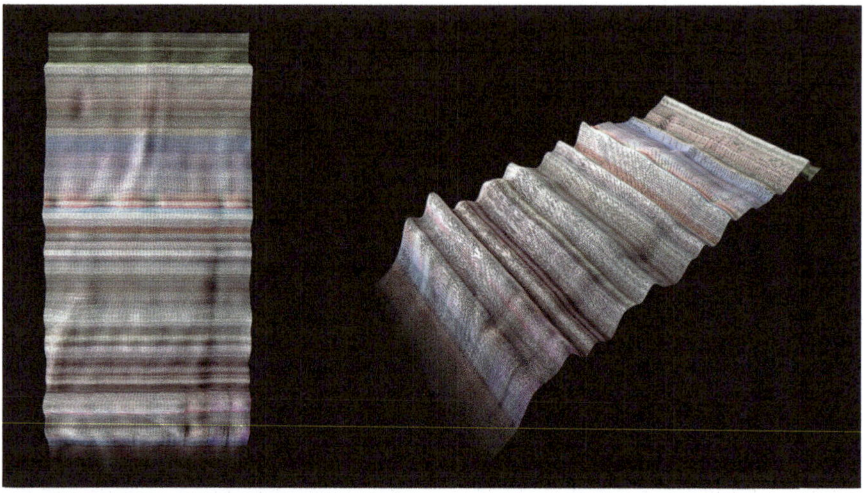

Fig. 13.12 Luminosity surface plot visualisations of the sum of images in a stack of Shinjuku district, Tokyo, Japan processed using *ImageJ's* Interactive 3D Surface Plot plugin. (Original image: Tokyo Motion/Shutterstock.com)

luminance is defined as weighted or unweighted average of the colours (Ferreira and Rasband 2011). The advantage of this approach, however, is that the combining of processes adds high-level quantitative support data to other qualitative data, thus generating a new hybrid mode of urban analysis that draws upon a broad variety of complex and unedited urban conditions.

13.4 The Material City

In the essay *Too Blue*, Brian Massumi (2002) argues that colour cannot be quantified because its complex properties resist its reduction to a single idea. This is because the idea of a colour held in the memory exceeds the *testable* meaning of the word. He goes on to explain that, as a correlate of colour, brightness is an equally uncontrollable phenomenon, dismissing the exclusion of its aberrational forms, such as glare and diffraction, from current modes of representation as a reductive and normalising approach. "The 'anomalies' of vision can't be brushed aside for the simple reason that they are what is *actually* being seen" (Massumi 2002, p. 162). For Massumi, ambiguity within the perceptual field thus opens up the potentially limitless production of affective conditions in which urban dwellers reside and which are an indispensable part of any data-gathering process in this space.

With the city's qualitative visual properties now readily translatable into data, a new approach to the design and manufacture of its material surfaces also becomes possible. The emergence of an indexical relationship between the digital image and the urban landscape now means that the image not only *informs* future form, but form can affect the numeric values within the image. However, for affect to be truly affective, in the sense that it is "*other than* conscious knowing" (Gregg and Seigworth 2010, p. 1) and about multiplying the ambiguity and complexity of urban conditions, then it is only through a combination of the capacity of the material surface to involve the full spectrum of viewed conditions, including its aberrations, and the visioning technology that present these conditions to a global audience in an unedited form, that the data for a comprehensive picture of urban space for analysis is possible.

13.4.1 The Urban Surface as Qualitative Colour

The generative capacity of the *space-time* image stacks made visible by *ImageJ* as discrete sectional views is further extended by its ability to abstract image content as temporal patterns of colour and brightness. In a departure from conventional data-assessment visualisations, here complex urban conditions unfold as a single strip or a multi-tiered colour profile of the recomposed urban landscape (Fig. 13.13).

Just as they offer a high degree of scrutiny in a medical context, so can individual *slices* or images from the different axes of any image stack be extracted for design-related analysis using the *Re-slice* tool design. Therefore, broadly speaking, given the quantum of activated flow in Shibuya Crossing, the progression of colour and brightness in a stack of images can, in the same way, also be individually extracted and understood in this case as shifts in urban materiality and traffic flow. This type of mapping tool thus represents programmatic changes of all kinds; human and vehicular circulation patterns, as well as the effects of urban activation outside and inside buildings.

For the designer, this type of reconfigured image content also gives a precise insight into the more complex urban conditions to which an intervention might respond. These might include conditions associated with its visibility, such as its materiality (colour and texture) and its visibility over controlled intervals of time (brightness). As an example of this, a building might be required to stand in high contrast to its surrounding context, in which case a choice of materials and surface activation would be selected to function in opposition to that of its neighbours within a specific temporal frame. Similarly, a requirement for low visibility would

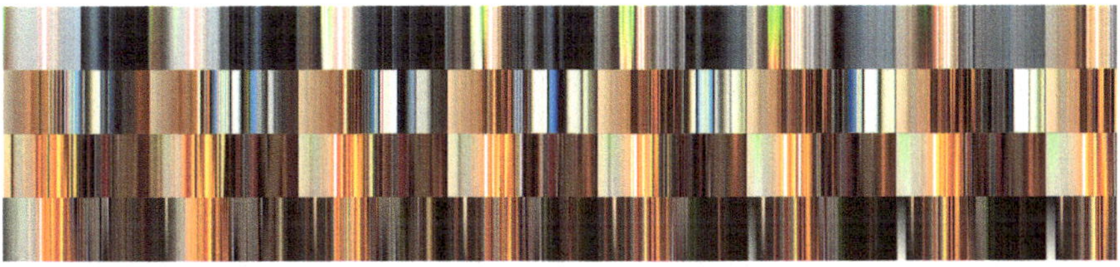

Fig. 13.13 Montage of image stack slices of Shibuya Crossing, Tokyo, reconfigured according to properties of colour and luminosity. (Original image: Forrest Brown/Shutterstock.com)

mean a selection of materials and surface activation that is indistinguishable from the building's immediate context. The same process can be used to understand different time spans and therefore can provide either a more detailed and specific level of information, such as an extended time span of 24 h. Applying this process according to the camera angle and location, the designer can identify precise temporal shifts in the city's material surfaces and how they interact progressively.

The extended capacity to explore the content of the various axes of an image stack axes is also offered by this software's previously mentioned *Z Project* function. The synthesis of the colour and brightness properties of the city are here presented in a single conflated and highly affective image that bears *ghostly* traces of the transitions in material and human activity which occurred in this particular space over a specified time span (Fig. 13.14). While on one hand the images offer a new insight into the continually evolving material character of the city, on the other they present composite data that can be readily quantified to support projective engagement in its future design functionality.

Furthermore, the global distribution of the Internet webcam network is such that this process can also be used to compare the conditions of one location with those of different locations at an international level. This facilitates the comparative assessment of urban space to be made within an identical temporal frame. This type of process would thus be able to deliver the means to make projective design decisions based upon this data. The capacity of the webcam's image-making network to support the ready cross-referencing of different urban conditions, both at a local and global level, thus provides the means whereby the complex conditions of modern life in one location can readily index and cross-pollinate those of another.

The abstract image or series of *colour profiles* of the city means that it is no longer recognisable in its traditional form. The new dominance of its qualitative aspects, in which the internal arrangement and hierarchy of image content is redistributed as colour and brightness, therefore also means that this process dismantles the capacity of pixel grouping to support any traditional urban narrative. This, and the deliberate inclusion of image artefacts such as blurring and colour aberrations, distance this type of urban picture from the highly curated properties of the promotional image, bringing a new type of urban visualisation into the design arena whereby the city's diverse conditions are made visible. Importantly, the unique

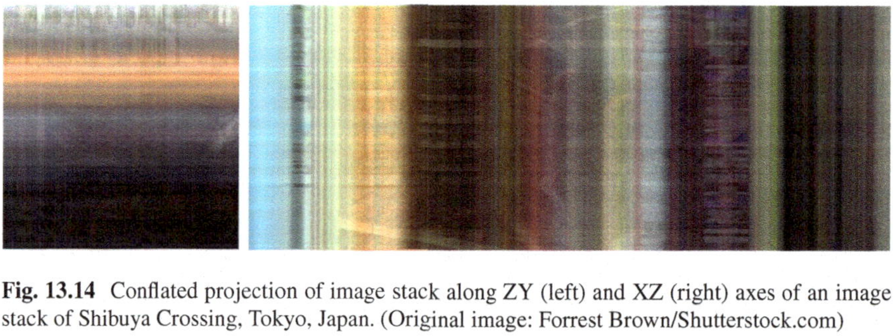

Fig. 13.14 Conflated projection of image stack along ZY (left) and XZ (right) axes of an image stack of Shibuya Crossing, Tokyo, Japan. (Original image: Forrest Brown/Shutterstock.com)

assemblies and compositions that make up this new qualitative urban landscape also connect the designer to correspondingly new and unique types of formal and material assemblies that reveal these previously hidden qualities. The ability to see the temporal evolution of this data further transforms the ways in which design intervention within urban space can therefore be addressed and understood.

13.4.2 The Urban Surface as Quantitative Chroma

In the same way that this software synthesises and presents a hybrid qualitative and quantitative data set of urban flow, so does it enable the same to be undertaken for urban materiality. The assessment of colour intensity and emission of any *viewed* urban space can be undertaken to a high degree of accuracy using traditional modes of colour weighting assessement that quantify the individual RGB colour channels in the image. If image colour content is traceable to the various differentiations in materiality throughout the captured space, then this is an accurate means of assessing and quantifying the contextual behaviour of physical surfaces located within that space.

The modelling of the colour content of urban space as a three-dimensional interactive made available by *ImageJ*'s Colour Inspector plugin allows the colour distribution of a space to be understood as an interactive model according to a variety of optional colour spaces. (Fig. 13.15). In design terms, this means that progressive material shifts in the city can be identified through a highly articulated temporal model, which further enables an intervention to be tested contextually.

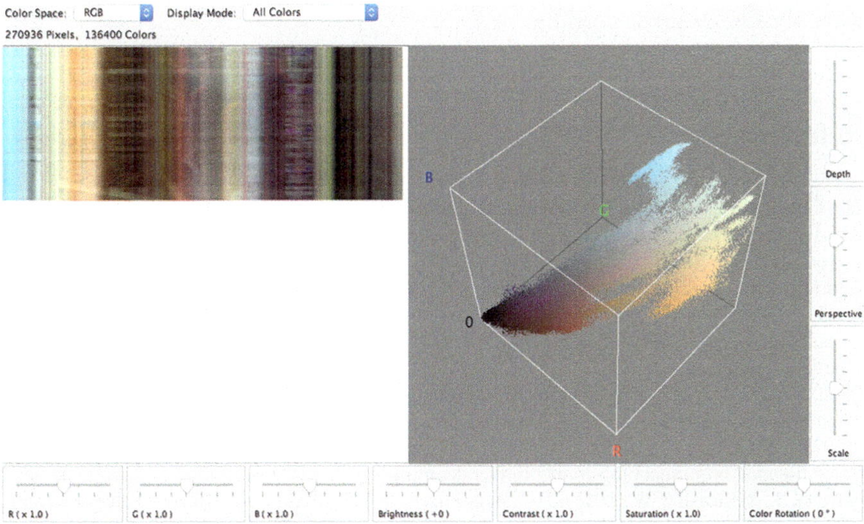

Fig. 13.15 *ImageJ*'s 3D Colour Inspector function showing progressive shifts in urban materiality over a prescribed interval of time

13.5 Conclusion

The generative capacities of the image are made possible by two key aspects of digital image-making: the pixel-based structure of the image and the image-making technology of the webcam. The ability to asign a numeric value to all types of urban conditions captured by the Internet webcam means that the image is a highly adaptable interface for the quantification and assessment of its real physical counterpart. In this respect, the *scaled-up* applicatiom of medical imaging software as an aurban analytical tool not only provides the designer with a temporal platform that can scrutinise the appropriateness of a proposed intervention in a constantly evolving and complex range of urban conditions, but the extension of its fine-grain, image-based analysis capabilities means that more ambiguous and often-disregarded properties of urban life are able to contribute to form part of a more comprehensive and wholistic data set.

Assessing the city terms of its more qualitative aspects of colour and light also transforms the ways in which design intervention within urban space can be approached. The inclusion of data about the evolution of a city's more qualitative aspects, of its programmatic activity and its material surfaces, radically shifts the type of design intervention that can be made here. The digital multiplication of urban space thus produces entirely new conditions for the data-gathering procedures used by those who design it. It also presents a completely new formal language to the discipline. Drawing upon the properties of the HVS as the terms of reference for formal discussion is a radical departure from traditional linear-based design language. Instead it is now the data associated with the relationship between an object's colour, brightness and shape that informs design decisions and the synthesis of quantitative and qualitative data that sets a new benchmark for the assessment of complex urban conditions.

References

21st Century Digital Art. http://www.digiart21.org/art/isee

Andrienko, N., & Andrienko, G. (2013). Visual analytics of movement: An overview of methods, tools and procedures. *Information Visualization, 12*(1), 3–24.

Andrienko, G., Andrienko, N., Bremm, S., Schreck, T., Von Landesberger, T., Bak, P., & Keim, D. (2010). Space-in-time and time-in-space self-organizing maps for exploring spatiotemporal patterns. *Computer Graphics Forum, 29*(3), 913–922. Blackwell Publishing Ltd.

Charcoal Design. http://www.charcoaldesign.co.uk/pipette

Chen, S. (2005). *Freeware vs Shareware vs Open Source* [Online]. Available: http://opensourcestrategies.blogspot.com.au/2005/09/freeware-vs-shareware-vs-open-source.html. Accessed 02/03 2013.

Color Blender. http://mabblog.com/colorblender.html

Ferreira, T., & Rasband, W. (2011). *The ImageJ user guide*. Bethesda: National Institutes of Health.

Ferreira, N., Poco, J., Vo, H. T., Freire, J., & Silva, C. T. (2013). Visual exploration of big spatio-temporal urban data: A study of New York city taxi trips. *IEEE Transactions on Visualization and Computer Graphics, 19*(12), 2149–2158.

Foley, J. D., Van Dam, A., Feiner, S. K., & Hughes, J. F. (2014). *Computer graphics: Principles and practice*. Upper Saddle River: Pearson Education Inc.
GigaPixelCam X10. https://www.earthcam.net/products/gigapixelcamx10.php
GNU Image Manipulation Program. http://www.gimp.org
Gregg, M., & Seigworth, G. J. (2010). An inventory of shimmers. In M. Gregg & G. J. Seigworth (Eds.), *The affect theory reader* (pp. 1–25). Durham: Duke University Press.
ImageJ. https://imagej.net/Fiji.
ImageJ: Image Processing and Analysis in Java. http://rsbweb.nih.gov/ij/.
Klette, R., & Rosenfeld, A. (2004). *Digital geometry: Geometric methods for digital picture analysis*. Amsterdam/Boston: Elsevier.
Kruegle, H. (2011). *CCTV surveillance: Video practices and technology*. Boston: Butterworth-Heinemann.
Kurgan, L. (2013). *Close up at a distance: Mapping, technology, and politics*. MIT Press.
Macarthur, J. (2000). From the air: Collage City, aerial photography and the picturesque. In M. Ostwald & J. S. Moore (Eds.), *Re-framing architecture: Theory, science and myth*. Sydney: Archadia Press.
Massumi, B. (2002). *Parables for the virtual: Movement, affect, sensation*. Durham: Duke University Press.
PixelMath Software. http://pixels.cs.washington.edu/PixelMath/pmdownload/request.php.
Poynton, C. (2012). *Digital video and HD: Algorithms and interfaces*. Amsterdam: Elsevier.
Raw Therapee. http://www.rawtherapee.com/.
Scheepens, R., Willems, N., Van de Wetering, H., Andrienko, G., Andrienko, N., & Van Wijk, J. J. (2011). Composite density maps for multivariate trajectories. *IEEE Transactions on Visualization and Computer Graphics, 17*(12), 2518–2527.
Scheepens, R., Hurter, C., Van De Wetering, H., & Van Wijk, J. J. (2016). Visualization, selection, and analysis of traffic flows. *IEEE Transactions on Visualization and Computer Graphics, 22*(1), 379–388.
Schindelin, J., Arganda-Carreras, I., Frise, E., Kaynig, V., Longair, M., Pietzsch, T., Preibisch, S., et al. (2012). Fiji: An open-source platform for biological-image analysis. *Nature Methods, 9*(7), 676.
Wongsuphasawat, K., & Gotz, D. (2012). Exploring flow, factors, and outcomes of temporal event sequences with the outflow visualization. *IEEE Transactions on Visualization and Computer Graphics, 18*(12), 2659–2668.
Zeng, W., Fu, C.-W., Arisona, S. M., Erath, A., & Qu, H. (2016). Visualizing waypoints-constrained origin-destination patterns for massive transportation data. *Computer Graphics Forum, 35*(8), 95–107.

Part VI
Socio-spatial Ecosystems

Chapter 14
Multimodal Accommodations for the Nomadic International Citizen [MANIC]

Kas Oosterhuis

Abstract In his book Towards A New Kind of Building and in this essay the author links current insights in astrophysics and natural physics to his theory of architecture which is based on the principles of swarm theory. He argues for the introduction of a personal time, which is the actual real time any person takes with him/her. The common notion of the fluidity of time is considered as an obsolete paradigm, while nature is seen as an extensive cellular automaton evolving is series of discrete steps. Gravity is seen as an emergent phenomenon as by-product of interacting information fields. From there the author builds the bridge to the connection of a universal ubiquitous booking system to the real time adaptivity of the game changing concept of multimodal accommodations for the nomadic international citizen. The nomadic citizen, freed from labour by the likewise ubiquitous robotic workforces, has been coined 50 years ago by the Dutch artist Constant Nieuwenhuys in his visionary project New Babylon. Architecture is entering the age of the 4th industrial revolution. Via spooky actions at a distance architecture meets the world of quantum unpredictability.

Keywords Personal time · No time · Quantum field · Information hubs · Emergent gravity · Spooky action at a distance · Nomadic · Computation · Ubiquitous · Multimodality · Pop-up loft · Internet of things and people · 4th industrial revolution

14.1 Personal Time

Being fascinated by the notion of time in relation to travel around the world, I have suggested in my book Towards A New Kind of Building (Oosterhuis 2011) to abandon the low-resolution time zones and replace it by real time personal time. Each

K. Oosterhuis (✉)
Qatar University, Doha, Qatar

Technical University Delft, Delft, The Netherlands
e-mail: koosterhuis@qu.edu.qa

N. Biloria (ed.), *Data-driven Multivalence in the Built Environment*, S.M.A.R.T. Environments, https://doi.org/10.1007/978-3-030-12180-8_14

person at whatever specific place would bear its own personal time. Using their prepared cell phones or laptops one caller would instantly see the personal time of the other party. Suppose one party types or says: "let's skype at 12.30" the other party would automatically see or hear that translated that into his/her personal time, which can be either slightly or completely different, depending on his/her position on earth. But they would immediately understand, and there would no longer be any confusion on what time zone one is referring to. This concept of personal would pay respect to the fact everyone, wherever in the universe, actually is the local and temporal centre of that universe. While the universe has no beginning nor an end, not a centre nor a boundary.

The big picture is that time zones must be seen as a relic from the earlier mechanistic world view, while we live in the age of the internet of things and people where everything is connected to everything else. These connections emerge from the level of the smallest constituting components, the smallest units, bodies, monads, the smallest input – processing – output machines, whereas physical distance is no longer a limiting factor. The new real time world view requires a reset of how we think of time. Time should be no longer be cut into low resolution fragments, but will be perceived in the highest possible resolution. Time is local and temporal, whereas each location, each object, each person, each planet is the centre of the universe, bearing its own unique experience of time.

14.2 No Time

In his intriguing, controversial and potentially influential book The End of Time (Barbour 1999) by Julian Barbour he boldly states that "There is no time", but a series of static instants, a unfathomable series of unique configurations. As Barbour puts it in simple terms: "I regard instants of time as real things, identifying them with possible instantaneous arrangements of all the things in the universe. They are configurations of the universe". His stance on the notion of time I find completely resonating with my vision of spatial arrangements of building components in time and place, which I will address later in this essay.

An almost absurd yet inevitable consequence of Barbour's theory of time is that the movements of bodies in space, i.e. atoms, molecules, cells, object, people, planets, galaxies are mere illusions of movement, caused by a vast series of minute changes in spatial configurations of minuscule fields of interaction. Imagine that every move you make, every bird that flies, every turn a wheel makes, are actually no movement of bodies in space, but reconfigurations of otherwise immobile interaction fields. I understand this as follows: as atoms [while the atom is not seen as a tangible unit but seen as an information field], quarks and more elementary fields of interaction constantly are exchanging packages of energy by interaction and dialogue, these fields in themselves do not move around with the speeds of light and beyond, but their interactions do. This can be understood as exchange of information. The repercussions of this idea are mind boggling. It basically means that the difference between ephemeral and solid is a change of information content and information exchange activity, on the basis of otherwise static interaction fields. It means that when a solid metal piece moves in space [as we humans perceive it] the space itself changes configuration from air into metal. Meaning that we ourselves and all things are in a constant transformation of information content on microscopic level, that we are recreating ourselves continuously at the speed of light or beyond that that speed, as in as of now unmeasurable small series of instances and interactions.

14.3 Emergent Gravity

Now Barbour has taken me there "in no time", his theory of no time does not stand isolated from other recent insights in natural physics. I am equally fascinated by theoretical physicist Erik Verlinde's theory of the emergent nature of gravity. In his revolutionary paper Emergent Gravity and The Dark Universe (Verlinde 2016) he states that "from a theoretical perspective, insights from black hole physics and string theory indicate that our 'macroscopic' notions of spacetime and gravity are emergent from an underlying microscopic description in which they have no a priori meaning." Erik Verlinde has a simple appealing reason why gravity has resisted all attempts to describe it as a fundamental force, because it isn't fundamental at all. He found that it might simply be an emergent property of space and time, much in the same way as elasticity is an emergent property of rubber. Gravity is here seen not as an elementary force but as the emergent result of other interactive fields of information. He basically states that all elementary forces are the result of information exchange. Which makes the universe a universal computer, and our world a computation. So, we are living in the Matrix after all. In an earlier paper published in 2010 Erik Verlinde writes: "Gravity is explained as an entropic force caused by changes in the information associated with the positions of material bodies."

14.4 Information Hubs

The reason that I am interested in his bold theory of emergent gravity is that it resonates with how I believe the interaction between things and people, between people and people, and between things and things like building components take place as to constitute a building assembly, in that statistically highly unlikely event where many different components from completely different origin and nature are flocking together to form a certain shape. I believe that all objects that we feel, see and make, including ourselves and our built environments, are in its essence a temporary crystallized form of information in the process of being exchanged, only experienced as such by the virtue of how we are constituted.

Imagine yourself to be so minuscule that you are navigating the space between the zooming information hubs of the electrons and the more Piranesi style spatial environments of the quark interactions. Now navigate from an atomic constellation that belongs to hard steel towards an atomic constellation that belongs to the domain of thin air. You would not even *notice* the difference, while the distances between the information knots are in both cases huge in relation to the tiny traveller. A Planck length traveller just floats in a seemingly empty ocean of subtle vibrations, devoid from any form of matter, probably only experiencing meaningless vibrating omnidirectional information exchange.

14.5 Quantumland

But our bodies are built in such a way that we do experience the difference between hard steel and thin air. We are equipped with sensorial organs, we feel by touch and radiation, we see the difference with our eyes, we smell, we hear the echoes. However, by sensing the way we sense we also are imprisoned in that way of experiencing. We cannot travel through steel, while the Planck length avatar can. We are bound to space land, while we cannot see nor feel quantum land. We can do no better than experience the shadows and echoes of the higher dimensions, like a flatlander will never be able to fully experience space land. Julian Barbour calls this other dimensional realm Platonia in his plea to understand the notion of time as a galactic number of discrete steps that nature is executing to create the illusion of time.

14.6 Nature is a Computation

Also, according to Stephen Wolfram nature is a computation, as he explains in his ground-breaking book “A New Kind of Science” (Wolfram 2002). He opposes abstract mathematics as the mathematical formulas are reversible by definition while the unfolding process of nature is not. He poses himself the question how can nature be described in terms of complex sets of cellular automata, basically as a huge executable file [.exe]. In the view of Wolfram nature takes discrete steps, numerous iterative steps running numerous sets of cellular automata, as to create complexity out of simple rules. Complexity based on simple rules is what is driving the swarm. Swarm behaviour is based on a set of simple rules that can be programmed applying simple algorithms. Based on his many attempts to create interesting patterns with cellular automata, Wolfram concludes that only some rules actually create complexity, while most rules create just very boring repetitive patterns, as running in circles, not getting anywhere.

I can draw with ease parallels to generative design procedures. There are many rules imaginable, but only certain specific rules create the circumstances for an intriguing further development of the design concept. This where science and the art of architecture meet. This is where natural physics, science and architecture meet. Emergence, complexity, simple rules. Complex yet not complicated.

The common idea behind the natural physics of Erik Verlinde, the new kind of science of Wolfram and the end of time of Julian Barbour is that our universe is unfolding in a series of discrete steps, whereas each step means a very small alteration of the previous step, culminating eventually in complexity, observed by people that are created along the same paths, and therefore only to be mutually experienced by those things and people that are caught in the same system. This is our spatial reality, albeit a very arbitrary and extremely limited spatial construct out of an endless number of possible quantum universes, driven by fields of information. By spatial I refer to the extreme limitation that space has with respect to the world of quantum. Space is not the ultimate frontier, it is our spacious prison. It can be easily imagined that endless other universal constructs are feasible, yet not visible and certainly not tangible by our bodily contraptions. What we see, feel and make, and what we are, are two sides of the same coin.

14.7 Spooky Action at a Distance

Albert Einstein noticed some hundred years ago a "spooky action at a distance", based on measurements executed by his colleagues of natural physics. The spooky action was labelled as such while no one could explain what exactly happened. It seemed that two seemingly unconnected elementary particles had an invisible connection, influencing each other's behaviour. Speculations were going adrift; higher dimensions were introduced to explain the phenomenon. There might be some form of shortcut through higher dimensions where one particle-wave is informed by the other, although substantial physical distances away. Perhaps in this higher dimension distances do not count, in perhaps much the same way as time does not exist outside our spacious galactic prison, as is explained by Julian Barbour. Or, as the theoretical physicist Juan Maldacena of Stanford University in California puts it "We are shadows at the edge of a higher dimensional universe".

14.8 The Highly Unlikely

Nature unfolding into complexity, defying the second law of thermodynamics, is in essence the same as the act of designing. Making a design and assembling a building is statistically a most unlikely event. According to the second law of thermodynamics systems tend to come to an equilibrium where the constituting parts mix to the max, until a homogeneous mix has been achieved. Nature as e know and design and construction as we know it are two sides of the same coin. There is nothing unnatural about any of the construct's humankind has made. Basically, the evolution of any product, from vehicles to homes, from homes to cities, from cities to the internet, they all work as the reverse of the second law of thermodynamics. They all work from a driving force within that constantly rearranges the configurations of information fields, which we perceive as matter, whether it be the formation of rocks, the emergence of organic life or the, the emergence of gravity, the invention of the internet.

In my practice the thrill started with the fax machine. You input information in a machine at one side, and the same information, albeit on a different carrier, comes out in exactly the same form at the other side of the globe. Spooky action at a distance! Now we have the Internet, which has changed our societal structures and the way we operate in our professions to the max. The project I will discuss more in detail in this essay the research project Multimodal Accommodations for the Nomadic International Citizen [MANIC] (Oosterhuis 2018) dealing with many of the fascinations as described above.

My profession is that of the architect, the designer, an author of the highly unlikely. I project events in the future, and as by some spooky action at a distance material, energy, ideas, cars, trucks move to one particular place on earth at one particular time as to assemble the swarm of building components to form that highly unlikely building. Some built constructs are more unlikely than others, while using more rare materials, more unique ideas, leading to new until then unexplored routes. The MANIC project is one such project, both in its virtual and in its physical existence. MANIC is a programmable building that is connected to the MANIC booking system.

14.9 Ubiquitous Booking

I believe that today almost everyone uses websites like booking.com to make reservations in remote cities. Spooky action at a distance! I share some information about myself with the system, and it results in being authorized to use a certain space in that remote city. We accept this as something natural, while it is in evolutionary terms a highly unlikely event. The system uses information exchange with the speed of light, travelling huge distances, often routed via detours, in small discrete packages of information. That info is subsequently received, processed and taken into effect in a set of physical actions at the other side. The complexity of this is extreme describing the process in minute detail as a computer programmer does, it will contain thousands of lines of code, driving many connected machines/servers. The speed of evolution is equally amazing, especially when we realize that the Internet and these booking systems are developed in the timespan of one generation of humankind.

The special evolutionary specification I will describe in this essay is a booking system that allow to book not only hotel room, but basically any type of space, for any period of time, at any place on earth of beyond. To achieve that a number of steps needs to be taken. One could begin by linking different types of booking to each other. Think of booking.com. Regus, cheap tickets, car rental, amazon, eBay, catering services, Uber, makerspaces, Fablabs, online fashion shops, delivery services etc. accessible from one portal. The basic authorization one needs is a credit card with sufficient allowance. One needs a key to access the services as to obtain the desired time and space, the digital version of your key to the door of your home and your car. Behind the door your personal time and space unfolds, no one unauthorized may enter without your permissions of without being punished for trespassing. Ownership and renting will merge into one system of booking.

Booking of time and space through a universal app connecting thousands of other apps may become an ubiquitous tool for every activity in your life, from having your morning coffee, transporting by automated vehicles to your workplace, for your leisure activities, anything. You are the managing director of your life, you are in control, based on your preference that you have shared with the ubiquitous booking system. You are connected via the ubiquitous booking system, which operates within the IoT&P, the Internet of Things and People, operating via complex spooky actions at a distance, active in another dimension as you own physical world. Everything is connected to everything else and anyone else. Some very simple rules are driving the connections.

14.10 Multimodality

I have written extensively on the concept of multimodality since my project Trans-Ports (Oosterhuis 2000), which I showed for the first time at the Architecture Biennale in Venice in the year 2000. Basically, Trans-Ports was a flexible adaptive structure that changes shape and content in real time. In the MANIC project I link this concept of multimodality to the ubiquitous booking system, facilitating the Nomadic International Citizen. The spaces are enhanced with adaptive programmable interiors that are directly connected to the settings and preferences of the authorized users. Users are the monads, basically anyone or anything that has an ID. Bodies, components, cells, proteins, quanta, they are the monads, interacting with their immediate neighbours regardless of their distance.

Suppose you book a working space for a period of 2 h in Doha. On the MANIC site you see a choice of venues, a choice of spaces, and a choice of interior arrangements. You make your choices, link it to your credit card and most likely connect it to other bookings for lodging, transport and catering. One can book everything in advance or take the chance to book other things later, depending on the level of adventurousness of the user. How much of your life do you really want to know in advance? Last minute bookings may get their discounts.

Once you have arrived at your destination, which is the MANIC building in Doha, the building knows your profile, recognizes you, welcomes you personally, and shows you the way to your venue, the working place for a period of 2 h. You may have invited other people to work with you, and you may have ordered your espresso, portion of dates and water. Before you arrive, the room will have reconfigured itself according to your pre-set preferences.

The high-resolution accommodation concept is expected to be ultimately profitable, since the intensity of the usage of the spaces may be doubled as compared to traditional functional zoning, which are based on function separation rather than function integration, and also as compared to existing mixed-use developments.

14.11 MANIC Loft

The system that I have designed earlier for a programmable and reconfigurable space is called the Pop-Up Loft (Oosterhuis 2017). A raised floor contains the foldable versions of tables, chairs, sofas, kitchen, bathtub and toilet. The sliding sectors of the walls contain the clothes, books and LED screen. From the ceiling comes the light to those spots where you wish to have the light. Also, from the ceiling come the separation walls to define the space into individual sectors. All is programmed when you were booking the space, and can be adjusted in real time using tan app on your tablet. Some of these features are already operational in the CitizenM (Citizen 2008) Hotels worldwide, but not the reconfigurability. CitizenM room are all exactly identical, while MANIC rooms are fully adaptive to its changing use.

The typical MANIC space (Fig. 14.1a, b) is a generous 48 m2 that can change from 48 m2 living room or a 48 m2 bedroom to a 48 m2 bathroom, or even 48 m2 toilet when you also sink the bathtub into the floor. When one functional object is not used it will sink automatically according to your preferred settings. The MANIC room is a programmable space that fluently adapts to your doings, yet you will be able at any time to interact with it and have it your own whimsical way. In the MANIC programmable space concept, no space remains ever unused, the space is in constant flux as to adapt to its actual form of usage. The 48 m2 MANIC loft can be subdivided in two equally large spaces of 24 m2, which in turn can be subdivide in 2 sections of 12 m2 each.

The MANIC concept allows for building in high densities while it typically uses only half of the space as compared to apartments and office space, where much of the space is not used during its day cycle. By programming the spaces, the overall density of number of spaces per the plot can be easily doubled within the same volume.

14.12 Porosity

Based on a recent ONL project called the Parametric Spatial Programming Tool [PSPT], the MANIC loft structures are designed using the parametric PSTP Porosity script, programmed in Rhino/Grasshopper. Porosity allows for planning spaces that are as of yet undefined in its function, and can be addressed to fulfil any function at any time in any of the programmable units. Porosity exploits the uncolonized space-time in between the bookings. In a certain moment of the day on one and the same

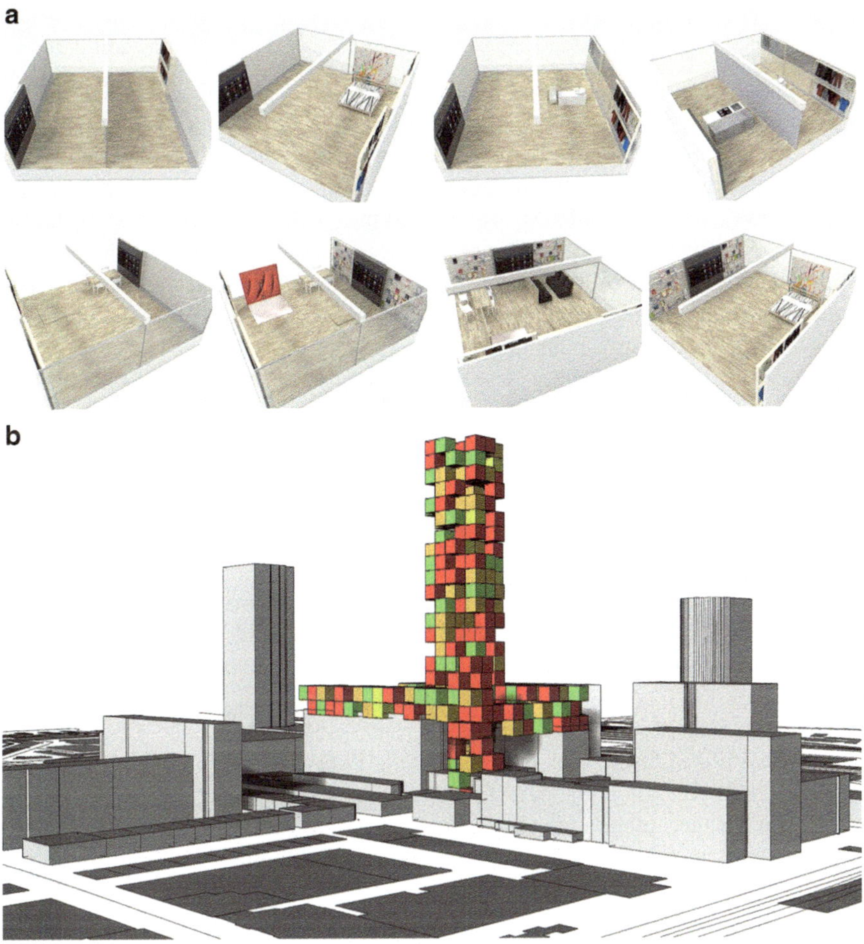

Fig. 14.1 (**a**) Programmable pop-up loft | ONL | Kas Oosterhuis 2012 (**b**) Parametric Spatial Programming Tool | ONL | Kas Oosterhuis 2018

floor, and in one and the same building, the units may be used for working, conferencing, dining, relaxing, sleeping, refreshing, lounging. The MANIC building reflects in itself the activities of a 24-hour city, never dull moment. The MANIC building itself is a straightforward structurally optimized steel structure, with an arrangement of up to 16 programmable units per floor arranged around a spacious atrium. By choosing this spatial lay-out, there is a possibility for an optimal visual and physical communication between the units, stimulating cultural exchange and knowledge transfer. The smallest units communicate with each other as to form spontaneous interest groups, dynamically changing position in the building and migrating in time.

14.13 New Babylon

The nomadic international citizen that lives in MANIC operated structures does not need a fixed living place, home is where he or she is at that moment in time and place. Much of the theoretical background of the new nomadic citizen has been developed in the late fifties by the Dutch artists Constant Nieuwenhuys. He develops in models, paintings and manifest writings the city New Babylon (Nieuwenhuys 1956) for the new nomads. Constant described New Babylon as a endless city "where land is owned collectively, work is fully automated and the need to work replaced with a nomadic life of creative play. New Babylon is inhabited by homo ludens, who, freed from labour, will not have to make art, for he can be creative in the daily practice of his life". Nomads are defined as anything or anyone that changes shape and content in real time, regardless of the speed of operation.

14.14 Architecture Meets Quantum

The interactions between information fields in the most intimate regions of our existence leading to such complex natural and neo-natural worlds as we are thriving in, and the interactions between people and things via the bidirectional information exchange via the Internet, between the MANIC booking app, the Porosity design tool and the MANIC loft structures bear a remarkable resemblance. One will lead its personal life in his/her personal time zone. Everyone will be the centre of the universe, defragmenting time in no time, gravitating towards people and places in a non-linear manner, often entangled with a partnering person, unfolding their lives and ambitions in a highly unlikely programmable environment, where information fields are clustered to form local and temporal information hubs, enabled by the spooky action at a distance of the MANIC ubiquitous booking system negotiating space and configurations of objects with the MANIC facilities and community.

Architecture is no longer a matter of stacking stones or assembling prefabricated parts. Architecture will be connected to the dynamic of the ubiquitous internet of things and people, until it becomes truly dynamic in itself. Architecture is entering the age of the 4th industrial revolution. Via the spooky actions at a distance architecture meets the world of quantum unpredictability.

References

Barbour, J. (1999). *The end of time* (p. 9). The Big Picture in Simple Terms, Oxford University Press.
Citizen, M. (2008). *Innovative hotel concept*. https://www.citizenm.com/content/innovative-rooms#
Nieuwenhuys, C. (1956–1974). *New Babylon*. The Hague: Gemeentemuseum.
Oosterhuis, K. (2000). *Programmable architecture*. Trans-Ports, L'Arcaedizioni. ISBN:978-8878381032.
Oosterhuis, K. (2011). *Towards a new kind of building* (p. 130). Versatile Time Zones, NAi Publishers.
Oosterhuis, K. (2017). *Pop-up loft*. Youtube https://www.youtube.com/watch?v=4nPAmVuviLk
Oosterhuis, K. (2018). *MANIC*. Qatar University Concept Development Grant.
Verlinde, E. (2016). *Emergent gravity and the dark universe* (p. 1 abstract). University of Amsterdam.
Wolfram, S. (2002). *A new kind of science*. Wolfram Media, ISBN: 1579550088.

Chapter 15
Understanding the Relationship Between Smart Cities and Entrepreneurial Ecosystems: The Case of Sydney

D. Cetindamar, T. Lammers, and N. Sick

Abstract Smart city literature is overdrawn with discussions on public services such as transportation while there is a need to broaden the analysis to understand the very rich dynamics of cities. In this chapter, the goal is to focus on the rise of technology-based entrepreneurs in cities which are creating emerging digital technologies. Cities have been a popular unit of analysis for technological development and economic activities due to their high dependency on immediate local context factors. Nowadays, the transformation of cities into "smart" has increased their role further – both for economic value and for technological growth. This paper aims to expand the smart city concept to an ecosystem approach where cities become hubs of digital technologies. By combining the previous literature on entrepreneurship and digital technologies within a particular urban context, this paper discusses how smart cities could be a solid base to build digital entrepreneurship ecosystems for sustainable, liveable and competitive cities. In particular, the paper provides a case study for Sydney by illustrating the interactions between smart cities and digital entrepreneurship ecosystems in practice. The chapter ends with a summary of findings and implications for both policy makers and digital entrepreneurs.

Keywords Digital technologies · Entrepreneurship ecosystems · Smart city · Digital entrepreneurship ecosystem

15.1 Introduction

The recent entrepreneurial literature provides several dynamic factors affecting the success of an entrepreneurial ecosystem (Stam 2015). However, researchers point out the role of local conditions and bottom-up processes and they advise customization of policies rather than copying successful policies applied in other regions such

D. Cetindamar (✉) · T. Lammers · N. Sick
School of Information, Systems and Modelling, University of Technology Sydney, Sydney, Australia
e-mail: Dilek.CetindamarKozanoglu@uts.edu.au; Thorsten.Lammers@uts.edu.au; Nathalie.Sick@uts.edu.au

N. Biloria (ed.), *Data-driven Multivalence in the Built Environment*, S.M.A.R.T. Environments, https://doi.org/10.1007/978-3-030-12180-8_15

as in Silicon Valley (Isenberg 2011). More importantly, they call policy makers for creating policies specified for digital entrepreneurial ecosystems rather than for entrepreneurship alone (Thurik et al. 2013). Agreeing with such a policy approach, this paper emphasizes the need for a city-based policy that integrates both entrepreneurship and technology policies to flourish and generate innovations for the overall performance of the digital entrepreneurial ecosystem.

Due to rapid urbanization, cities have become a major site of competition (Roger et al. 2015). As a United Nations (UN 2017) report summarizes, cities account for 70% of global gross domestic product in 2016. Thus, cities are becoming key platforms for policy makers. In parallel to increased economic importance of cities, policy makers are also expected to face new challenges arising from the radical transformation of cities into "smart cities" due to recent technological changes. The use of digital technologies for local government services (such as transportation, democratic transparency or clean energy) turns cities into smart ones. These developments put pressure on policy makers to catch-up with rapid technological changes in the digital arena.

Digital technologies such as big data analytics and 3-D printing are attracting attention from entrepreneurs and policy makers for different purposes. On the one hand, the phenomenon of unicorns, start-up companies valued at over US$1 billion, appeals entrepreneurs to start-up high technology companies. On the other hand, policy makers are attracted to host these companies in their countries, regions or cities from the perspective of economic value and social welfare. In addition, these digital technologies could deliver technologies to policymakers to effectively and efficiently manage their cities. The literature presents a number of studies on digital technologies and entrepreneurial policies carried out independently by disciplines ranging from operations management to entrepreneurship. By combining the previous literature on entrepreneurship and digital technologies within a particular urban context, this paper discusses how smart cities could be a solid base to build entrepreneurship ecosystems for sustainable, liveable and competitive cities. In particular, the paper provides a case study for Sydney by illustrating the dynamic interactions between smart city and digital entrepreneurship ecosystem in practice.

The paper has six sections. After this short introduction, Sect. 15.2 will give a quick overview on entrepreneurship literature related to entrepreneurship ecosystems. Then, Sect. 15.3 will present digital technologies and smart cities, followed with a section where we offer a conceptual framework that could combine entrepreneurship ecosystem approach for the utilization of digital technologies. Section 15.5 is the presentation of Sydney as a case of entrepreneurial ecosystem framework for competitiveness. The final section presents conclusions, discuss the implications of the findings for theory and practice, and derives a number of avenues for future research.

15.2 Literature on Regional Entrepreneurial Ecosystems

Entrepreneurship is the process by which individuals exploit opportunities for innovation (Schumpeter 1934), while ecosystem refers to the interconnectedness of organizations that are mutually dependent on each other's inputs and outputs (Stam 2015). The entrepreneurial ecosystem concept emphasizes that entrepreneurship takes place in a community of interdependent actors. Even though there are discussions around the use of entrepreneurial ecosystems, this paper will use it in a pragmatic manner to refer the interlinkages of complex and dynamic actors (Oh et al. 2016). Considering that entrepreneurship is an important source of innovation, productivity growth and employment (World Economic Forum 2013), many countries are searching for ways of supporting their local conditions to create an amiable environment for entrepreneurship to flourish in a competitive world.

Seemingly paradoxical, there is a revival of emphasis on regions and on the importance of geography in economics in the twenty-first century despite the extent to which globalisation has turned our world into a "global village" (Henderson 1995). In this context, the entrepreneurial ecosystem approach has commonalities with other established concepts, in particular regional innovation systems (Cooke 1992) and regional innovation management (Kriz et al. 2016). Similar approaches highlighting the importance of the regional environment as a driver of innovation are industrial districts, industrial clusters, and innovative milieus (Asheim et al. 2011). These concepts are grounded in Marshall's work (Marshall 1898) on industrial districts where economic value results from the interplay of institutions, agglomeration economics and cooperation of firms. The original definition of industrial district is the spatial concentration of firms operating in one particular industry in a town or a few neighbouring small towns where especially small firms cooperate with each other and are embedded in the local community (Richardson 1995).

The attractiveness of a region is a function not only of geographical and socio-economic factors taken in isolation, but also of a complex interplay of external economies characteristic of a prior industrial agglomeration (Richardson 1995). For example, the sources of agglomeration economies arise from local concentration of customers, which reduce overhead and infrastructure costs; economies of scale in production or distribution; sufficient demand to warrant the provision of specialized infrastructure; and deep and diversified pool of workers sufficient to realize a more specialized local division of labour. In the same way, these economies are product of the use of specialized equipment and services; opportunities for bulk purchasing; joint research; organized markets for finished products; reduced cost of negotiating and monitoring contracts; and existence of specialized brokers or specialized machinery producers (Henderson 1995; Marshall 1898).

Agglomeration economies refers to the unit cost reductions of a firm arising from internal and external economies when it is located together with relatively dense clusters of other firms or specialized resources rather than located elsewhere. These economies fall into one of the following three groups (Hoover 1975). The first one, internal economies, is related to the idea of economies of scale and caused by the increase of the firm scale of production at one point. The second one, localization economies, is externalities associated with the presence of many other producers in the same industry or sector. The last one, urbanization economies, is externalities associated with the co-presence of firms from diverse industries. In other words, urbanization economies are applicable to all firms in all industries, arising from the enlargement of the total economic size of that location for all industries taken together. Over time, agglomeration economies have become the crucial element for regional and economic policies (Hoover 1975). Along these lines, Leydesdorff and Deakin (2011) pointed out that cities are "key components of innovation systems" because of their dense networks between academia, industry and government. Cities thus provide exceptional circumstances for collaborations across the triple helix as an essential prerequisite for regional development (Katz and Wagner 2014).

Cities/metropolitan areas are not only the base for the accumulation of ubiquitous assets, economic, physical, as well as networking (Newman 2017), but they are the implementation arena for many digital technologies. In the past, there have been studies on the economic development around technologies developed and utilized at cities that forms the base of a rich literature on Technopolis (Phillips 2006). It seems history repeats itself with new digital technologies. The goal for policy makers could be to find ways to identify the potential industrial clusters in their cities and then to support entrepreneurship ecosystems around them in order to efficiently utilize digital technologies.

15.3 Literature on Digital Technologies and Smart Cities

Digital technologies are general-purpose technologies and have the potential to change all aspects of production, consumption, and government services in our daily life. They will have a massive impact on entrepreneurship ecosystems not only by providing new capabilities and business models but also by affecting their environment and its surrounding regulating frameworks (see Fig. 15.1). Current trends in digital technology development include the Internet of Things (IoT), enhanced

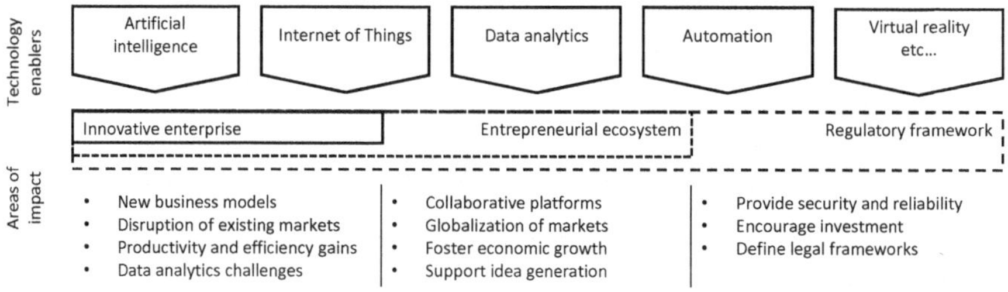

Fig. 15.1 Dimensions of digital technology impact

data analytics, artificial intelligence (AI) and virtual reality. Companies increasingly realize that digital transformation will become an imperative in today's competitive market (Newman 2017). Currently, the pace of change provoked by digital technologies is not only accelerating, but also widening. For example, it will not only enable people to increase their capabilities but also increase organizational innovation as well as integrate whole ecosystems and supply chains (Groopman et al. 2017). These macro trends will bring with them massive regulatory challenges to provide stability on topics such as AI and cyber security (Dia 2016; Hellwig 2017). Research goes as far as claiming that advances in digital technology could automate half of today's work by 2055 (Manyika et al. 2017).

Originally created in the context of manufacturing in Germany, the term Industry 4.0 describes a new trend of automation and data exchange enabled through the IoT, cyber-physical systems and cloud-computing (Jasperneite 2012). This technological shift will have a significant impact on global competitive frameworks, as companies change to become integrated networks with high automation levels and real-time data access (Brettel et al. 2014). Increasing technologically enabled customer demands put further pressure on organisations' competitiveness (Kumar 2017). The impacts of this shift go beyond manufacturing. It will provide business opportunities and challenges in areas such as logistics, smart services IT infrastructures, and workforce management (Schlaepger et al. 2014). Thus, policy makers should consider the ways of integrating digital technologies into their ecosystem plans.

For this purpose, the smart city approach provides a valid starting point to design digital entrepreneurial ecosystems. The concept of smart cities arose from smart specialisation strategies for regions, where (1) the competitive advantages of the region is identified, (2) R&D and innovation efforts are targeted in these areas, and (3) based on that, a vision for regional innovation is developed (OECD 2013). Smart cities apply these principles on a city (metropolitan) level, mostly with a focus on IT as an enabler (Caragliu et al. 2011). Having just emerged with the rise of IT, there is no coherent definition of a smart city yet, but rather common elements of existing smart city concepts (Chourabi et al. 2012). However, key elements consist of a technology-based infrastructure, a closely connected network of partners, a creative class, and an urban development plan for economic and social sustainability (Hollands 2008).

15.4 Digital Entrepreneurial Ecosystems as a Competitive Advantage of Smart Cities

Big cities around the world are trying to leverage on their advantages and overcome their city-specific challenges to attract start-ups and provide an optimal breeding ground for digital entrepreneurship. The use of digital technologies to generate competitive advantage is, among others, a critical factor affecting the success of an entrepreneurial ecosystem. However, researchers point out the role of local conditions and bottom-up processes and they suggest customization of policies for the respective entrepreneurial regional economy (Stam 2015; Thurik et al. 2013). Thus, a comprehensive policy should integrate both entrepreneurship and technology policies in order to flourish and generate innovations for the overall performance of the ecosystem.

The geographical unit for ecosystems could be city, region, nation, or even a group of countries such as the European Union. This paper chooses the city as a feasible unit of analysis. However, it is necessary to note that city does refer to the metropolitan area in the geographical sense. There are three main reasons for choosing the city level as the scope of investigation for policy makers. First, due to the trend of rapid urbanization, there are abundant entrepreneurial opportunities. The United Nations (2017) project the number of people living in cities to reach to more than 6 billion people. City population represents not only customers, but also workforce, innovators, and entrepreneurs. Second, digital technologies are diffusing rapidly at cities as previous technologies have done (Phillips 2006). As discussed in section three, cities have also become the major unit of competitiveness and therefore policy makers at cities race with each other to build smart cities to gain competitive advantage (Roger et al. 2015). Third, city level analysis helps to consider a well-defined unit of location for understanding social, historical, and political fabric, which creates the base for an entrepreneurial ecosystem (Thurik et al. 2013; Roger et al. 2015).

A word of caution, concentrating on city level does not limit understanding the links among different layers of policies. Just on the contrary, it might sharpen the views of the policy makers to see each city and its own networks with other regional layers. In fact, many cities do not compete with local cities alone, but rather with global cities in other countries and they try to be a hub for global supply chains by collaborating with some other global cities (Cetindamar and Gunsel 2012). By doing so, they become a source of innovation and entrepreneurship at a global level. The more cities are strengthened, the more they contribute to local and national economic growth. However, it gets complicated and policy makers should be equipped to have a rich approach to grasp dynamics of their cities.

In summary, to create a competitive environment for flourishing digital entrepreneurial ecosystems, there is an urgent need to align cities' entrepreneurial and technology policies. Since this area is still largely unexplored, we pose the following questions, which might help to refine this area of research:

1. How could we observe the connection among digital technologies, entrepreneurial ecosystems, and smart cities?
2. What are the possible mechanisms in aligning policy agendas around digital technologies, entrepreneurial ecosystems, and smart cities?

To provide a first set of answers to these questions, we follow a bottom-up approach with a case study of the city of Sydney. Insights into Sydney's digital entrepreneurial ecosystem, its context, structure, success factors and challenges starting point to identify the connections between digital technologies and entrepreneurial ecosystems on city level.

15.5 The Case of Sydney: Digital Entrepreneurial Ecosystem

15.5.1 Background and Context

Sydney is particularly suitable to demonstrate how the dynamic relationships between different factors should help to flourish a city-level digital entrepreneurial ecosystem. Historically, Australian cities have not been at the forefront of strategic investment in smart city infrastructures. Australian city leaders have realised this and are currently making smart cities a serious policy focus (The Committee for Sydney 2017). As a key financial hub for Asia Pacific, Sydney has the opportunity to become a world-leading city of urban innovation and data ecosystems. Currently counted between 1300 and 2100, Sydney hosts Australia's highest concentration of technology start-ups (Startup Genome 2017). This amounts to 64% of Australia's tech start-ups (NSW Government 2012). Also, Sydney has very good access to skills, creativity and talent relevant to digital entrepreneurship ecosystems. In 2017, Sydney's population recorded the highest score of all Australia's capital cities for digital inclusion. This score was also substantially higher than the score for rural New South Wales (Thomas et al. 2017). This is in line with the perception of 58% of people in Sydney, who think that their city is digitally advanced (the highest number of all Australian cities) and that digital technologies can help overcome city-specific infrastructural challenges such as housing affordability and congestions in the case of Sydney (EY Sweeney 2017). On city-level, proximity of individuals to exchange knowledge and drive innovations remains important in the digital era. This is specifically true for Sydney, currently holding the number 1 ranking of knowledge cities in Australia (Pratchett et al. 2017).

15.5.2 Competitive Positioning

The ability as a city to provide an ideal ecosystem for digital technology entrepreneurship is of high political relevance. Currently, aspects of this ability are being measured using different metrics ranging from broad country to city-specific as well as from emphasising entrepreneurship environments to emphasising digital technologies and smart city aspects. Table 15.1 provides an overview of key indices, their focus and (if applicable) how Sydney performs in them.

Sydney is positioned as the number one knowledge city in Australia according to the KCI. It has the highest KC (24.16) and KE (23.68) among the 25 Australian cities. Sydney is already saturated in its knowledge capability compared to other cities in Australia. However, there are still some areas for Sydney to make improvements in terms of Knowledge Industries, Knowledge Mobility and Smart Work.

Many of the existing indices (such as the above) however do not focus or entail information on digital business and entrepreneurship. If they do, the information provided is rather generic and in the form of a simple overview. What is currently

Table 15.1 City rankings
Selected indices for digital entrepreneurship environments and the ranking of Sydney

Index	Context	Focus[a]	Measured categories	Rank
International city rankings				
Startup Ecosystem Report (Startup Genome 2017)	Analyses ecosystems with best chance of global success for early-stage start-ups	EE	Performance	17/55 *(TOP 20 ranked)*
			Funding	
			Market reach	
			Talent	
Innovation Cities Index (2thinknow Global Innovation Agency 2017)	Tests cities with potential as an innovation economy based on key pre-conditions	EE	Cultural assets	14/500
			Human infrastructure	
			Networked markets *(162 indicators in three clusters)*	
Smart Cities Index (EasyParkGroup 2017)	Measures metropolises at the forefront of smart urban growth through digitalization	DTR	Transport and mobility	12/100
			Sustainability	
			Governance	
			Innovation economy	
			Digitalization	
			Living standard	
			Expert perception	
Domestic city rankings				
Digital Inclusion Index (Thomas et al. 2017)	Measures level of digital inclusion across Australian population focussing on household and personal use digital technologies	DTR	Access	1
			Affordability	
			Digital ability	
Knowledge City Index (Pratchett et al. 2017)	Measures knowledge cities as future drivers of prosperity	EE	Knowledge capital (capacity, mobility, digital access)	1/25
			Knowledge economy (industries, income, smart work)	

[a]*EE* Entrepreneurship Ecosystem, *DT* Digital Technology Readiness

missing, in fact, is a systematic analysis of factors affecting a city's competitiveness in the digital age – with a view on how the urban start-up ecosystem responds and interacts with specific technologies. This is where we need to distinguish between tech in smart city and tech to be developed.

15.5.3 Discrepancies Between Smart Entrepreneurial and Digital Technology Strategies

As indicated by the selected indices, digital infrastructure as well as entrepreneurial ecosystems are important for a good position as a competitive digital entrepreneurial ecosystem. Compared to other OECD nations, framework conditions in Australia are already more favourable to the creation of innovative start-ups, new business models, and new services enabled by digital technologies. Considering that ecosystem of digital technologies could further push the ongoing transformation of economies and societies (OECD 2017), policy makers in Australia are developing numerous policies and strategies around digital technologies, smart cities and entrepreneurship. With a focus on Sydney, we will summarize some of these policies and strategies and try to point out their discrepancies.

1. Digital and entrepreneurship strategies

Four major initiatives regarding digital and entrepreneurial policies take place at different policy layers and might be summarized as follows. First, the Australian federal government is currently in the process of drafting a digital strategy and has already identified opportunities for small and medium-sized businesses to embrace digital innovation to drive customer value, improve their services and unlock their potential as core questions going forward (Australian Government 2017a).

Second, the NSW state government has identified growing Sydney's Digital Precinct as a key driver. This precinct is meant to bring together industry leaders, entrepreneurs in emerging technologies and relevant research and academic partners to develop an 'innovation ecosystem' for the whole state (City of Sydney 2016).

Third, the City of Sydney has translated these general concepts and outcomes into two distinctive strategies – the Sydney Digital Strategy and the Sydney Tech Start-up plan. The Sydney Digital Strategy is very broad and covers various aspects of the city such as infrastructure, education/literacy, community and business. Within the business section, reference is made to the Tech Start-ups Action Plan (e.g." Continue to deliver the City of Sydney Tech Start-ups Action Plan to enable local businesses to grow into global businesses."). It is also highlighted that the digitisation of existing business is key for success, which is an area worth exploring in much more detail. In terms of education, there is no specific information provided which skills we should focus on when developing school and university curricula to feed into specific technologies in tech start-up environment. The Tech Start-ups Action Plan, despite the dynamic and hands-on name, as well only delivers a rough understanding of what the action plan for Sydney will look like. The first half of the lengthy document is spent on explaining and presenting tech start-ups as well as on describing the current status in Sydney. After an analysis of the barriers and pitfalls for growing tech start-ups in Sydney, a high-level overview of the resulting activities is given. The actions are specified later on, but the timeframe and the type of action indicate that the outcomes are still too generic to draw a vivid picture of how exactly Sydney will be set on track towards a digital entrepreneurial ecosystem.

Fourth, at the Sydney city level, the Start-up Ecosystem Report aims to lay the ground for entrepreneurship (Startup Genome 2017).

- Not-for-profit group TechSydney has been established to turn Sydney into a world-class hub,
- Atlassian set record 4.4bn evaluation for Au tech firm, Afterpay went IPO and is worth more than 100m,
- Sydney is one of the most globally connected startup ecosystems, but its market reach is held down by its relative lack of foreign customers,
- Sydney ecosystem ranks on the global top 5 in global connectedness showing a deep understanding of global business models and international markets,
- 44% of Sydney based startups report that they are offering a product that is the first of its kind in relation to gloibal average of 34%,
- Sydney ranks outside the top 20 and only slightly above the global average in terms of its early stage funding over startup, indicating an opportunity for growth.

2. Smart cities

Similar to the digital and entrepreneurship initiatives, there are some influential initiatives regarding smart cities. Two of them deserve to be mentioned here. First, Wethecity is an international movement whose Sydney arm was established in 2013. This think thank group built a number of strategies for the city of Sydney (The Committee for Sydney 2017). Accordingly, Sydney has the opportunity to be a world leader in building the data-smarts if a sound Smart Sydney strategy if followed; a Smart city commissioner could be established; a government backed smart city team could be formed and a new financial tool could be developed (something called "Smart city impact bonds"). Some of the suggestions seem to be working. For example, a government commission (the Greater Sydney Commission) and a civic organization (the Committee for Sydney) were established in 2015. The former one has no particular project in smart cities topic, while the second one is as an independent think tank with task forces and has an interest in smart cities. In addition, thanks to the NSW Government and the Committee of Sydney, the 'Knowledge Hub' initiative called Piivot was established at the University of Technology Sydney in order to build Sydney's reputation as a global innovation and tech hub.

Second, the Australian Government prepared "The Smart Cities Plan" in 2016 in order "to position Australian cities to succeed in the 21st Century economy by supporting productive, accessible, liveable cities that attract talent, encourage innovation and create jobs and growth" (Australian Government 2016). As a follow-up to this plan, in 2017, the Australian government decided to fund 52 smart cities projects with a total of AU$28.5 million in shared funding. Interestingly, Australia has a minister with a title of Cities and Digital Transformation. However, having one title does not necessarily bring the integration of these two strategies together. In other words, the plan aims to invest in smart city infrastructure (a total budget of AU$50 million), collect data on cities, and utilize technologies especially in transport, communications and energy efficiency.

The Smart Cities Plan has some goals that might be linked to entrepreneurship. For example, it targets to build job clusters drawing on a deep pool of skilled labour and to support active participation of research institutions through business partnerships with leading research institutions, including universities, health facilities and government bodies such as the CSIRO.

The Australian Government launched a set of performance data on cities in December 2017 (Australian Government 2017b). The section on innovation and digital opportunities, the only criteria used are: LinkedIn contacts by location and Workers in knowledge intensive services. These two metrics might be some indicators however far more than indicative for any policies or comparison of cities in terms of their performance.

15.5.4 A Proposal to Overcome Strategic Discrepancies

Relating back to the literature analysis, we can identify two major shortcomings in Sydney's strategic planning. First, the entrepreneurial and the technology strategy are only marginally aligned. Second, there is no reference made to existing technological capacities Sydney can build on to develop a custom-tailored digital entrepreneurial ecosystem. The two shortcomings are closely intertwined as a deep understanding of a city's digital technological capabilities is a crucial building block to align entrepreneurial and technology strategy. This assumption is based on the concept of technological relatedness, whereby new and even disruptive industries build on existing local technological knowledge bases (Tannery 2016). Therefore, our suggestion is to first identify the digital technological capacities in a city to supply critical information such as technological strengths of the city, evolution of the city's technological base over time, and key actors in each technology field. Building on the identified technological strengths, entrepreneurial and technology strategy can be aligned in a second step and combined to a roadmap towards a digital entrepreneurial ecosystem.

In order to assess technological capabilities, patent analysis has proven to be a powerful tool. Using patent analysis, not only the technological knowledge base can be specified, but also the complementarity of technological knowledge needed to generate technological innovation (Golembiewski et al. 2015). Another advantage of patent analysis is the flexible level of detail, so that capacities concerning individual digital technologies can be assessed. Thus, the different specific technologies that Sydney companies are involved in can be identified and used as a basis to focus and detail as well as interconnect technology and entrepreneurial strategies on city level.

Tanner (2016) showed using patent analysis that the fuel cell industry across Europe grew out of existing regional technological knowledge bases. We thus argue that in order to fuel a digital entrepreneurial ecosystem, a city should build on existing technological capabilities in the digital arena. If urban companies and universities are e.g. strong in artificial intelligence, the digital entrepreneurial ecosystem should be built around this strength instead of spreading out into a range of digital technologies. The focal technology nurtures the whole ecosystem, e.g. university courses can be designed around the focal theme, providing custom-tailored graduates for local employers in industry and academia. Furthermore, the study revealed that the regional variety of knowledge required for an interdisciplinary field such as fuel cells (e.g. chemistry, material science, and engineering) also contributed to the emergence of the new industry. This recombination of knowledge from different fields is also required in the digital arena, as digital technologies need to be for specific applications such as smart infrastructure.

15.6 Concluding Remarks

This paper has outlined some of the recent studies regarding smart cities, entrepreneurship ecosystems and digital technologies. Even though smart city aims to resolve various urban problems (public service unavailability or shortages, traffic, over-development, pressure on land, environmental or sanitation shortcomings and other forms of inequality) through ICT-based technology connected up as an urban infrastructure, it also contributes to the creation of a better, more sustainable city, in which people's quality of life is higher, their environment more liveable and their economic prospects stronger (Lee et al. 2014). All these contribute to the attraction of cities to become hubs for entrepreneurs and creative people. However, the link between entrepreneurial ecosystems and smart cities is waiting to be established by policy makers and entrepreneurial leaders. To do so, they need to go one level deeper (to the level of specific technologies, such as blockchain, AI, etc) to understand the digital technology capacities of cities and their potential impact on the city level entrepreneurial ecosystems. On this level, a city can create a lifecycle following the triple helix to provide the environment, infrastructure, education for start-ups to then develop the technologies which then feed back into the city.

A systemic perspective of in-depth patent analysis could be instrumental in finding ways of how best to align digital technologies with entrepreneurial capabilities at local ecosystems. This local data could prevent to pursue unrealistic trends set by global hype on some digital technologies in general. Thus, we believe that a closely connected analysis of individual digital technologies could be of high significance in two direct ways. First, both managers and entrepreneurs might improve their utilization of digital technologies by understanding the complex relationships between digital technologies and entrepreneurs. For example, the commercialization of science has been a national priority in Australia (e.g. the Australian Government's Science and Research Priorities). The effective adoption of digital technologies at companies/start-ups could result not only in immediate economic benefits alone, but it could also generate many spill over effects. One such spill over effect is the transfer of digital capabilities to other sectors in the city environment, contributing to the further smartization of cities. Another one is the increased collaboration among business and researchers of innovation ecosystems at cities.

Second, policy makers could improve their policies by addressing the complementary needs of education, industrial, innovation and technological policies at the city level. For example, they might plan educational programs at their cities according to future expectations at manufacturing industries and digital technologies. This could be helpful in generating inclusive cities by reducing the digital divide in skills as well as addressing STEM concerns and development of women occupations in manufacturing industries. Thus, the potential policy changes in industry and technology programs could contribute to any country's competitiveness capacity that will capture digital technology opportunities, thus enabling the long-term success for their economy and welfare.

This chapter is dedicated to highlight the relationship between smart cities and entrepreneurial ecosystems. After theoretically discussing this relationship, this paper presents the case of Sydney by underlying the need for integrating new tools to generate data on quantifying this relationship. We believe that future research might contribute in two major ways. First, studies could conduct a detailed patent analysis for each digital technology. Second, patent analyses could be used to develop potential scenarios for building connections between technologies and digital entrepreneurship environment at city level.

References

2thinknow Global Innovation Agency. (2017). *Innovation cities index.* https://www.innovation-cities.com/innovation-cities-index-2016-2017-global/9774

Asheim, B. T., Smith, H. L., & Oughton, C. (2011). Regional innovation systems: Theory, empirics and policy. *Regional Studies, 45*(7), 875–891.

Australian Government. (2016). *Smart cities plan.* https://cities.infrastructure.gov.au/smart-cities-plan

Australian Government. (2017a). *The digital economy: Opening the conversation.* https://industry.gov.au/innovation/Digital-Economy/Documents/Digital-Economy-Strategy-Consultation-Paper.pdf

Australian Government. (2017b). *The national cities performance framework.* https://smart-cities.dashboard.gov.au/all-cities/overview

Brettel, M., Friederichsen, N., Keller, M., & Rosenberg, M. (2014). How virtualization, decentralization and network building change the manufacturing landscape: An industry 4.0 perspective. *International Journal of Mechanical, Industrial Science and Engineering, 8*(1), 37–44.

Caragliu, A., Bo, C. D., & Nijkamp, P. (2011). Smart cities in Europe. *Journal of Urban Technology, 18*(2), 65–82.

Cetindamar, D., & Gunsel, A. (2012). Measuring the creativity of a City: A proposal and an application. *European Planning Studies, 20*(8), 1–18.

Chourabi, H. et al. (2012). *Understanding smart cities: An integrative framework.* Paper presented at the 45th Hawaii international conference on system sciences, 4–7 January, Hawaii, the USA.

City of Sydney. (2016). Digital strategy. City of Sydney, Sydney. http://www.cityofsydney.nsw.gov.au/__data/assets/pdf_file/0005/288167/Digital-Strategy.pdf.

Cooke, P. (1992). Regional innovation systems: Competitive regulation in the new Europe. *Geoforum, 23*(3), 365–382.

Dia, H. (2016). *Who (or what) is behind the wheel? The regulatory challenges of driverless cars.* The conversation. https://theconversation.com/who-or-what-is-behind-the-wheel-the-regulatory-challenges-of-driverless-cars-55434

EasyParkGroup. (2017). *Smart cities index.* https://easyparkgroup.com/smart-cities-index/

EY Sweeney. (2017). *Digital Australia, state of the nation.* Sydney: Ernst & Young Australia.

Golembiewski, B., vom Stein, N., Sick, N., & Wiemhöfer, H.-D. (2015). Identifying trends in battery technologies with regard to electric mobility: Evidence from patenting activities along and across the battery value chain. *Journal of Cleaner Production, 87*, 800–810.

Groopman, J., Lieb, R., Owyang, J., & Szymanski, J. (2017). *Three macrotrends impacting the journey to 2030.* Kaleido insights. http://www.kaleidoinsights.com/jeremiah/report.pdf

Hellwig, C. (2017). *New perspectives on cyber security: The regulatory challenge.* Global Risk Insights. https://globalriskinsights.com/2017/05/new-perspectives-cyber-security-regulatory-challenge/

Henderson, J. V. (1995). Not a funeral but a wake: Regional science in perspective. *International Regional Science Review, 17*(3), 333–336.

Hollands, R. G. (2008). Will the real Smart City please stand up? *City, 12*(3), 303–320.

Hoover, E. M. (1975). *An introduction to regional economics* (2nd ed.). New York: Alfred A. Knopf.

Isenberg, D. J. (2011). Introducing the entrepreneurship ecosystem: Four defining characteristics. *Forbes*. Available at http://www.forbes.com/sites/danisenberg/2011/05/25/introducing-the-entrepreneurship-ecosystemfour-defining-characteristics/

Jasperneite, J. (2012). *Was hinter Begriffen wie Industrie 4.0 steckt.* Computer Automation. http://www.computer-automation.de/steuerungsebene/steuern-regeln/artikel/93559/0/

Katz, B., & Wagner, J. (2014). *The rise of innovation districts: A new geography of innovation in America.* Washington, DC: Brookings Institute.

Kriz, A., Molloy, C., Kriz, A., & Sonntag, S. (2016). All Australian regions are not born equal: Understanding the regional innovation management sandpit. *Technology Innovation Management Review, 6*(6), 11–23.

Kumar P. A. (2017). *Customer experience trends in digital transformations.* CapGemini. https://www.capgemini.com/2017/11/customer-experience-trends-in-digital-transformations/

Lee, J.-H., Hancock, M. G., & Hu, M.-C. (2014). Towards an effective framework for building smart cities: Lessons from Seoul and San Francisco. *Technological Forecasting and Social Change, 89*, 80–99.

Leydesdorff, L., & Deakin, M. (2011). The triple-Helix model of smart cities: A neo-evolutionary perspective. *Journal of Urban Technology, 18*(2), 53–63.

Manyika, J., Chui, M., Miremadi, M., Bughin, J., George, K., Willmot, P., & Dewhurst, M. (2017). *A future that works: Employment, automation and productivity.* San Francisco: McKinsey Global Institute.

Marshall, A. (1898). *Principles of economics* (4th ed.). London: Macmillan.

Newman, D. (2017). *Top 10 trends for digital transformation in 2018.* Forbes CMO Network. https://www.forbes.com/sites/danielnewman/2017/09/26/top-10-trends-for-digital-transformation-in-2018/#358985ee293a

NSW Government. (2012). *NSW digital economy – Industry action plan.* https://www.industry.nsw.gov.au/__data/assets/pdf_file/0004/53725/digital_economy_iap_final_20121213.pdf

OECD. (2013). *Innovation-driven growth in regions: The role of smart specialisation.* Paris: OECD.

OECD. (2017). *Digital economy outlook.* Paris: OECD Publishing. https://read.oecd-ilibrary.org/science-and-technology/oecd-digital-economy-outlook-2017_9789264276284-en#page1.

Oh, D. S., Phillips, F., Park, S., & Lee, E. (2016). Innovation ecosystems: A critical examination. *Technovation, 54*, 1–6.

Phillips, F. (2006). *Social culture and high tech economic development: The Technopolis columns.* London: Palgrave Macmillan.

Pratchett, L, Hu, R, Walsh, M, Tuli, S (2017). *The knowledge city index – A tale of 25 cities in Australia.* University of Canberra. http://www.canberra.edu.au/research/faculty-research-centres/nexus-centre-for-research/research-progeammes/research-programs/research-areas/

the-knowledge-city-index-a-tale-of-25-cities-in-australia/kci-files/A-Tale-of-25-Cities-in-Australia-PDF.pdf

Richardson, H. W. (1995). Economies and diseconomies of agglomeration. In H. Giersch (Ed.), *Urban agglomeration and economic growth*. Kiel: Springer.

Roger, M., Florida, R., Pogue, M., & Mellander, C. (2015). Creativity, clusters and the competitive advantage of cities. *Competitiveness Review, 25*(5), 482–496.

Schlaepger, R., Koch, M., & Merkofer, P. (2014) *Industry 4.0 – Challenges and solutions for the digital transformation and use of exponential technologies*. Deloitte Report, Switzerland. https://www2.deloitte.com/content/dam/Deloitte/ch/Documents/manufacturing/ch-en-manufacturing-industry-4-0-24102014.pdf

Schumpeter, J. A. (1934). *The theory of economic development*. Cambridge, MA: Harvard University Press.

Stam, S. (2015). Entrepreneurial ecosystems and regional policy: A sympathetic critique. *European Planning Studies, 23*(9), 1759–1769.

Startup Genome. (2017). *Global startup ecosystem report*. https://startupgenome.com/thank-you-enjoy-reading/

Tannery, A. N. (2016). The emergence of new technology-based industries. *Journal of Economic Geography, 16*, 611–635.

The Committee for Sydney. (2017). *#Wethecity3 – Towards a data-driven and responsive Sydney* (Issues Paper 19).

Thomas, J, Barraket, J, Wilson, C, Ewing, S, MacDonald, T, Tucker, J & Rennie, E, (2017). *Measuring Australia's digital divide: The Australian digital inclusion index 2017.* RMIT University, Melbourne, for Telstra. https://digitalinclusionindex.org.au/wp-content/uploads/2018/03/Australian-Digital-Inclusion-Index-2017_v2.pdf

Thurik, R., Stam, E., & Audretsch, D. (2013). The rise of the entrepreneurial economy and the future of dynamic capitalism. *Technovation, 33*(8–9), 302–310.

UN. (2017). *World cities report 2016*. New York: UN.

World Economic Forum. (2013). *Entrepreneurial ecosystems around the globe and company growth dynamics*. Davos: World Economic Forum.

Chapter 16
Urban Wellbeing in the Contemporary City

Nimish Biloria, Prasuna Reddy, Yuti Ariani Fatimah, and Dhrumil Mehta

Abstract The concept of *well-being* in the contemporary city refers to people's ability to live healthy, creative and fulfilling lives. In this chapter, the intent is to understand theoretical perspectives about well-being research, essentially objective and subjective health and well-being of individuals in modern urban society. The emphasis is given to "non-medical" factors to determine the term by complex interactions between social, cultural, physical environments and individual behaviours. The chapter further indicates the tools and techniques adopted by researchers for measuring well-being emphasising the capability approach by Amartya Sen and Luc Boltanski's approach on critical capacity. As a conclusion, based on the views and measures, the chapter suggests that addition of citizen science methodologies have potential utility for bridging objective and subjective perspectives of health and well-being, and influencing urban planning and design.

Keywords Wellbeing · Health · Urban environments · Measurement tools · Citizen science

16.1 Introduction

The term *well-being* has a complex and multi-faceted nature. While *well-being* is a widely used term in academic, public sector and commercial arenas, it can be defined and measured in a variety of ways (Dodge et al. 2012; Alatartseva and Barysheva 2015). Definition and measurement are further confounded by terms that

N. Biloria (✉) · D. Mehta
Faculty of Design Architecture Building, University of Technology Sydney, Sydney, Australia
e-mail: nimish.biloria@uts.edu.au; Dhrumil.D.Mehta@student.uts.edu.au

P. Reddy
Faculty of Science, Engineering and Technology, Swinburne University of Technology, Hawthorn, VIC, Australia
e-mail: preddy@swin.edu.au

Y. A. Fatimah
Institute of Technology Bandung, Bandung, Indonesia

N. Biloria (ed.), *Data-driven Multivalence in the Built Environment*, S.M.A.R.T. Environments, https://doi.org/10.1007/978-3-030-12180-8_16

are used interchangeably with *well-being* such as "quality of life", "happiness", or "life satisfaction" (Dodge et al. 2012; Ballas 2013). Typically, in studies investigating well-being in the urban context, *well-being* is equated with "mental health" (Evans 2003; Bond et al. 2012) or considered synonymous with "health" (Koohsari et al. 2013). Some studies exploring well-being in built environments define *well-being* as a combination of health and comfort, or health, comfort and happiness (Bluyssen 2010).

At its broadest level, the concept of *well-being* refers to people's capacity to live healthy, creative and fulfilling lives. In the late 1990s, psychologists Kahneman, Diener and Schwartz (Kahneman et al. 1999) proposed a new science of well-being focused on explaining positive states of mind and subjective assessments of emotions and quality of life. Social scientists have since shown great enthusiasm in understanding the nature and determinants of well-being.

Two conceptual approaches dominate well-being research: the objective approach examines the objective components of a good life; the subjective approach explores people's subjective evaluations of their lives. The objective approach defines well-being in terms of quality of life indicators such as material resources, income and housing, and social attributes, such as education, health, and social networks. This approach to well-being is exemplified in Amartya Sen's work about how to measure poverty and economic inequality (Sen 1973, 1992), and its extension to the capabilities that individuals should have to live fulfilling lives (Sen 1999). This approach is also the basis of Michael Marmot's seminal work *Social Determinants of Health* (Marmot et al. 2008) that has demonstrated the complex social, cultural, political and economic factors that contribute to the pronounced health inequalities in modern urban society.

The objective approach to well-being informs national and international statistical indicators such as the OECD's Better Life initiative, and the United Nations Development Programme Human Development Index. Social indicators frameworks attempt to measure societal development and quality of life using aggregate measures of income, education, employment, housing, security, health, social inclusion, and environmental quality. It is recognised that objective well-being is not equally distributed. For example, recent longitudinal analyses of inequalities in objective well-being in Australia show that gender, age, class and ethnicity are sources of categorical inequality (Western and Tomaszewski 2016).

Considerable academic work exists in the behavioural and social sciences which seeks to define *well-being* from a subjective perspective. Two key definitions can be identified in this well-being research: hedonic well-being (Diener et al. 2018) and eudaimonic well-being (Deci and Ryan 2008; Ryff and Singer 2008). Hedonic or subjective well-being (SWB) relates to happiness and perceived quality of life; well-being is conceptualised and measured using people's subjective overall life evaluations. The concept of SWB falls within the hedonic perspective that defines wellness or happiness as being fundamentally about maximising pleasure and avoiding or minimising pain. The independent facets of SWB most often researched are life satisfaction, positive affect and negative affect. Conceptualisation of SWB is discussed further in scholarly work on measurement of well-being (Kahneman and Krueger 2006).

Definitions of *well-being* have expanded to move beyond life satisfaction and affect to a meaningful interaction between individuals and their physical and social environment, such that well-being includes cognitive, physical, and mental health, as well as psychosocial well-being and the meeting of basic needs. Eudaimonic well-being relates to a fuller psychological concept of one's life having purpose and individuals having the capabilities to function effectively to this end, known as self-determination (Ryan and Deci 2011) or flourishing (Shah and Marks 2004). From the eudaimonic perspective, one lives in accordance with one's "true self" focusing on meaning in life and self-realisation. Individuals are considered to be "well" if they have opportunities to realise their full potential. Capabilities theory proposes that the opportunity to reach the potential of each individual depends on related factors such as living conditions, socioeconomic status, access to education and health care. Less attention has been paid in the urban health literature to eudaimonic well-being, but there is growing interest in capabilities theory in conceptualisation of well-being in the built environment (Watson 2018).

Subjective well-being has aroused interest in many disciplines, particularly psychology, economics, geography, and sociology (Clark et al. 2008; Diener 2000; Schwanen and Atkinson 2015). Subjective well-being is defined as people's overall cognitive and affective evaluations of their lives (Diener et al. 2003). The cognitive element refers to broad appraisals, such as judgments about life satisfaction in global terms (life as a whole), and in domain terms (in specific areas of life such as work and relationships). The affective element refers to emotions, moods and specific feelings that reflect how people are reacting to or experiencing the events and circumstances in their lives (Diener et al. 2018). The different facets of subjective well-being are separable in factor analyses and have distinctive associations with other variables. The life satisfaction component represents a cognitive evaluation of various life domains (including health, finances, job, leisure, relationships) across a relatively long time period. The other two components are usually interpreted as affective emotions within a shorter time period. Positive Affect (PA) includes the person's desirable or pleasant emotions, such as contentment, enjoyment, and gratitude. Negative Affect (NA) refers to feelings experienced as unpleasant, such as anger, guilt, shame, worry, and sadness.

A large body of research has demonstrated that the three components of subjective well-being: life satisfaction, PA and NA, are independent factors that should be measured and studied separately. Further, these facets of well-being are separable in terms of what influences them, and in turn, what they influence (Diener et al. 2017).

16.2 Determinants of Health and Well-Being

Researchers have suggested several domains that may affect people's subjective well-being. At the individual level, predictors of subjective well-being include temperament, income and supportive social relationships. Higher subjective well-being has been associated with good health and longevity, better social relationships, work performance and creativity. Positive emotions seem to be influenced by strong social relationships (Tay and Diener 2011) and negative emotions seem most related to internal and social conflicts (Stoeva et al. 2002). Individual life satisfaction is also strongly related to chronically accessible evaluations of one's health, income, and the quality of one's work (Schimmack and Oishi 2005). Healthier people are happier and more satisfied with their lives. Good health is associated with greater subjective well-being, while setbacks in health have negative effects (Ngamaba 2017).

At the community and societal levels, there are both universal and unique predictors of subjective well-being. Across diverse cultures, life satisfaction is positively associated with satisfaction of autonomy, relatedness, and competence needs (Church et al. 2013). Fulfillment of the basic needs featured in Maslow's theory has predicted higher life satisfaction across data from over 100 countries (Tay and Diener 2011). At both individual and national levels, income and household financial satisfaction are drivers of happiness and life satisfaction (Diener et al. 2013; Kahneman and Deaton 2010).

Research evidence suggests that subjective well-being is malleable at both the individual and societal level. Studies assessing the health and behaviours of groups with varying levels of subjective well-being show that high subjective well-being can lead to a number of beneficial outcomes, including improved health, supportive social relationships, work productivity and citizenship (Diener et al. 2013, 2015). People higher in subjective well-being are more likely to enact healthy behaviours such as exercising, not smoking, and wearing seat belts (Diener et al. 2015). A number of studies suggest a positive association between social connections and SWB is because people greatly value the quality of their social relationships; people who are higher in SWB are also more prosocial in their behaviour (Tenney et al. 2016).

Subjective well-being is strongly shaped by the objective conditions of people's lives. Social well-being theory, self-determination theory and other theories of human nature maintain that understanding what is meant by the "good things of life" is not universal; our understanding and evaluations of happiness and satisfaction depend on our cognitive and social capital, which are influenced by sociohistorical factors such as culture, religion, work, and intergenerational transfer. Capabilities theory proposes that the opportunity for individuals to reach their full potential depends on objective factors such as socioeconomic conditions, education and employment. According to proponents of capabilities theory, gender equality, trust, community engagement and freedom are among the conducive conditions a society should possess to provide opportunities for people to realise their full potential and to achieve the good things of life.

Recent longitudinal studies examining relationships among a broad number of well-being measures have reported evidence of strong positive associations between objective well-being and subjective life satisfaction (Western and Tomaszewski 2016). These strong linkages imply that if objective differences in well-being can be addressed, subjective well-being indicators such as life satisfaction and happiness can be improved for many people (Bellani and D'Ambrosio 2011).

16.3 Studying Well-Being in the Urban Context

A substantial amount of research has been conducted on the relations between urban environments and the broader concept of *health and well-being* among several disciplines, including public health, epidemiology, urban planning and the social sciences. Many of these studies has followed conceptual models aligned with social determinants of health (SDH) which propose that health is determined not only by biological factors but also by complex interactions between social, cultural and economic factors, the physical environment and individual behaviours (Northwood et al. 2018; Solar and Irwin 2010). These "non-medical" factors or social determinants of health account for 75% of the factors that influence health (Kirby n.d.). The SDH framework outlines how social, economic and political mechanisms (the context) produce a set of socioeconomic positions where populations are stratified hierarchically according to education, occupation and income, gender and ethnicity (structural determinants).

The context in the SDH conceptual model includes governance, macroeconomic policies, social policies, public policies and cultural and societal values (Solar and Irwin 2010). For example, the design and implementation of social policies on housing would be studied within the SDH framework as influencing the health and well-being of individuals in their urban communities. Where people live and work affects their health and chances of leading flourishing lives. Communities and neighbourhoods that ensure access to basic goods, that are socially cohesive, that are designed to promote good physical and psychological wellbeing, and that are protective of the natural environment are essential to health equity (Marmot et al. 2008).

There are a number of different institutions with projects worldwide that are concerned with the challenges posed by rapid global urbanisation, such as increasing socioeconomic disparities and increasing environmental stressors on health and wellbeing. The International Council for Science (ICSU) has a "Science plan on Health and Wellbeing in the Changing Urban Environment" that places importance on planning to meet the challenges of rapidly growing urban environments and "shaping cities for health" (Rydin et al. 2012). The London School of Economics and Political Science (LSE) has a project on "Cities, health and wellbeing"; the World Health Organization focuses on "national healthy cities networks" in Europe (World Health Organization Regional Office for Europe n.d.), and the Healthy People 2020 organisation monitors "health-related Quality of Life and Well-Being" in the United States (Healthy People 2020 n.d.). The major recommendations from these institutions are that we need to reduce inequalities in health outcomes, and build capacity at regional and national levels to promote improvements in urban health and wellbeing.

A recent study conducted a systematic review of published literature on objective and subjective measurement on health-related well-being in an urban context (Krefis et al. 2018). The authors used a conceptual model that relates determinants to four different sectors – individual, society, stressors, and morphology – and associates these to objective and subjective indicators of health-related urban well-being. Objective indicators included information from external sources such as census data, income, crime rates, and environmental factors such as green space, noise or air pollution. Subjective indicators of urban health and well-being were largely based on social survey data and self-reported information such as subjective health status, mental health and emotional aspects of health. The literature search, which was focused on studies conducted in European cities or cities located in northern America, showed that subjective urban health and well-being was mostly measured by using the 12-item General Health Questionnaire (GHQ-12) and the short-form Warwick Edinburgh Mental Well-being Scale (WEMWBS) respectively.

The systematic review (Krefis et al. 2018) found that most studies on relations between urban environments and health and well-being describe or analyse either associations between urban determinants and health in general, specific urban determinants and health, or associations between urban environments and well-being. Fewer studies have investigating diseases and urban health and well-being. Traffic noise for instance, is known to be associated with several health outcomes, such as hypertension (Babisch et al. 2014). Air pollution has been associated with hospital admissions for cardiovascular and respiratory diseases (Bravo et al. 2017). Respondents to the US General Social Survey reported greater subjective well-being when surveyed on days with lower air pollution within their local area (Levinson 2012). The authors noted that there is a lack of interdisciplinary approaches that highlight the complexity or urban health and well-being, particularly the complexity of urban structures and dynamics and their influence on health and well-being.

Studies focused on associations between urban environments and health and well-being show the great importance of public parks (Larson et al. 2016) and green space usage (Bertram and Rehdanz 2015) to promote better health and well-being. The objective quantity of green space within a geographical territory has been found to be related to indicators of health and well-being, such as self-reported general health (Maas et al. 2006), mental health (Van den Berg et al. 2010), physical health (Pereira et al. 2013) and well-being (Krekel et al. 2016). Several reviews have addressed the influence of the urban neighbourhood environment on walkability (Saelens and Handy 2008; Talen and Koschinsky 2013), which has been shown to be associated with better physical health and quality of life (Inoue et al. 2010; Jaskiewicz and Besta 2014). Experimental and longitudinal studies show that people living in areas with more green space tend to have higher subjective well-being (Hartig et al. 2003; Velarde et al. 2007; MacKerron and Mourato 2013). One reason for these beneficial effects could be that communal green spaces facilitate positive social interactions which are associated with subjective well-being (Sandstrom and Dunn 2014). Place attachment has also been considered important to the overall well-being of an individual (Lewicka 2011); people may develop emotional attachment to urban green space, which may be conducive to their health and well-being. These and other studies add to the growing recognition that subjective spatial factors may be more important for well-being than objective ones; in the same manner as socio-economic and social capital factors are more important than spatial factors overall (Ala-Mantila et al. 2018).

16.4 Measuring Well-Being

Many of the tools and techniques for measuring well-being consider the term to denote that something is in a good state (Veenhoven 2007). It refers to the condition of an individual or group of people in their social, economic, psychological, spiritual and medical situation. It is a broad construct mainly divided into two large realms: objective and subjective well-being. Objective well-being is based on material, tangible and quantitative indicators that measure aspects of education, physical and built environment, community and economy (Measurement of Well-Being n.d.). The focus is on measuring hard facts in terms such income in dollars, living accommodation in square meters and other aspects like educational attainment, safe neighbourhoods, security and stability. Subjective well-being, on the other hand, focuses on soft matters such as satisfaction with income, and perceived adequacy of dwelling (Veenhoven 2007). It is based on an individual's perspective and gives importance to one's mental judgement, emotions and reactions of their own life.

Since the definition of "well-being" is a multidimensional construct, the fundamental challenge to measure it is the extent of diverse perceptions, disagreements over its definition and theoretical basis (Dodge et al. 2012; Deci and Ryan 2008; Linton et al. 2016). It is problematic as some investigators approach the topic from the perspective of basic human needs, while others investigate the capabilities of an individual, or give importance to individual preferences rather than the market behaviour (Linton et al. 2016). These multiple theories and varying perceptions have influenced the development and range of well-being measurement instruments (Linton et al. 2016). With the presence of ambiguity due to differing perspectives on the topic, absence of a universally accepted measure and a little guidance on the specificity of instruments within the growing number of instruments available, researchers have had to select the instruments familiar to them within their particular discipline, what is most often used by others or to create yet another new instrument (Linton et al. 2016).

Researchers Linton, Dieppe and Lara developed a "PRISMA" diagram that evaluates a systematic framework that includes a relation between themes, dimension and instruments (Linton et al. 2016). Themes represent a broader spectrum in terms of mental, social, physical, spiritual, economic well-being as mentioned above, dimensions are well-being aspects that clusters around these themes and instrument are measurement tools that investigate the dimension to locate it in one of the categories. For example, Keller's Symptom Questionnaire measures friendliness representing social and mental well-being where the questionnaire is the instrument, an aspect of friendliness is the dimension and social and mental characteristic are the themes of well-being. Based on this approach, they have listed around 100 measuring tools that also correspond with many of the measurement tools that Jarden presents in his 'Positive Psychological Assessment Workbook' (Jarden 2012).

The chapter lists an inventory of measuring tools based on the following identified themes:

Mental well-being concentrating on thoughts and feelings of an individual about their state of life is measured by tools such as the Happiness Measures, The Satisfaction with Life Scale, The gratitude questionnaire, The flourishing Scale, The Short Grit Scale, The Depression, Stress, Anxiety Scale, Brief Resilience scale, The Curiosity and Exploration Scale. These tools assess subjective qualities in terms of perceived happiness, life satisfaction as a whole, things an individual is proud of, positive relations, feeling of competence, perseverance and passion for long-term goals, the perception of social isolation, ability to recover from stress respectively (Jarden 2012).

Functional Assessment of Cancer Therapy-General Population†, Quality of Life Index-Generic, Quality of Life Inventory, and Valued Living Questionnaire evaluate social qualities in terms of family and partner relations. Kellner's Symptom Questionnaire, Warwick-Edinburgh Mental Well-Being Scale-Short and Social Well-being Scale, The loneliness Scale, and Quality of Life Inventory look at other aspects of friendliness, parenting and social actualisation, and perception of social isolation, in order to understand people's connection in their local and wider community (Linton et al. 2016).

For a broader understanding of subjective well-being, spiritual well-being plays a vital role that is concerned with meaning and connection to high power than oneself. For example, Spiritual Well-Being Scale measures existential well-being while Jarel Spiritual Well-Being Scale, Serenity Scale-Brief, Quality of Life Inventory weighs intangible notions of faith, inner haven, self-responsibility and philosophy of life. Other reflective characteristics of religious well-being, search for meaning, and self-discovery are found in instruments such as the Meaning in Life Questionnaire, The Spirituality Scale, and Valued Living Questionnaire (Linton et al. 2016).

Activities and functioning theme look at the relationship between time and action, in other words, involvement in specific activities to fill one's time and ability to undertake these tasks. The tools to determine this include 15D, Positive Mental Health instrument, CASP-19 (Control, Autonomy, Self-realisation and Pleasure), ICECAP-O, Quality of Life Inventory, Valued Living Questionnaire, Life Satisfaction Questionnaire-9, Nottingham Health Profile that measures the idea of control, creativity, eating, recreation, work and the time spent on vacations (Linton et al. 2016). Researcher Anadante Hadi Pandyaswargo also involves a time use study along with the participatory survey while conducting research in Indonesia for well-being. She uses a time-use diary that demonstrates how much time in a day each person is using activities, how often the activities are performed during weekdays and on weekends and which of the kind of basic needs (water, food, energy, jobs, and community environment) are involved in each activity. The objective of this time-use is to get information on how people use their time such as the presence of others, means of transportation, for whom the activities are done, emotional states, utilities involved. The intention behind this measure is to understand the relation where the time defines the intensity of satisfaction and the quality of each need.

External conditions and pressures in terms of environmental and socioeconomic concerns such as income and financial security is an important factor not only confined to an individual but also represents wellbeing of a community, city and a country. 'Social equality index' assesses income statistics on registration of taxes and salaries. 'Index of Social progress' involves safety in the streets, political stability rule of law, unemployment (Veenhoven 2007). 'Economic Global Liveability Index' measures hard facts regarding infrastructure, environment, education through factors like financial security, the efficiency of public transport services, carbon footprint and literacy rate (Rozek et al. 2018). Besides these, other quantitative index includes 'Global Food security' providing a worldwide perspective on most and least vulnerability to food, 'Global Innovation Index' that particularly measures the innovations in the above sectors mentioned.

The tools measuring subjective well-being or measuring from an individual perspective involves verbal and written questionnaires as the main methodology while tools looking at well-being from a global point of view or objective well-being use government, institutional and demographic data. Also, some of these tools weigh more than one theme as in the case of Quality of Life inventory that surveys social and spiritual well-being as well as activities and functioning of an individual. Taken together, the weight of different themes through dimensions and tools and its property to overlap gives a better overview of a multidimensional "well-being".

Measuring well-being from a capability approach is a great challenge. The capability approach proposed by Amartya Sen extends the subjective well-being position that "well-being" is not only confined to a human's basic needs of food, shelter, work, wealth and education but the intangible qualities of feelings of satisfaction, pleasure or happiness form an integral part of larger understanding of one's capacity to attain these goals. But this approach, has two problems which he states as 'physical-condition neglect' and the 'valuation neglect'. The term 'physical-condition neglect' represents the adaptable nature of human beings in any condition, that is, the poor and sick can be relatively happy same as the rich and healthy individual. The term 'valuation neglect' means that valuing is a reflective activity that is what is worth as a long-term goal where happiness or sadness are evidences to achieve that objective (Richardson and Schokkaert 2019). Thus, the argument, in his capability approach is that by giving books to someone who cannot read or providing someone with a car at a place with poor infrastructure does not solve the problem of well-being but rather it is important to focus on what people can effectively be and willing to be, that is, on their capability (Richardson and Schokkaert 2019; Robeyns 2003).

To practise this approach in the space of capabilities, it is more important to understand its core concepts and the intrinsic differences between them. Three essential concepts proposed in Sen's approach are the following:

- Functioning and Capabilities: "A functioning is an achievement, whereas a capability is the ability to achieve. Functionings are, in a sense, more directly related to living conditions, since they are different aspects of living conditions. Capabilities, in contrast, are notions of freedom, in the positive sense: what real opportunities you have regarding the life you may lead" (Sen 1987). He explains this definition by giving a classic example of comparison between two persons who don't eat enough to enable the functioning of being well-nourished. "The first person is a victim of a famine in Ethiopia, while the second person decided to go on a hunger strike in front of the Chinese embassy in Washington to protest against the occupation of Tibet. Although both persons lack the functioning of being well-nourished, the freedom they had to avoid being hungry is crucially distinct' (Robeyns 2003). In this example, both lack the achievement of being well nourished, the difference is that the protestor has the capability to achieve it but makes the choice of not to, while the famine victim lacks in terms of choice or opportunity, claiming that well-being only in terms of functioning is insufficient and it also includes freedom (Richardson and Schokkaert 2019). In other words, it is a combination of action and desire, that is the effective opportunity they want to engage in and be whom they want to be, influenced by its personal, social and environmental characteristics they are living in.

- Importance of Human Diversity: "Investigations of equality, theoretical as well as practical, that proceed with the assumption of antecedent uniformity (including the presumption that 'all men are created equal') thus miss out on a major aspect of the problem. Human diversity is no secondary complication (to be ignored, or to be introduced 'later on'); it is a fundamental aspect of our interest in equality" (Sen 1992). In other words, "Indeed, if human beings would not be diverse, then inequality in one space, say income, would more or less be identical with inequality in another space, like capabilities" (Robeyns 2003). He gives an example of a man and woman who have equal access to higher education, receives the same scholarship, and want to enable certain functionings in terms of being self-esteem, ambitious, independent and so on. But since the woman is discriminated in the labour market, she may not be able to achieve capability as the man in spite of having similar functioning. The point he is trying to make is that characteristic in terms of prejudices, social norms, habits and traditions need to be acknowledged in the space of capabilities.
- Basic and General Capabilities: The term Basic Capabilities that Sen is referring to is the freedom to achieve basic necessities for survival and escape poverty. In other words, "not so much in ranking living standards, but in deciding on a cut-off point for the purpose of assessing poverty and deprivation" (Sen 1987). The term is crucial to study to differentiate poverty analysis as a part of well-being analysis in developing countries whereas the more affluent countries would focus on capabilities that are less necessary for survival.

Looking at these core concepts, the approach gives more importance to opportunity than outcome, preferences and possibilities than acceptance thereby challenging the notion of neo-liberalist and utilitarian policies. Sen mentions that "if a person with low capability well-being is contented with her situation and requires only low levels of resources to reach high utility levels, then the capability approach will assess her capability level, and disregard her utility level" (Robeyns 2003; Alkire 2015). This ideology is clearly reflected in Bhutan's Innovative extension for Gross Happiness Index than Gross Domestic Product. This extension conceptualizes deprivation cut off as a sufficiency cut off, the poverty cut off as happiness threshold and the national index in positive terms, that is wellbeing, rather than poverty challenging the ideology of utility and resources (Alkire 2015). To further understand this concept, sufficiency cut off is the datum in terms of attainment of his or her achievement. For instance, if a student has studied for 30 years where the cut off is 21 years, then it will be viewed as 21 years of sufficient education. Hence, it looks at the idea of equivalence which dissolves the hierarchical notion of being above or below. Another interesting aspect is the happiness threshold which states that "though many people are not wealthy they have achieved a kind of flourishing, fulfilment, and richness to life that is important. Though many are illiterate or have material challenges that need not necessarily be decisive for their happiness" (Alkire 2015) thereby giving greater importance to freedom of choice than acceptance.

Critical Capacity Approach proposed by Luc Boltanski and Laurent Thevenots: The term critical capacity means the ability to make your own decision with a legitimate justification of that selection/choice. Their theory explores the grammar of justification; the core element is that legitimate justification of what is right and wrong to say and to do must follow the common moral orders dominating the specific social situation. "These orders of worth are a set of social conventions that people can draw on, each with its own set of evaluative criteria and the related conception of 'the common good' "(Thorslund and Lassen 2016; Boltanski and Thevenot 2006). These concepts of worth represent the different worlds that we exist and co-exist in, that is, World of inspiration focusing on passion, creativity, dreams, enthusiasm, feelings and excitement, the Domestic world where the personal relationship in terms of generation, tradition, and hierarchy becomes the key element of justice and qualities of being distinguished, straightforward, faithful and have a character is being evaluated (Boltanski and Thévenot 1999). The other world represents the market world where the quantitative value for money is the judging criteria as the actions are inspired by the materialistic things. Competition, rivalry, vale, desire, selfishness becomes the key elements of justice (Thorslund and Lassen 2016) while the civic world focuses on the notion of human will as the citizen look for a common good than mere personal interest. The uniqueness of this world is to give important to beings who are not individual beings but are collective ones representing immaterial objects in terms of rules, codes and procedures. The industrial world 'is based on the efficiency of beings, their performance, their productivity, and their capacity to ensure normal operations and to respond usefully to needs' (Thorslund and Lassen 2016; Boltanski and Thevenot 2006) while The World of Renown relies on the response and reactions of the public to determine one's success where the ability to visible, getting attention, being recognised and famous are the qualities of worthy beings. As a whole, they claim that the modern society is not a single social order but an interwoven complex entity of these multiple orders in one single space and that same persons have, on the same day and in the same social space use different devices for assessment in form of justification, including the reference different types of worth, when they shift from one situation to another. To further understand this, he gives an instance of a school examination aiming at the pupil's capabilities can be said to be mainly industrial. In this situation, he states that one can criticise the pupil of displaying his family status and wealth of the market world or criticise the teacher by accusing him or her on signs of luxury that is not relevant in this situation. Hence, the situation is criticised as unfair because the kind of wroth relevant inside one world has been carried to the other devaluing the agenda for which the test was meant for. Hence, by inter-crossing the six worlds mentioned above, a matrix can be drawn up to chart the most frequent criticisms in our society as "without this capacity, human relationships would simply be impossible" (Boltanski and Thévenot 1999).

16.5 Citizen Science Participatory Research in Urban Settings

Given these many views and measures of well-being, how can we capture the best of objective and subjective aspects of individual and collective well-being? Recent research focused on health literacy and citizen science methodologies may be a pathway to assessing subjective well-being in urban context.

The good health of all its citizens is one of the most effective indicators of a city's sustainable development. Health literacy entails knowledge, motivation, and competencies of citizens to access, understand, appraise, and apply information to manage health and interact with services related to health and well-being. Health literate citizens are an asset for communities and the cities at large – not only do they have resources to take personal responsibility for their own health and well-being, they can become involved as citizens in social and political processes that address health inequalities in access to care (Sorensen 2018).

One approach for mobilising multi-level efforts to improve citizens' health literacy and improve their environments to enhance health and well-being, is to engage in a process of citizen science. It is a participatory research approach involving members of the public working closely with research investigators to initiate and advance scientific research projects.

Increasingly, participatory approaches have been used to form meaningful citizen engagement in urban planning and health promotion strategies to improve built environment outcomes. For instance, citizen science and other participatory approaches have been utilised to make ecological observations, such as conducting air quality monitoring, and address a wide range of health and environmental justice challenges in community settings (Downs et al. 2010). Citizen science methodologies have embraced new technologies and community-academic partnerships in fields such as community mapping to document community conditions both spatially and visually to assist community residents in influencing place-based decision making. Participatory approaches such as photovoice use photographs to raise awareness about critical community issues and advance policy change.

A recent study of environmental hazards in an urban environment using a citizen science approach was able to demonstrate that community-based knowledge can contribute to and extend scientific enquiry, as well as help residents to leverage action to address community concerns (Jelks et al. 2018). Another recent study (Chrisinger and King 2018) developed a methodology to integrate geospatial technology with biometric sensing within a previously developed, evidence-based citizen science protocol, called "Our Voice" to identify objective and perceived elements of the built environment that contributed to participants' subjective well-being. The researchers noted that such approaches present opportunities to engage the community members in collecting and analysing their own geospatial and biometric data to increase their understanding of their local environments and activate potential environmental improvements.

There is growing interest in the use of technologies, such as the "internet of things" (IoT), to measure and improve health and well-being of urban populations (Kamel Boulos and Al-Shorbaji 2014; Kamel Boulos et al. 2015). Citizens are connected via sensors and devices with the Internet, with the aim of improving their health and well-being. For instance, the health of older people in Barcelona, Spain has been targeted via a smartphone (Alcaraz 2014) that aims to create stronger networks, and "Games for Health" have been developed in Finland (Holopainen et al. 2016).

An innovative investigation called Urban Mind (Bakolis et al. 2018) used a novel smartphone-based tool to monitor the impact of nature on mental well-being in real-time and real-world urban environments. The researchers found that short-term exposure to specific natural features, such as being outdoors, seeing trees, hearing birds singing, seeing the sky, and feeling in contact with nature, has measurable beneficial effects on mental well-being. In addition, the researchers reported a lagged effect, that is, the beneficial effects could still be observed after several hours, even if the participant was no longer outdoors and no longer had access to nature.

These investigations represent successful examples of citizen science methodologies in urban environments and their findings have potential implications from the perspectives of health and well-being, urban planning and design. The data derived from these participatory approaches provide a much-needed evidence base that could inform future investments and policies on urban planning and design aimed at improving the health and well-being of populations within the built environment (Bakolis et al. 2018). Citizen science approaches combined with geospatial mapping maximise ecological validity because data are collected in real-world environments. Further, such designs allow for investigating the greater complexities of urban health and well-being using objective and subjective measures that capture dynamic information.

16.6 Conclusions

The various definitions and views around the term *well-being* addressed in this Chapter, show strong linkages between objective and subjective well-being. Addressing objective differences can improve the subjective well-being of an individual in terms of the individual's health, life satisfaction and happiness. The definition has expanded beyond conveying elementary human needs to include cognitive, physical, mental as well as psychological well-being in order to understand factors which influence the holistic development of an individual. Accordingly, the studies suggest that subjective factors are equally or sometimes more important for well-being than simply the objective ones. Further, the research shows that 75% of "non-medical" factors in terms of complex interaction between social, cultural, economic and physical environment have more influence on the health of an individual's behaviour than biological factors. Spatial factors, especially the socio-economic and social capital factors, become important determinants of health and well-being in an urban context. The tools measuring subjective well-being investigating the broad spectrum of mental, social, physical, spiritual well-being mentioned above mainly involve verbal and written questionnaires as the main methodology whereas objective well-being uses government, institution and demographic datasets. Also, theoretically, the capability approach proposed by Amartya Sen gave emphasis to the notion of opportunity rather than outcome, possibilities rather than acceptance or in other words, the extension to capabilities that individuals should have to live fulfilling lives. Hence, taken together, the weight of different themes through tools, perspectives and its property to overlap gives a better overview of a multidimensional nature of "well-being".

Considering the acknowledged views on well-being, measures of well-being and recent research around health literacy, we further suggest the addition of citizen science based participatory methods as an effective tool to understand well-being in the contemporary city. A participatory approach where citizens can closely work with research investigators to uncover urban problems and prospects as opposed to being a volunteer for post-processing urban solutions, citizen science methodology can prove to be a vital resource for informing future investments and policies aimed at improving health and well-being of populations within the built environment. The approach emphasises a process-oriented methodology with a combination of scientific data to give more accurate and dynamic information to investigate the complexities revolving around the well-being of an individual. Understanding well-being from a holistic and humanistic perspectivewill benefit from the introduction of such participatory and democratic methodologies.

References

Ala-Mantila, S., Heinonen, J., Junnila, S., & Saarsalmi, P. (2018). Spatial nature of urban well-being. *Regional Studies, 52*(7), 959–973. https://doi.org/10.1080/00343404.2017.1360485.

Alatartseva, E., & Barysheva, G. (2015). Well-being: Subjective and objective aspects. *Procedia – Social and Behavioral Sciences, 166*, 36–42. https://doi.org/10.1016/j.sbspro.2014.12.479.

Alcaraz, T. G. (2014). *Could new technology help older people in Barcelona create stronger networks?* Available online: https://www.hteguardian.com/cities/2014/oct/28/could-new-technology-help-older-people-in-barcelona-create-stronger-networks

Alkire, S. (2015). *Capability approach and well-being measurement for public policy* (*OPHI Working Paper 94*). New York: Oxford University Press. https://doi.org/10.1093/oxfordhb/9780199325818.013.18.
Babisch, W., Wolf, K., Petz, M., Heinrich, J., Cyrys, J., & Peters, A. (2014). Associations between traffic noise, particulate air pollution, hypertension, and isolated systolic hypertension in adults: The KORA study. *Environmental Health Perspectives, 122*(5), 492–498. https://doi.org/10.1289/ehp.1306981.
Bakolis, I., Hammond, R., Smythe, M., Gibbons, J., Davidson, N., Tognin, S., & Mechelli, A. (2018). Urban mind: Using smartphone technologies to investigate the impact of nature on mental well-being in real time. *Bioscience, 68*(2), 134–145. https://doi.org/10.1093/biosci/bix149.
Ballas, D. (2013). What makes a 'happy city'? *Cities, 32*, S39–S50. https://doi.org/10.1016/j.cities.2013.04.009.
Bellani, L., & D'Ambrosio, C. (2011). Deprivation, social exclusion and subjective well-being. *Social Indicators Research, 104*(1), 67–86. https://doi.org/10.1007/s11205-010-9718-0.
Bertram, C., & Rehdanz, K. (2015). The role of urban green space for human well-being. *Ecological Economics, 120*, 139–152. https://doi.org/10.1016/j.ecolecon.2015.10.013.
Bluyssen, P. M. (2010). Towards new methods and ways to create healthy and comfortable buildings. *Building and Environment, 45*(4), 808–818. https://doi.org/10.1016/j.buildenv.2009.08.020.
Boltanski, L., & Thévenot, L. (1999). The sociology of critical capacity. *European Journal of Social Theory, 2*(3), 359–377. https://doi.org/10.1177/136843199002003010.
Boltanski, L., & Thevenot, L. (2006). *On justification*. Princeton: Princeton University Press.
Bond, L., Kearns, A., Mason, P., Tannahill, C., Egan, M., & Whitely, E. (2012). Exploring the relationships between housing, neighbourhoods and mental wellbeing for residents of deprived areas. *BMC Public Health, 12*, 48. https://doi.org/10.1186/1471-2458-12-48.
Bravo, M. A., Ebisu, K., Dominici, F., Wang, Y., Peng, R. D., & Bell, M. L. (2017). Airborne fine particles and risk of hospital admissions for understudied populations: Effects by urbanicity and short-term cumulative exposures in 708 U.S. counties. *Environmental Health Perspectives, 125*, 594–601. https://doi.org/10.1289/EHP257.
Chrisinger, B. W., & King, A. C. (2018). Stress experiences in neighbourhood and social environments (SENSE): A pilot study to integrate the quantified self with citizen science to improve the built environment and health. *International Journal of Health Geographics, 17*, 17. https://doi.org/10.1186/s12942-018-0140-1.
Church, A. T., Katigbak, M. S., Locke, K. D., et al. (2013). Need satisfaction and well-being. Testing self-determination theory in eight cultures. *Journal of Cross-Cultural Psychology, 44*(4), 507. https://doi.org/10.1177/0022022112466590.
Clark, A. E., Frijters, P., & Shields, M. A. (2008). Relative income, happiness, and utility: An explanation for the Easterlin paradox and other puzzles. *Journal of Economic Literature, 46*(1), 95–144. https://doi.org/10.1257/jel.46.1.95.
De Neve, J. E., Diener, E., Tay, L., & Xuereb, C. (2013). The objective benefits of subjective well-being. In J. Helliwell, R. Layard, & J. Sachs (Eds.), *World happiness report 2013* (pp. 54–79). New York: UN Sustainable Development Solutions Network.
Deci, E. L., & Ryan, R. M. (2008). Hedonia, eudaimonia, and well-being: An introduction. *Journal of Happiness Studies, 9*(1), 1–11. https://doi.org/10.1007/s10902-006-9018-1.
Diener, E. (2000). Subjective well-being: The science of happiness and a proposal for a national index. *American Psychologist, 55*, 34–43. https://doi.org/10.1037/0003-066X.55.1.34.
Diener, E., Oishi, S., & Lucas, R. E. (2003). Personality, culture, and subjective well-being: Emotional and cognitive evaluations of life. *Annual Review of Psychology, 54*, 403–425. https://doi.org/10.1146/annurev.psych.54.101601.145056.
Diener, E., Tay, L., & Oishi, S. (2013). Rising income and the subjective well-being of nations. *Journal of Personality and Social Psychology, 104*(2), 267–276. https://doi.org/10.1037/a0030487.

Diener, E., Kanazawa, S., Suh, E. M., & Oishi, S. (2015). Why people are in a generally good mood. *Personality and Social Psychology Review, 19*(3), 235–256. https://doi.org/10.1177/1088868314544467.

Diener, E., Heintzelman, S. J., Kushlev, K., Tay, L., Wirtz, D., Lutes, L. D., & Oishi, S. (2017). Findings all psychologists should know from the new science on subjective well-being. *Canadian Psychology/Psychologie Canadienne, 58*(2), 87–104.

Diener, E., Lucas, R. E., & Oishi, S. (2018). Advances and open questions in the science of subjective well-being. *Collabra: Psychology, 4*(1), 15. https://doi.org/10.1525/Collabra.115.

Dodge, R., Daly, A., Huyton, J., & Sanders, L. (2012). The challenge of defining wellbeing. *International Journal of Wellbeing, 2*(3), 222–235. https://doi.org/10.5502/ijw.v2i3.4.

Downs, T. J., Ross, L., Mucciarone, D., Calvache, M. C., Taylor, O., & Goble, R. (2010). Participatory testing ad reporting in an environmental-justice community of Worcester, Massachusetts: A pilot project. *Environmental Health, 9*, 34. https://doi.org/10.1186/1476-069X-9-34.

Evans, G. W. (2003). The built environment and mental health. *Journal of Urban Health, 80*(4), 536–555. https://doi.org/10.1093/jurban/jtg06.

Hartig, T., Evans, G. W., Jamner, L. D., Davis, D. S., & Garling, T. (2003). Tracking restoration in natural and urban field settings. *Journal of Environmental Psychology, 23*(2), 109–123. https://doi.org/10.1016/S0272-4944(02)00109-3.

Healthy People 2020. (n.d.) *Health-related quality of life and well-being*. Available online: https://www.healthypeople.gov/2020/topics-objectives/topic/health-related-quality-of-life-well-being

Holopainen, A., Arpola, T., & Wuorisalo, J. (2016). *Games for health – Finland*. Available online: https://de.slideshare.net/gamesforhealthfinland/health-tuesday-games-for-health-finland

Inoue, S., Ohya, Y., Odagiri, Y., Takamiya, T., Ishii, K., Kitabayashi, M., Suijo, K., Sallis, J. F., & Shimomitsu, T. (2010). Association between perceived neighbourhood environment and walking among adults in 4 cities in Japan. *Journal of Epidemiology, 20*(4), 277–286. https://doi.org/10.2188/jea.JE20090120.

Jarden, A. (2012). Positive psychologists on positive psychology: Introduction. *International Journal of Wellbeing, 2*(2), 70–71. https://doi.org/10.5502/ijw.v2i2.1.

Jaskiewicz, M., & Besta, T. (2014). Is easy access related to better life? Walkability and overlapping of personal and communal identity as predictors of quality of life. *Applied Research in Quality of Life, 9*(3), 505–516. https://doi.org/10.1007/s11482-013-9246-6.

Jelks, N. O., Hawthorne, T. L., Dai, D., Fuller, C. H., & Stauber, C. (2018). Mapping the hidden hazards: Community-led spatial data collection of street-level environmental stressors in a degraded, urban watershed. *International Journal of Environmental Research and Public Health, 15*, 825. https://doi.org/10.3390/ijerph15040825.

Kahneman, D., & Deaton, A. (2010). High income improves evaluation of life but not emotional well-being. *Proceedings of the National Academy of Sciences, 107*(38), 16489–16493. https://doi.org/10.1073/pnas.1011492107.

Kahneman, D., & Krueger, A. B. (2006). Developments in the measurement of subjective well-being. *Journal of Economic Perspectives, 20*(1), 3–24.

Kahneman, D., Diener, E., & Schwarz, N. (Eds.). (1999). *Well-being: The foundations of hedonic psychology*. New York: Russell Sage Foundation.

Kamel Boulos, M. N., & Al-Shorbaji, N. M. (2014). On the internet of things, smart cities and the WHO healthy cities. *International Journal of Health Geographics, 13*, 10. https://doi.org/10.1186/1476-072X-13-10.

Kamel Boulos, M. N., Tsouros, A. D., & Holopainen, A. (2015). Social, innovative and smart cities are happy and resilient': Insights from the WHO EURO 2014 International Healthy Cities Conference. *International Journal of Health Geographics, 14*, 3. https://doi.org/10.1186/1476-072X-14-3.

Kirby, M. J. L. (n.d.) *The health of Canadians: The federal role. Final report on the state of the health care system in Canada* (Volume 6: Recommendations for reform 2002). Available at http://www.parl.gc.ca/Content/SEN/Committee/372/soci/rep/repoct02vol6-e.pdf

Koohsari, M. J., Badland, H., & Giles-Corti, B. (2013). (Re)Designing the built environment to support physical activity: Bringing public health back into urban design and planning. *Cities, 35*, 294–298. https://doi.org/10.1016/j.cities.2013.07.001.

Krefis, A. C., Augustin, M., Schlunzen, K. H., Obenbrugge, J., & Augustin, J. (2018). How does the urban environment affect health and well-being? A systematic review. *Urban Science, 2*(1), 21. https://doi.org/10.3390/urbansci2010021.

Krekel, C., Kolbe, J., & Wustemann, H. (2016). The greener, the happier? The effect of urban land use on residential well-being. *Ecological Economics, 121*, 117–127. https://doi.org/10.1016/j.ecolecon.2015.11.005.

Larson, L. R., Jennings, V., & Cloutier, S. A. (2016). Public parks and wellbeing in urban areas of the United States. *PLoS One, 11*, e0153211. https://doi.org/10.1371/journal.pone.0153211.

Levinson, A. (2012). Valuing public goods using happiness data. The case of air quality. *Journal of Public Economics, 96*, 869–880. https://doi.org/10.1016/j.pubeco.2012.06.007.

Lewicka, M. (2011). Place attachment: How far have we come in the last 40 years? *Journal of Environmental Psychology, 31*(3), 207–230. https://doi.org/10.1016/j.jenvp.2010.10.001.

Linton, M. J., Dieppe, P., & Medina-Lara, A. (2016). Review of 99 self-report measures for assessing Well-being in adults: Exploring dimensions of Well-being and developments over time. *BMJ Open, 6*(7), e010641. https://doi.org/10.1136/bmjopen-2015-010641.

Maas, J., Verheij, R. A., Gronewegen, P. P., de Vries, S., & Spreeuwenberg, P. (2006). Green space, urbanity, and health: How strong is the relation? *Journal of Epidemiology and Community Health, 60*(7), 587–592. https://doi.org/10.1136/jech.2005.043125.

MacKerron, G., & Mourato, S. (2013). Happiness is greater in natural environments. *Global Environment Change, 23*(5), 992–1000. https://doi.org/10.1016/j.gloenvcha.2013.03.010.

Marmot, M., Friel, S., Bell, R., Houweling, T. A. J., & Taylor, S. (2008). Closing the gap in a generation: Health equity through action on the social determinants of health. *Lancet, 372*(9650), 1661–1669.

Measurement of Well-Being. https://www.hsph.harvard.edu/health-happiness/research-new/positive-health/measurement-of-well-being/

Ngamaba, K. H. (2017). Determinants of subjective well-being in representative samples of nations. *The European Journal of Public Health, 27*(2), 377–382. https://doi.org/10.1093/eurpub/ckw103.

Northwood, M., Ploeg, J., Markle-Reid, M., & Sherifali, D. (2018). Integrative review of the social determinants of health in older adults with multimorbidity. *Journal of Advanced Nursing, 74*, 45–60. https://doi.org/10.1111/jan.13408.

Pereira, G., Christian, H., Foster, S., Boruff, B. J., Bull, F., Knuiman, M., & Giles-Corti, B. (2013). The association between neighbourhood greenness and weight status: An observational study in Perth Western Australia. *Environmental Health, 12*, 49. https://doi.org/10.1186/1476-069X-12-49.

Richardson, H. S., & Schokkaert, E. (2019). How do we measure well-being? *The Conversation*. September 19, 2018. Accessed 30 Sept, 2018. https://theconversation.com/how-do-we-measure-well-being-70967

Robeyns, I. (2003). *Valuing freedoms: Sen's capability approach and poverty reduction* (A. Sabina Ed.), Oxford/New York: Oxford University Press, vii 340 pages. *Economics and Philosophy, 19*(2), 371–377. https://doi.org/10.1017/S0266267103231229.

Rozek, J., Giles-Corti, B., & Gunn, L. (2018). 'The World's most Liveable City' title isn't a measure of the things most of us actually care about. *The Conversation*. September 13, 2018. Accessed 30 Sept 2018. https://theconversation.com/the-worlds-most-liveable-city-title-isnt-a-measure-of-the-things-most-of-us-actually-care-about-101525

Ryan, R., & Deci, E. (2011). A self-determination theory perspective on social, institutional, cultural, and economic supports for autonomy and their importance for well-being. In *Human autonomy in cross-cultural context* (pp. 45–64). Berlin: Springer.

Rydin, Y., Bleahu, A., Davies, M., Davila, J. D., Friel, S., de Grandis, G., et al. (2012). Shaping cities for health: Complexity and the planning of urban environments in the 21st century. *Lancet, 379*, 2079–2108. https://doi.org/10.1016/S0140-6736(12)60435-8.
Ryff, C. D., & Singer, B. H. (2008). Know thyself and become what you are: A eudaimonic approach to psychological well-being. *Journal of Happiness Studies, 9*(1), 13–39. https://doi.org/10.1007/s10902-006-9019-0.
Saelens, B. E., & Handy, S. L. (2008). Correlates and intervention of walking behavior built environment correlates of walking: A review. *Medicine and Science in Sports and Exercise, 40*, S550–S566. https://doi.org/10.1249/MSS.0b013e31817c67a4.
Sandstrom, G. M., & Dunn, E. W. (2014). Social interactions and well-being: The surprising power of weak ties. *Personality and Social Psychology Bulletin, 40*, 900–922. https://doi.org/10.1177/0146167214529799.
Schimmack, U., & Oishi, S. (2005). The influence of chronically and temporarily accessible information on life satisfaction judgments. *Journal of Personality and Social Psychology, 89*(3), 395–406. https://doi.org/10.1037/0022-3514.89.3.395.
Schwanen, T., & Atkinson, S. (2015). Geographies of wellbeing: An introduction. *The Geographical Journal, 181*(2), 98–101. https://doi.org/10.1111/geoj.12132.
Sen, A. (1973). *On economic inequality*. Oxford: Clarendon Press.
Sen, A. (1992). *Inequality re-examined*. Oxford: Clarendon Press.
Sen, A. (1999). *Development as freedom*. Oxford: Oxford University Press.
Sen, A. (1987). *The standard of living: The Tanner lectures*. Cambridge: Cambridge University Press.
Shah, H., & Marks, N. (2004). A wellbeing manifesto for a flourishing society. *Journal of Public Mental Health, 3*(4), 9–15. https://doi.org/10.1108/17465729200400023.
Solar, O., & Irwin, A. (2010). *World Health Organization: A conceptual framework for action on the social determinants of health*. Social Determinants of Health Discussion Paper 2 (Policy and Practice). Available at: http://www.who.int/social_determinants/publications/9789241500852/en/
Sorensen, K. (2018). Health literacy: A key attribute for urban settings. In V. E. Papalois & M. Theodosopoulou (Eds.), *Optimizing health literacy for improved clinical practices* (pp. 1–16). Hershey: IGI Global.
Stoeva, A. Z., Chiu, R. K., & Greenhaus, J. H. (2002). Negative affectivity, role stress, and work-family conflict. *Journal of Vocational Behavior, 60*(1), 1–16. https://doi.org/10.1006/jvbe.2001.1812.
Talen, E., & Koschinsky, J. (2013). The walkable neighborhood: A literature review. *International Journal of Sustainable Land Use and Urban Planning, 1*(1), 42–63.
Tay, L., & Diener, E. (2011). Needs and subjective well-being around the world. *Journal of Personality and Social Psychology, 101*(2), 354–365. https://doi.org/10.1037/a0023779.
Tenney, E. R., Poole, J. M., & Diener, E. (2016). Does positivity enhance work performance?: Why, when, and what we don't know. *Research in Organizational Behavior, 36*, 27–46. https://doi.org/10.1016/j.riob.2016.11.002.
Thorslund, C. A. H., & Lassen, J. (2016). Context, orders of worth, and the justification of meat consumption practices. *Sociologia Ruralis, 57*, 836–858. https://doi.org/10.1111/soru.12143.
Van den Berg, A. E., Maas, J., Verheij, R. A., & Groenewegen, P. P. (2010). Green space as a buffer between stressful life events and health. *Social Science & Medicine, 70*(8), 1203–1210. https://doi.org/10.1016/j.socscimed.2010.01.002.
Veenhoven, R. (2007). Subjective measures of Well-being. In *Human well-being* (pp. 214–239). London: Palgrave Macmillan. https://doi.org/10.1057/9780230625600_9.
Velarde, M. D., Fry, G., & Tveit, M. (2007). Health effects of viewing landscapes: Landscape types in environmental psychology. *Urban Forestry & Urban Greening, 6*(4), 199–212. https://doi.org/10.1016/j.ufug.2007.07.001.

Watson, K. J. (2018). Establishing psychological wellbeing metrics for the built environment. *Building Services Engineering Research & Technology, 39*(2), 232–243. https://doi.org/10.1177/0143624418754497.

Western, M., & Tomaszewski, W. (2016). Subjective wellbeing, objective wellbeing and inequality in Australia. *PLoS One, 11*(10), e0163345. https://doi.org/10.1371/journal.pone.0163345.

World Health Organization Regional Office for Europe. (n.d.) *National healthy cities networks in the WHO European region – Promoting health and well-being throughout Europe*. Available online: http://www.euro.who.int/_data/assets/pdf_file/0011/285995/Healthy-Cities-promoting-health-and-equity.pdf

Part VII Conclusions

Nimish Biloria

This first volume of the S.M.A.R.T. Environments Book series titled Data Driven Multi-Valence in the Built Environment focuses on the identification, ingestion, implications and accountability of variable urban data within the contemporary city. These are showcased via a variety of case studies and reviews exemplified through seventeen chapters in the book. Multiple stakeholders ranging from Government authorities, Industry players, Academicians as well as Citizens and the vitality of the data produced and processed by them in variable forms are thus explored in this volume. In doing do, the book specifically maintains its multi-disciplinary nature and attempts to bring together the disciplines of Built Environment, Urban Health, Urban Infrastructure, Smart energy, Spatial economics as well as Human Centric design under a bigger banner of Multivariance of Urban Data. This multi-disciplinary nature alongside the multi-scalar aspect, which prominently runs throughout the book serves as a good example of underpinning the importance of a wholistic focus on evolving Smart Environments. The book, apart from presenting the implications of technical tools and techniques for the contemporary city, is also instrumental in understanding the inferences of economic policies, the vitality of participatory design systems and the value of democratic governance in order to manage the complex metabolism of today's urbanised cities. The book serves as both, a critique on the current state of smart cities globally as well as a discussion board for generating new socio-technical realities for empowering the citizen.

The book not only focuses on drawing attention to data sources while professing on multiple ways in which data interoperability and relational modelling of variable data sets can be fruitful in gaining a deeper understanding of the city, but also brings forth a critical viewpoint focusing on contemporary challenges in managing, mining

N. Biloria (✉)
Faculty of Design Architecture and Building, University of Technology Sydney, Sydney, Australia

N. Biloria (ed.), *Data-driven Multivalence in the Built Environment*, S.M.A.R.T. Environments, https://doi.org/10.1007/978-3-030-12180-8

and mediating within the existing operations of the city while being transparent and participatory in essence. The book thus deliberately does not focus specifically on issues pertaining to data standards, data security, data protocols and network typologies but rather focuses on front-end applications such as Intelligent transport systems, Smart City control centres, City dashboards, Image processing workflows and associated tangible interfaces in the form of social and spatial robotics, physiological support systems, 3d printed customized bio-synthetic devices and bio-tech focused energy generation systems etc. Besides this, the book also encourages active debate around the condition of the urban from a social, technical as well as economic perspective. All of these narratives in the form of Scientific Chapters however, maintain their focus on the central premise of the book concerning the role of Data and its usage in the contemporary city from the aforementioned social, economic, political and technical viewpoints.

The book, a first in the series, not only outlines the extensive body of research being conducted globally within the domain of smart environments but also opens up a variety of questions pertaining to urban data, data sciences and its applicability for democratic governance, urban planning and place making. Some of these questions will be addressed in subsequent books which adhere to a more focused singular agenda per volume such as Smart Health and Wellbeing, Smart Energy, Smart Built Environment and Smart Urban computing. However, as the rate at which the availability of open data and the means to harness this data increases exponentially, the need for empirical evidence-based research in order to understand our Cities within this data rich context. This book and the next four volumes hope to actively contribute to this rich debate around understanding the City and the new political, cultural, economic and technical realities that this multivariance of data and its inter-operability brings to the urban context.

Printed by Printforce, the Netherlands